TRAUMA AND RESILIENCE IN THE LIVES OF CONTEMPORARY NATIVE AMERICANS

Indigenous Peoples around the world and our allies often reflect on the many challenges that continue to confront us, the reasons behind health, economic, and social disparities, and the best ways forward to a healthy future. This book draws on theoretical, conceptual, and evidence-based scholarship as well as interviews with scholars immersed in Indigenous wellbeing, to examine contemporary issues for Native Americans. It includes reflections on resilience as well as disparities. In recent decades, there has been increasing attention on how trauma, both historical and contemporary, shapes the lives of Native Americans. Indigenous scholars urge recognition of historical trauma as a framework for understanding contemporary health and social disparities.

Accordingly, this book uses a trauma-informed lens to examine Native American issues with the understanding that even when not specifically seeking to address trauma directly, it is useful to understand that trauma is a common experience that can shape many aspects of life. Scholarship on trauma and trauma-informed care is integrated with scholarship on historical trauma, providing a framework for examining contemporary issues for Native American populations.

It should be considered essential reading for all human service professionals working with Native American clients, as well as a core text for Native American studies and classes on trauma or diversity more generally.

Hilary N. Weaver, DSW (Lakota) is a Professor and Associate Dean for Academic Affairs in the School of Social Work, University at Buffalo (State University of New York). She received her BS from Antioch College in social work with a cross-cultural studies focus and her MSW and DSW from Columbia University. Her teaching, research, and service focus on cultural issues in the helping process with an emphasis on Indigenous populations. Dr Weaver received funding from the National Cancer Institute to develop and test a culturally grounded wellness curriculum for urban Native American youth—the Healthy Living in Two Worlds program. She is a member of NASW and CSWE, and currently serves as President of the Indigenous and Tribal Social Work Educators' Association (formerly American Indian Alaska Native Social Work Educators' Association). Dr Weaver has presented her work regionally, nationally, and internationally, including presenting at the Permanent Forum on Indigenous Issues at the United Nations in 2005–2008 and 2013–2018.

TRAUMA AND RESILIENCE IN THE LIVES OF CONTEMPORARY NATIVE AMERICANS

Reclaiming our Balance, Restoring our Wellbeing

Hilary N. Weaver

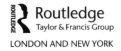

Routledge
Taylor & Francis Group

LONDON AND NEW YORK

First published 2019
by Routledge
2 Park Square, Milton Park, Abingdon, Oxon OX14 4RN

and by Routledge
711 Third Avenue, New York, NY 10017

Routledge is an imprint of the Taylor & Francis Group, an informa business

British Library Cataloguing in Publication Data
A catalogue record for this book is available from the British Library

Library of Congress Cataloging-in-Publication Data
A catalog record has been requested for this book

ISBN: 978-1-138-08828-3 (hbk)
ISBN: 978-1-138-08829-0 (pbk)
ISBN: 978-1-315-10996-1 (ebk)

Typeset in Bembo
by Taylor & Francis Books

CONTENTS

INTRODUCTION

> Our ancestors did a Hansel and Gretel for us. Our job is to pick up the breadcrumbs and find our way home.

These words have echoed through my mind repeatedly since I heard them spoken at the Indigenous Voices in Social Work conference in Darwin, Australia, in 2015. Indigenous Peoples around the world and our allies often reflect on the many challenges that continue to confront us, the reasons behind health, economic, and social disparities, and the best ways forward to a healthy future. The simple statement above goes beyond an acknowledgement of contemporary challenges and provides an affirmation that what we need to move forward in a positive way is available to us.

This book draws on theoretical, conceptual, and evidence-based scholarship as well as interviews with scholars immersed in Indigenous wellbeing, to examine contemporary issues for Native Americans. It includes reflections on resilience as well as disparities. In recent decades, there has been increasing attention on how trauma, both historical and contemporary, shapes the lives of Native Americans. Indigenous scholars urge recognition of historical trauma as a framework for understanding contemporary health and social disparities. The multigenerational grieving associated with massive collective trauma leaves a lingering sadness that continues to envelop many Native people (Peacock, 2011).

Accordingly, this book uses a trauma-informed lens to examine Native American issues with the understanding that even when not specifically seeking to address trauma directly, it is useful to understand that trauma is a common experience that can shape many aspects of life. Scholarship on trauma and trauma-informed care is integrated with scholarship on historical trauma, providing a framework for examining contemporary issues for Native American populations.

While the primary focus of this book is on Native Americans, Indigenous Peoples in various parts of the world share commonalities in their sense of rootedness in their traditional territories and histories of colonization and dispossession. The boundaries that define the United States divide tribal territories and split communities and families. Based on these imposed boundaries, different citizenship statuses were conferred on members of some Indigenous communities. Thus, who is considered Native American—rather than Aboriginal Canadian or Indigenous Mexican—is arbitrary. Indigenous Peoples transcend national boundaries.

While many people have strong preferences, there is no clear consensus on the use of various labels, such as Native Americans, American Indians, Indigenous Peoples, First Nations Peoples, and Aboriginal Peoples. Some terms are more common in some regions. For example, First Nations and Aboriginal are familiar terms in Canada; Aboriginal is commonly used in Australia; Native American is commonly used in the United States (particularly in regions like the Northeast); and American Indian is also commonly used in the United States (particularly in regions like the Southwest). Historically, the US federal government has primarily used the terms Indian and American Indian.

Throughout this book, when referring to the Native people of the United States, the terms Native American and American Indian are used interchangeably. The original term used is preserved in quotes. Indigenous may refer to any original inhabitants, regardless of current national boundaries, including people in the United States. It is important to note that, following significant activism, the United Nations has recognized the importance of Indigenous Peoples (collective entities) and not simply Indigenous people (multiple individuals). Therefore, throughout this text, capitalization is used to recognize this status.

The importance of understanding trauma

The prevalence of trauma across all the United States, regardless of age, gender, socioeconomic status, race, ethnicity, or sexual orientation, has led to its recognition as a major public health concern (SAMHSA, 2017). While trauma is common across populations, it has a disproportionate impact on some populations. Indigenous people, poor people, and populations of color are at particular risk of trauma exposure (SAMHSA, 2017). In the case of Native Americans, there may also be interplay between elements of Indigenous cultures and trauma exposure that influence the impact of trauma and its sequelae (Brave Heart et al., 2012; Evans-Campbell, 2008; Vernon, 2012).

Trauma can be conceptualized as a wound inflicted upon the mind or, as Duran (2006) understands it, as a soul wound. It can also be understood as a narrative of interconnected experiences that have an ongoing impact on wellbeing (Vernon, 2012). In other words, trauma often does not just go away or get better spontaneously. Telling and retelling stories of atrocities can give voice to traumatic wounds and validate this reality for both those who have experienced them and their communities (Vernon, 2012). The trauma literature emphasizes the importance of storytelling in terms of acknowledging what happened as both a prerequisite and a component of healing. This can have great therapeutic value for trauma survivors. It can also be meaningful for family members and descendants to understand what happened and how this may shape behaviors, values, and other aspects of survivors' lives. However, while speaking about traumatic experiences can be validating and therapeutic, there are also times when this process can be painful and retraumatizing. Encouragement to disclose traumatic experiences must be done with thoughtfulness, sensitivity, and attention to its potential therapeutic value or harm.

There is increasing recognition that trauma is intergenerational in nature. What happened in one generation can have a lasting impact on subsequent generations. As research establishes connections between various behavioral and public health concerns and trauma, it is apparent that policy makers, and indeed all of us, can benefit from a greater understanding of trauma and its impacts. Trauma can lead to both personal and communal strains on the body and mind and has been linked to violence, substance misuse, and other concerns (Myhra & Wieling, 2014; SAMHSA, 2017).

Historical trauma theory posits that cumulative emotional and psychological wounding can be experienced by groups and transmitted across generations within communities (SAMHSA, 2017). Incorporating individual, familial, and communal dimensions of trauma and trauma responses is a necessary element of understanding the complex, long-term effects of multiple, devastating historical events with impacts at multiple levels. The historical trauma framework provides a mechanism for this multidimensional endeavor (Evans-Campbell, 2008).

Many Native American groups have a concept of Seven Generations—a sense that contemporary people are nestled within a framework of past and future generations. Some Native American traditions conceptualize this as counting backward to ancestors seven generations ago and forward to the next seven generations of people yet to be born. Some count backwards for three generations, forward for three, and see the people of today as nested in the middle. Either way, contemporary Native Peoples are connected to both past and future generations.

Contemporary Native Peoples continue to exist with remnants of sovereignty, land, culture, and language, specifically because our ancestors planned for us and for our contemporary needs. Likewise, we have a responsibility to plan for future generations so the environment, both physical and social, is nurturing, sustaining, and capable of meeting our needs. This sense of wellbeing, firmly grounded within a framework of those who came before and those who will come after, reinforces a sense of intergenerational connection. In turn, awareness of the devastation that happened in past generations can make contemporary Native people keenly aware of ancestral pain and displacement and internalize the consequences of past trauma. Indigenous philosophies of interdependence among people, other living beings, and the natural world mean that the suffering of any of these entities has far-reaching consequences (Vernon, 2012).

The concept of historical trauma has the potential to reframe understandings of a range of social and health issues in Native American communities (Hartmann &

Gone, 2014). It provides a framework to understand current problems in Indigenous communities through the lens of past atrocities associated with colonization. The importance of understanding this context was promoted by Indigenous clinicians who were able to draw on both their clinical experiences in Native American communities and psychological theories of trauma and trauma treatment (Hartmann & Gone, 2014).

Trauma and the contemporary social environment

There is a growing realization that, rather than being rare, trauma is experienced by many people over the course of their lifetimes. Lifetime trauma exposure is particularly prevalent among Native Americans, where exposure rates have become a significant public health concern (Beals et al., 2013). The impact of adverse childhood events (ACEs) and post-traumatic stress disorder (PTSD) are reviewed in the next chapter.

Trauma is often the result of violence. Native Americans continue to be one of the most victimized groups in the United States (Myhra & Wieling, 2014). The high levels of violence in many Native American communities puts Native people at greater risk of trauma exposure and PTSD than other Americans (Beals et al., 2013). Likewise, Native Americans experience high rates of trauma sequelae. High rates of PTSD in Native American populations result from higher rates of exposure to traumatic events (Beals et al., 2013). The majority of PTSD cases in Native women are the result of interpersonal trauma, most notably sexual and physical abuse, while PTSD in Native men is more evenly distributed among different types of trauma (Beals et al., 2013). It is also noteworthy that experiencing a traumatic event early in life may have greater implications than a traumatic event experienced during adulthood (Myhra & Wieling, 2014).

It can be difficult for clinicians and researchers to distinguish between the impact of individual and collective trauma. Likewise, ongoing trauma and stressors cannot easily be separated from intergenerational trauma and subsequent individual and community dysfunction, including learned helplessness and internalized oppression (Myhra & Wieling, 2014). Complex trauma is common in Native American communities where the risk of experiencing or witnessing a traumatic event and developing PTSD is compounded by multiple persistent traumatic life events (Myhra & Wieling, 2014).

Indigenous women and girls are not only at high risk of physical and sexual violence but societal and governmental indifference. Lack of awareness of the large numbers of missing and murdered Indigenous women compounds trauma for their families and communities. A 2004 Amnesty International report focused on the "Stolen Sisters"— missing and murdered Aboriginal women in Canada. The report identified factors that create a climate of heightened risk of violence for Indigenous women. These factors include social and economic marginalization, combined with a history of government policies that have undermined Indigenous families and communities. These, in turn, pushed many Native women into dangerous situations, including extreme poverty, homelessness, and prostitution. Violence motivated by racism and fueled by societal indifference to the safety of Indigenous women is exacerbated by a climate that allows perpetrators to go unprosecuted (Amnesty International, 2004).

Furthermore, Indigenous Peoples' connection to land leads many Native Americans to experience exploitation of land, water, and other natural resources as a form of violence against the earth; the wellbeing of the earth being directly connected to the wellbeing of these people. These values and beliefs are illustrated by recent confrontations near Standing Rock Reservation around extending the Dakota Access Pipeline (DAPL) under Lake Oahe, a primary water source for people in the region, both Indigenous and non-Indigenous (University of Arizona Rogers College of Law, 2018).

Key principles

There are several key principles that undergird this book, including recognition of Indigenous sovereignty, human rights, and social justice, and recognition of colonial dynamics and the need for decolonization. These principles have clear implications for Indigenous wellbeing. Accordingly, they have direct applications in social work and other helping professions.

Indigenous Peoples existed on these lands prior to the arrival of people from other continents. We had our own social institutions and forms of governance that were recognized in treaties signed with foreign powers. Although subsequent laws infringed on Indigenous Peoples' ability to exert complete control over all aspects of their lives, many aspects of sovereignty remain, including rights to self-governance, determining tribal membership, and, in most cases, not to be subjected to state authority within reservation boundaries.

Government-to-government relationships between tribes and the federal government continue. It is important to recognize political relationships between tribes and state and federal governments to avoid the misconception that Indigenous Peoples are simply a minority group. By not fully understanding and recognizing the importance of sovereignty, helping professionals have unwittingly contributed to colonial distress.

Native Americans are both Indigenous nations and racialized minorities in the United States—a complexity that is missed by many scholars who do not recognize how the colonizer–Indigenous relationship is integrally connected to, and distinct from, how the settler society relates to other groups. Racism and colonialism share a foundation of White supremacy. Dismantling colonialism requires dismantling racism and vice versa. Failing to address either allows structural inequities to persist and flourish (Klopotek, Lintinger & Barbry, 2008).

While sovereignty is often discussed as a legal concept, it is important to understand it also as the inherent right of Indigenous Peoples to direct their future. It is the foundation for tribal nation-building efforts and mirrors professional values of self-determination. Helping professionals need to have a solid understanding of Indigenous sovereignty to work effectively with Indigenous nations and Peoples.

Reframing professional aims in ways that center sovereignty strengthens an ability to assist Indigenous clients (Cavalieri, 2013).

Infusing a sovereignty perspective includes awareness about the impact of ongoing colonial structures. The helping professions are rooted in Western worldviews and knowledge to the extent that clinicians may be unaware of how these informed their training and their practice (Cavalieri, 2013). For example, the belief that the individual is the basic social unit underlies much of Western thought and may go unquestioned by human service professionals grounded in Western professional education. On the other hand, Indigenous Peoples may bring a different worldview that prioritizes the collective.

Individualistically focused theories and interventions can privilege individual autonomy over interconnectedness—an important value in Indigenous societies. Native Americans often espouse a collective sense of identity that ties an individual's wellbeing to that of their community. Interventions that prioritize individual functioning over family, community, and tribal wellbeing can be counterproductive and exacerbate survivors' or thrivers' guilt (Cavalieri, 2013).

An absence of social justice has been at the heart of Native/non-Native interactions from the beginning. Many colonial interactions demonstrated no recognition of Indigenous Peoples' status as human beings. It is important for helping professionals to understand the role of legislation in shaping the lives of Native Americans in order to proceed from a foundation of social justice that recognizes the impact of trauma (Turner & Pope, 2009). Human rights principles are concerned not only with violence itself but also with the official response to violence (Amnesty International, 2004). Indeed, laws and policies have sanctioned maltreatment of Indigenous Peoples in both the United States and Canada (Turner & Pope, 2009). Human rights principles recognize the inherent dignity and worth of every human being (Amnesty International, 2004). This is the antithesis of the dehumanization that is a necessary and inherent component of colonization.

Social work is a profession built on a foundation of recognizing human rights and striving for social justice. Likewise, professionals from other backgrounds such as community psychology and transcultural nursing recognize the centrality of these principles to effective work with Indigenous populations.

Social justice and human rights concerns arise when helping professionals provide substandard or culturally inappropriate services to Indigenous Peoples. Helping professionals may inadvertently provide biased treatment by using Western or mainstream standards as a norm to which all others are compared. It is imperative to examine how theories, research, and therapeutic processes can be grounded in Western thought and values and thus continue to employ colonial dynamics (Cavalieri, 2013).

It is also noteworthy that evidence-based treatments developed in other populations may not be transferable to Native Americans. Making evidence-based practice models standard for Indigenous Peoples is a colonial practice (Cavalieri, 2013).

In choosing to use non-Indigenous theorizations and approaches, social work replicates colonial tendencies and aligns with the root causes of many social inequalities rather than seeking to eliminate them. In other words, social work continues to pursue the rhetoric of social justice but not its realization for Indigenous communities.

(Johnston-Goodstar, 2013, p. 4)

Indigenous Peoples may have different understandings and beliefs than their mainstream counterparts. For example, the American Psychiatric Association's *Diagnostic and Statistical Manual* (DSM) uses a medical model based on a Western understanding of beliefs and behaviors. On the other hand, in Indigenous cosmology all beings have spirits, and relationships often take priority over individual needs. There are few of the clear, dualistic distinctions, such as human/nonhuman, animate/inanimate, and disordered/healthy, that are found in Western ideas (Cavalieri, 2013). Western assumptions about progress are also frequently at odds with Indigenous worldviews.

It is also important for helping professionals to understand colonization, decolonization, and how colonial dynamics can continue to play a role in helping processes (Cavalieri, 2013). Historically, this included the imposition of Western forms of education and healthcare as well as policies that undermined governance structures, denied religious freedom, and systematically stripped Indigenous Peoples of land and other resources. Colonial dynamics are perpetuated when Indigenous understandings of health, wellbeing, and family structures continue to be undermined by helping professionals, educators, and policy makers.

By privileging time and progress as the organizers of therapeutic experiences, therapists can displace location as an important organizer of experience for Tribal peoples ... It also ignores that for most, if not all, Tribal peoples, historical traumas have been brought about over physical places that have had deep significance to the Tribe. Thus, it may be important for mental health professionals to develop their understanding of meaningful places that impact clients' health, whether those are Tribally defined or idiosyncratic. Listening for the role that place plays in the lives of AIAN [American Indian Alaska Native] clients moves away from colonial restructuring that emphasizes when things happened over where things happened.

(Cavalieri, 2013, p. 33)

Colonization systematically deters Indigenous expressions of culture and governance and is ultimately internalized and self-perpetuating (Cavalieri, 2013). It is important to decolonize human services and infuse respect for sovereignty and self-determination in helping processes. Incorporating sovereignty into discussions of Indigenous wellness both resists colonial processes and affirms the rights of Indigenous people to self-determination (Cavalieri, 2013). Decolonization is a process of active resistance to colonialism and exploitation of Indigenous minds, bodies, and lands. In "working toward decolonization, we are not relegating ourselves to a status as victim, but rather we are actively working toward our own freedom to transform our lives and the world around us" (Waziyatawin & Yellow Bird, 2012, p. 3). Decolonization is an important pathway to eliminating physical health and mental health disparities.

The global context

The United Nations monitors a variety of indicators of wellbeing for Indigenous populations. The experiences of Native Americans are often similar to those of Indigenous Peoples in other parts of the world. Indigenous Peoples typically experience significant health and social disparities compared to non-Indigenous Peoples, including high rates of poverty, disease, and violence. These disparities are rooted in colonial histories and ongoing marginalization (Hansen, Jepsen & Jacquelin, 2017).

After years of debate, the United Nations passed the Declaration on the Rights of Indigenous Peoples (United Nations, 2008). It is noteworthy that the International Federation of Social Workers, working from UN draft documents, developed and passed its own policy statement on Indigenous Peoples in 2005 (Weaver & Congress, 2009). Both the United Nations and the International Federation of Social Workers documents can serve as guidelines for human service providers in supporting sovereignty and decolonization for Indigenous Peoples. The United Nations has also established an annual Permanent Forum on Indigenous Issues, where Indigenous delegates from around the world share concerns and recommendations.

Terminology

The literature on trauma and Native Americans uses a variety of related and overlapping terms, such as historical trauma, intergenerational trauma, and colonial trauma response. While individual scholars typically describe how they use these terms, there is inconsistency as to which are preferred and how they are defined. The most common term—historical trauma—is the primary term used in this text, but other terms and concepts are employed as necessary to clarify distinct ideas.

Although raised by some scholars in the 1970s, the concept of historical trauma in Native American populations received little attention until the work of Maria Yellow Horse Brave Heart in the mid-1990s. As per Brave Heart,

> *Historical trauma* (HT) is defined as cumulative emotional and psychological wounding across generations, including the lifespan, which emanates from massive group trauma ... Historical trauma theory frames lifespan trauma in the collective, historical context, which empowers Indigenous survivors of both communal and individual trauma by reducing the sense of stigma and isolation. The *historical trauma response* (HTR) has been conceptualized as a

constellation of features associated with a reaction to massive group trauma. *Historical unresolved grief*, a component of this response, is the profound unsettled bereavement resulting from cumulative devastating losses, compounded by the prohibition and interruption of Indigenous burial practices and ceremonies.

(Brave Heart et al., 2011, p. 283)

Confusion has resulted when the term historical trauma has been used to refer to both the distress itself and a causal explanation of that distress (Cavalieri, 2013). Historical trauma response may add clarity by focusing on the response to group trauma. Likewise, the term historical unresolved grief has led to confusion. The term was intended to indicate that trauma was introduced historically but is not necessarily relegated to the past (Cavalieri, 2013). Some clinicians and scholars prefer the term colonial trauma response as a conceptualization that is inclusive of microaggressions and individual traumatic experiences as well as those the group experienced in the past.

While scholars continue to refine definitions and theories, there is general agreement that four key components underlie historical trauma:

1. Injury from colonial subjugation and dispossession.
2. The collective nature of this injury and resulting impairment.
3. The cumulative and synergistic effects of these injuries and ongoing oppression.
4. And transmission of these injuries to subsequent generations resulting in legacies of risk and vulnerability to behavioral health problems until such time as healing can occur *(Hartmann & Gone, 2014)*.

Historical loss is another concept imbedded in historical trauma (Tucker, Wingate & O'Keefe, 2016). This involves expending cognitive resources thinking about the consequences and impact of multiple losses associated with colonization. These losses include land, Native Peoples, culture, language, and traditional spiritual practices. Historical loss thinking can involve dwelling on the consequences of forced acculturation and relocation with a negative repetitive thinking style (Tucker et al., 2016).

My standpoint

I am Lakota and a social worker. I have focused my career on making the social work profession responsive to the needs of diverse populations, particularly Indigenous Peoples. I approach this work both as a scholar and as a community member. I live in an urban Native American community and raise my children within this multicultural context, grappling with many of the issues addressed in this book, such as challenges with educational systems. I have extensive experience within governing structures of Indigenous organizations, including service as President of the Board of Directors of Native American Community Services of Erie and Niagara Counties (my home community) and President of the Indigenous and Tribal Social Work Educators' Association, a national organization in the United States. I was honored to receive the latter organization's American Indian Elder of the Year award in 2017—the youngest person ever to receive this award. I provided a keynote address for the International Indigenous Voices in Social Work conference in Darwin, Australia, in 2015 and have spoken at the United Nations Permanent Forum on Indigenous Issues ten times between 2005 and 2018. The content of this book is presented through my dual perspectives as a scholar in this area and my experiences as a Lakota person who has lived much of my life in Haudenosaunee Territory, within the urban Native American community of Buffalo, New York.

Overview of the book

This book bridges scholarship on trauma with information on the historical and contemporary experiences of Native Americans. Theoretical foundations and empirical support for current scholarship on trauma, including intergenerational or historical trauma, are described in Chapter 1. While not a clinical text, the book draws on clinical literature to inform understandings of Indigenous Peoples and issues. This is done to help readers understand manifestations of trauma, both historical and contemporary, in Native American populations. The book includes a concise history of Native Americans (Chapter 2) as well as a description of contemporary issues facing these populations (Chapter 3). The second half of the book explores the impact of trauma in the lives of Native Americans, including specific chapters devoted to child and family wellbeing (Chapter 4), elders and veterans (Chapter 5), education (Chapter 6), health (Chapter 7), and community wellbeing (Chapter 8). This content is informed by interviews with leading scholars in these areas. Although the book focuses on the experiences of Native Americans, global connections are made throughout.

Although this book is divided into chapters with specific themes, it is important to recognize that the topics are interrelated rather than separate and independent of one another. The content weaves in and out, with different parts of the story coming to the fore in different chapters, while other parts recede into the background, providing the necessary context for fuller understanding. In this sense, the chapter on child and family wellbeing (Chapter 4) informs the reader's understanding of the material in the chapter on health (Chapter 7) and vice versa. The same can be said of the other chapters.

This book is filled with the stories of contemporary Indigenous Peoples, informed by historical events and policies that shaped current circumstances. These stories are filled with shifting nuances, always changing, growing, and subject to interpretation. They are not without ambiguity. Multiple things can be true within the same time and space: trauma and resilience, strength and vulnerability, loss and continuity. It is possible for multiple people to read the same words and each have a different "take away," often based on what they need to learn at that moment in their lives. It is my hope that readers will gain whatever they need from this book.

1

EXAMINING THE IMPACT OF TRAUMA

Trauma can have a significant and lasting impact on individuals, families, and communities. This chapter reviews how trauma is defined and how its impacts were originally recognized and conceptualized. Trauma theory, prevalence, and treatment are reviewed, including discussions of post-traumatic stress disorder (PTSD), adverse childhood events (ACEs), trauma-informed care (TIC), and resilience.

The chapter also provides background information on the major tenets of historical or intergenerational trauma, including theoretical development, empirical support, and critiques of these theories. Finally, it includes a review of the major implications of historical trauma for individuals, communities, and service providers as well as a discussion of resilience and healing.

Early explorations of trauma

The term trauma is used to describe both something that has happened and the lasting impact of distressful event(s). From a clinical perspective, in order to be considered trauma, the event (or series of events) must be accompanied by a real or perceived threat of death or serious injury resulting in overwhelming fear, terror, hopelessness, and/or helplessness (Wilson, Pence & Conradi, 2013). Perceptions can be subjective. In other words, what may be experienced as threatening and terrifying by one person may be regarded differently by another. Individuals display unique responses to highly stressful events. These individualized responses can be shaped by factors including past experiences, genetics, and available support networks.

Early ideas about trauma were influenced by the work of Sigmund Freud. The psychoanalytic theory he championed posited that symptoms are the result of repressed childhood trauma (Lewis, 2012). Psychoanalysis was proposed as treatment for alleviating resulting neuroses.

The field of psychiatry grew in prominence as it sought ways to understand the impact of combat stress and the psychological symptoms of veterans returning from World War I. Clinicians began to understand and explore the psychological ramifications of warfare, so-called shell shock, as an alternative to attributing symptoms to personal weakness (Fueshko, 2016). Explorations of combat-related post-traumatic stress continued as veterans from other conflicts, such as World War II, the Korean War, and the Vietnam War, returned to their communities, often significantly changed by their experiences.

By the mid-1980s, the mental health community recognized that what they had learned about the stress experienced by combat veterans and resulting psychological symptoms had relevance for understanding the symptoms of people who had experienced violent crimes and other major traumatic life events. In 1985, the International Society for Traumatic Stress was founded. This association of professionals sought answers for how best to understand and assist clients who had experienced various types of trauma. Subsequent decades saw a major expansion of theory and research on trauma and its impacts (Wilson et al., 2013). Focus on trauma is now one of six strategic initiatives of the Substance Abuse and Mental Health Services Administration (SAMHSA).

Historical trauma

Growing understandings of trauma have opened the door for explorations of how trauma experienced by past generations may have a lingering impact. Intergenerational continuity has often been explored through parent-to-child transmission of behaviors and wellbeing. For example, mental illness or substance abuse can affect the ability to parent, which in turn can result in the manifestation of problems in children. Maladaptive parenting has been linked to adverse child outcomes, thus perpetuating a cycle of trauma (Walls & Whitbeck, 2012).

The life-course perspective emphasizes interdependence and informs how historical events can shape lives across generations (Walls & Whitbeck, 2012). Themes of historical experiences and intergenerational transmission of behaviors offer a conceptual foundation for examining how historical trauma has an ongoing impact across generations (Walls & Whitbeck, 2012).

The concept of historical trauma has resonated with many people, including some who embrace it as an explanation of their own experiences. One Native American elder described the impact of traumatic historical events by stating:

> Your mind, your body, and your spirit don't know what to do with it. So you dwell on it. And to relieve that, you go to alcohol or some kind of addiction. As you do it, you destroy yourself and your whole being.
>
> *(Grayshield et al., 2015, p. 301)*

This study of elders' perceptions revealed they believed that historical trauma includes a genetic component whereby trauma such as that resulting from forced

attendance at boarding schools was transmitted to subsequent generations. Historical trauma was also seen as the root of internalized oppression (Grayshield et
al., 2015). Elders believed that historical trauma is connected to contemporary
problems with alcohol, substance abuse, and food. They also associated historical
trauma with loss of culture and language as well as community discord and youth
being sedentary and at risk of cyberbullying. They emphasized the need to focus
on the positive and raise awareness of historical trauma. They found hope in
returning to cultural and spiritual traditions and learning tribal languages (Grayshield et al., 2015).

Theoretical development of historical trauma and related concepts

The field of behavioral health has an evolving understanding of psychological
trauma as well as how trauma can be inflicted. Researchers are continuing to
learn more about the effects of trauma on the brain and the implications of
childhood trauma for ongoing risks. Other research examines the impact of
trauma that occurred in past generations. Historical trauma theory, originally
developed to explain the residual impact of the Jewish Holocaust on the children of survivors, expanded to incorporate the impact of trauma on entire
communities, particularly communities of color (SAMHSA, 2016). Indeed, the
concept of historical trauma is relevant to understanding the experiences of
many populations that have experienced colonization, oppression, and genocide
(Mohatt et al., 2014).

Scholars use various terms in addition to historical trauma to describe contemporary implications of trauma experienced by past generations. There is an
underlying consensus that this phenomenon consists of a collective wounding that
can lead to symptoms in contemporary members of the affected group, even
though they may not have experienced the original traumatizing events directly
(Mohatt et al., 2014). Historical oppression has been defined as "the chronic, pervasive, and intergenerational experiences of subjugation that, over time, have been
imposed, normalized, and internalized" (Burnette, 2015, p. 531).

Historical trauma is not just an explanatory framework for reactions to past events
but a lens for understanding contemporary issues and disparities. The historical trauma
narrative connects the collective histories of traumatic events to contemporary
experiences of individuals and communities. Past and present narratives function as
layers. These stories grounded in socially endorsed memory blend with present suffering and resilience (Mohatt et al., 2014).

Historical trauma can be expressed as unresolved grief resulting from events that
have not been adequately acknowledged, expressed, or addressed. Disenfranchised
grief results when losses are not publicly voiced or acknowledged. For example, the
massive population decimation resulting from colonization is often omitted from
history texts or dismissed as irrelevant. Internalized oppression occurs when people
integrate the views of the oppressor and perpetuate a cycle of self-hatred and
negative behaviors (SAMHSA, 2014).

Evans-Campbell (2008) proposed the Colonial Trauma Response (CTR) as a way to explore interactions between historical and contemporary trauma in Native Americans. The connection between colonization and trauma is a defining feature of CTR. In particular, contemporary discrimination or microaggressions experienced by an individual may connect him or her to a larger historical event and an associated sense of trauma and injustice (Evans-Campbell, 2008).

Contemporary conceptualizations of the impact of trauma on Indigenous populations over time build on earlier foundations that examine the impact of colonization. The work of Paulo Freire is particularly relevant. His work examines how oppression associated with colonization becomes internalized and self-perpetuating, leading to horizontal violence and sub-oppression; striking out at those with similar levels of power or less (Burnette & Figley, 2017).

The scholar most closely associated with the development of historical trauma theory is Maria Yellow Horse Brave Heart. Dr. Brave Heart's career direction was influenced by Native American activism in the 1970s that drew attention to broken treaties and massacres. After feeling overwhelming grief while looking at historical photos, she began to theorize about the contemporary implications of large-scale historical events that devastated Indigenous Peoples (Deschenie, 2006). As a clinician, she developed interventions to address historical trauma and evaluated their effectiveness, thus moving the knowledge base forward in this area. Other scholars, such as Evans-Campbell, Gone, Whitbeck, and Burnette, have developed substantial scholarship that continues to build on and refine her work.

In Burnette's conceptualization of historical oppression, she emphasizes the compounding effects of contemporary oppression. This framework reflects the ongoing, pervasive, intergenerational experiences of oppression that have become normalized and incorporated into the day-to-day lives of Native people. While building on historical trauma theory, historical oppression takes into account specific local contexts. Not all Native people had identical experiences with colonization or contemporary oppression. It is important to consider proximal factors that continue to perpetuate specific acts of discrimination, microaggressions, poverty, and marginalization (Burnette & Figley, 2017). Burnette's work is notable in that much of it is grounded in the experiences of Indigenous Peoples of the Delta Region of the United States, an often overlooked area.

Ideas about the intergenerational transmission of trauma are grounded in family systems theories (Coleman, 2016). Historical trauma scholars also draw on attachment theory to explain insecure or ambivalent attachment and anxiety disorders in descendants of trauma survivors (Mohatt et al., 2014). The disruptive nature of colonization processes impeded culturally grounded grieving and protective processes, leading to unresolved grief, increased risk of health disparities, and various psychosocial issues (Brave Heart et al., 2011; Mohatt et al., 2014).

The minority stress model, developed by Meyer, posits that the stress of racism and discrimination experienced by marginalized groups affects health and mental health outcomes (Coleman, 2016). This model integrates psychosocial theory, particularly the association between stress and illness, political and economic theories to account for structural determinants of health, and social and ecological systems theories to explain multiple influences on health and wellbeing (Mohatt et al., 2014). Mohatt and colleagues expand this framework to add a narrative level. They view historical trauma as a public narrative. How the story is remembered and told (or not told) influences the ongoing, contemporary impact of the event.

Core concepts

There are several core concepts that underlie historical trauma and related theories. These theories emphasize the extensive victimization and pervasive trauma-generating experiences that happened to Native Americans. They also emphasize the communal or collective nature of many of these experiences. Such experiences have an impact across generations and at multiple levels, including individuals, families, and communities. There is also recognition of synergy between contemporary trauma and unresolved historical traumatic events. Indeed, the term *historical* trauma can be misleading, given the prevalence of ongoing racist practices, ideologies, and colonial efforts (Burnette & Figley, 2017; Coleman, 2016).

Another key aspect of historical trauma is that it remains unresolved. Past events have a continuing impact on survivors as well as subsequent generations. This continuing impact is characterized by emotional, behavioral, and thought patterns that impair the physical, psychological, and social wellbeing of individuals or groups (Grayshield et al., 2015). Mourning is an important communal experience that starts the path to healing. Past prohibition of many traditional forms of grieving prevented adequate mourning of losses for many Indigenous Peoples, thus preventing resolution and perpetuating related problems (Deschenie, 2006).

> Traumatic experiences are cumulative. If one generation does not heal, problems are transmitted to subsequent generations. In some form, this cultural trauma affects every Native person. It sculpts how we think, how we respond emotionally. It affects our social dynamics and, at the deepest level, impacts our spirituality. Intergenerational trauma has wounded us deeply … There were times in my life that I wondered "Is there something wrong with me? Is there something wrong with us? What did we do to cause all of this to happen?" The truth is there is nothing wrong with Native people; we are perfectly normal people responding to an abnormal history.
>
> *(Brokenleg, 2012, p. 10)*

Evidence of the devastating effects of historical trauma caused by genocide and forced acculturation policies has been mounting. Historical trauma causes anger, depression, guilt, anxiety, internalized oppression, and impaired parenting (Walls & Whitbeck, 2012). There are associations between historical and contemporary trauma. In Brave Heart's conceptual model, historical trauma and historical trauma response are intertwined with lifetime traumatic events, both related to unresolved grief, PTSD, depression, and substance abuse (Brave Heart et. al., 2011). Native

American children and Sami children in Norway make connections between their current experiences with trauma and historical and intergenerational trauma related to histories of colonization and marginalization (Nicolai & Saus, 2013). Additional research is needed to untangle complex relationships between the effects of historical trauma and current stressors, such as poverty, health disparities, and discrimination (Walls & Whitbeck, 2012).

Historical trauma is collective and can have a compounding effect when trauma from different times, including across generations, becomes internalized in an individual. Descendants of those who suffered historic atrocities continue to identify with ancestral suffering (Evans-Campbell, 2008). The culturally based emphasis on ancestral ties, combined with ongoing reminders of colonization, may enhance vulnerability. This leads to a continuing impact on individuals' and families' health, mental health, and identity.

How people and cultures respond to traumatic events is more meaningful than details of the events themselves (Mohatt et al., 2014). Although there are differences in how individuals experience events, historical trauma narratives are grounded in real injustices or disasters. There are clear empirical links between thinking about historical loss and mental health indicators. The public narrative of historical loss is a contemporary stressor with specific, measurable health implications (Whitbeck et al., 2004).

A narrative conceptualization of historical trauma acknowledges atrocities while shifting the focus to how historical events are represented and connected to contemporary health outcomes and local contexts (Mohatt et al., 2014). For example, it is an undisputed fact that many Native children were taken from their families and communities and sent to boarding schools. Contemporary narratives describe the disruption of this forced removal of children, which resulted in the loss of traditional parenting practices, harming the parenting ability of subsequent generations, leading to health disparities.

The complex interaction between past trauma, resilience, and recent trauma is not easily understood in terms of a linear relationship. For example, Quechua women in Peru display notable resilience, in spite of experiencing a continuum of violence, including recent armed conflict and social inequalities (Suarez, 2013). It is important to recognize this strength and see women as contributing to rebuilding societies post-conflict, rather than viewing these women simply as victims.

The ongoing impact of historical trauma

Historical trauma can have a multitude of ongoing implications for wellbeing. For instance, it can have an impact on psychological, social, and biological functioning. Estrada (2009) links historical trauma to socioeconomic status. Traumatic experiences can lead to lower education and unemployment, factors that, in turn, can lead to poverty. It is also important to note that trauma can have different impacts on different individuals and Peoples. There can be intertribal or regional differences in experiences with and expressions of historical trauma (Burnette & Figley, 2017; Brave Heart et al., 2011).

As previously noted, unresolved intergenerational trauma is frequently compounded by contemporary trauma (Brave Heart et al., 2011). In addition to historical trauma being widespread and generating significant distress and mourning in Native American populations, it is noteworthy that the events are often intentionally perpetrated by outsiders. This intent is integral to understanding historical trauma and how it interacts with ongoing oppression. Many atrocities that have happened to Native people can be considered as genocide (Evans-Campbell, 2008).

Initial documentation of intergenerational trauma came from psychiatrists, psychologists, and medical professionals working with Jewish Holocaust survivors and their families. Clinical studies of survivor syndrome documented

> a wide range of affective and emotional symptoms transmitted over generations: distrust of the world, impaired parental function, chronic sorrow, inability to communicate feelings, an ever-present fear of danger, pressure for educational achievement, separation anxiety, lack of entitlement, unclear boundaries, and overprotectiveness within a narcissist family system.
>
> *(Braga, Mello & Fiks, 2012, p. 135)*

Empirical studies and clinical findings are divided about the long-term psychological implications of the Holocaust (Iliceto et al., 2011). One study found grandchildren of Holocaust survivors have a similar affective temperament to their peers, including self-perception and measures of hopelessness. They may, however, be more irritable and angry, and have a more negative perception of others (Iliceto et al., 2011).

Psychological trauma is associated with a loss of trust in fellow human beings (Dionne & Nixon, 2014). The unresolved grief resulting from historical trauma can be characterized as a soul wound (Duran, 2006) or an injury to the spirit (Smith, 2003). Thinking about historical losses requires cognitive energy and time; thus, this type of thinking is linked to negative mental health outcomes (Tucker, Wingate & O'Keefe, 2016). Interventions must be grounded in an understanding of the magnitude of losses, both historical and contemporary, as well as an understanding of traditional grief resolution to address grief and loss effectively in Indigenous populations (Brave Heart et al., 2012).

Internalized oppression is a manifestation of historical trauma (Durham & Webb, 2014). When past trauma is unacknowledged or unresolved, it can be passed to subsequent generations, leading to a sense of psychological loss (Durham & Webb, 2014). Historical trauma frames health disparities (Brave Heart et al., 2012). People who have experienced trauma can be retraumatized by multiple exposures to traumatic events (SAMHSA, 2016), leading to a compounding effect. Intergenerational transmission of trauma contributes to contemporary health and social disparities, including high rates of child abuse and neglect (McQuaid et al., 2015).

Native American adults with a stronger sense of ethnic identity are more likely to think about historical losses (Tucker et al., 2016). A study of Native college students found that more than 20 percent thought about historical losses at least monthly, with the most prevalent thoughts related to loss of culture. More than one-third thought about this particular loss monthly or more (Tucker et al., 2016).

Historical trauma has an impact on individuals, families, and communities. These are distinct but interrelated areas. In addition to individuals and families experiencing the effects of trauma, they may live within impacted communities, so the social environment may have more dysfunction and fewer supports (Evans-Campbell, 2008). It is important to understand context. Research that looks only at social problems, such as interpersonal violence, without considering the context of historical oppression risks overlooking the underlying causes of social and health disparities while stigmatizing Indigenous Peoples for these disparities (Burnette, 2015). The community impact of historical trauma may be the most insidious but also the least studied and understood effect (Evans-Campbell, 2008).

Trauma and diverse populations

Just as the development of historical trauma theory began with other groups before being more fully developed with Indigenous populations, it continues to have broad applicability, particularly with marginalized populations. For example, Estrada (2009) connects historical trauma with the Mexican American experience. Scholars like Coleman (2016) have identified a post-traumatic slave syndrome whereby African Americans carry the burden of historical trauma as well as contemporary threats to their safety and wellbeing. The hypervigilance, anger, and exaggerated responses associated with PTSD can be contextualized as normal responses to historical trauma and other abnormal situations experienced by African Americans (Coleman, 2016).

Racial minorities in the United States are at greater risk of developing PTSD, yet the DSM does not consider intergenerational trauma, discrimination, or racism as contributing factors in development of the disorder. Coleman (2016) explored how PTSD in African American military personnel can be better understood by incorporating more complex and inclusive frameworks. A broader understanding of PTSD can incorporate intergenerational trauma theories and subsequent coping mechanisms. This broader conceptualization can also enable explorations of the relationship between racial discrimination, high stress levels, and PTSD (Coleman, 2016).

Historical trauma is an issue for many Indigenous Peoples beyond the United States. The commonality of colonization, displacement, ongoing resistance, and resilience creates a bond among Indigenous Peoples around the world. Peoples with significant histories of collective trauma and contemporary marginalization develop narratives of historical trauma. These cultural narratives can sustain psychological wounds in ways that inhibit psychological growth. They may also support resilience with narratives of survival through adversity. Such positive narratives may empower Indigenous Peoples to manage contemporary oppression (Mohatt et al., 2014).

Likewise, there are many non-Indigenous Peoples who struggle with the impact of historical and contemporary trauma. There continue to be many wars, displacements, and refugee-producing situations around the world. Refugees may experience PTSD symptoms of numbness, dissociation, and anxiety. They are likely to transmit this trauma to their children through direct means, including corporal punishment, as well as indirectly, through being psychologically distant and having less involvement in family activities. Children of survivors of genocide in Rwanda, Nigeria, Cambodia, Armenia, and the former Yugoslavia all have distinct pathological symptoms (Braga et al., 2012).

Being a child soldier is associated with both experiencing and perpetrating violence. As former child soldiers mature and have children of their own, researchers have identified a further opportunity to examine intergenerational transmission of trauma. A qualitative study in Burundi found parents who are former child soldiers transmit stress to their children. These children are attuned to their parents' distress and try to comfort them. Being a former child soldier carries societal stigma, which also reinforces intergenerational trauma (Song, Tol & Jong, 2014).

Implications of traumatic exposure

While traumatic events can have a lasting and substantial impact on individuals, families, and communities, it is important to note that responses to trauma vary substantially. Early trauma can be particularly influential in causing later vulnerabilities to behavioral and psychological problems (McQuaid et al., 2015). Trauma can have profound effects on development and impede coping abilities.

People with strong support systems, resilient qualities, and no previous exposure to trauma may not experience mental health concerns as a result of trauma. Others, however, experience significant, ongoing difficulties (SAMHSA, 2017). Experiencing multiple traumatic events can have a snowball effect, increasing risk factors for social, behavioral, health, and mental health concerns (Maschi, Viola & Morgen, 2014). For example, many people who are homeless or receiving mental health services have trauma histories (Kelly et al., 2014).

After a traumatic event, an individual may feel powerless and fearful, have recurrent feelings of hopelessness, and be constantly vigilant. They may feel shocked, betrayed, dehumanized, unsafe, and unable to trust. Trauma can affect multiple life domains and relationships, often leaving the traumatized individual isolated with feelings of shame, guilt, and rage (Kelly et al., 2014).

There is often a cyclical phenomenon where a traumatic event causes symptoms, resulting in impairments that increase the risk of additional trauma. In particular, experiencing violence can be traumatic, and this trauma can increase the risk of an individual becoming violent toward her/himself or others (Kelly et al., 2014). This, in turn, may lead to involvement with the criminal justice system or involuntary psychiatric hospitalization—settings where additional trauma and triggering situations are likely. Trauma histories can be associated with aggression and criminal behavior as well as developmental adversity and mental health issues. Cumulative adversity affects subsequent psychosocial functioning (Stinson, Quinn & Levenson, 2016). It is important to recognize trauma as a deeper issue and not just treat symptoms. Awareness of the dynamics of trauma can lead to the development of coping strategies, such as recognizing and avoiding triggering situations (Brokenleg, 2012).

In addition to having an impact on individuals, trauma has shaped society (Brokenleg, 2012). Times of great social upheaval provide opportunities for examining societal trauma. For example, examining the unique historical circumstances of what it meant to grow up during the Great Depression informs an understanding of how this influenced the work patterns, values, and health of people who lived through this era. Recognizing the societal impact of trauma sets the stage for exploring Indigenous experiences in colonial settler societies (Walls & Whitbeck, 2012).

Human service providers need a comprehensive understanding of trauma and the different ways this can be manifested (Goodman, 2013). Native Americans tend to have close-knit, large family networks. Such deep connections to large numbers of people may lead to frequent, multiple losses, including the deaths of close attachment figures. This intense positive attachment can be a risk factor for prolonged grief (Brave Heart et al., 2012).

Indigenous Peoples may live in a context of heightened vulnerability. An epidemiological study explored interactions between historical and lifetime trauma, cultural connections, risk factors, and resilience among young, urban Indigenous drug users. Drugs are often used as a coping mechanism for historical and lifetime trauma. Drug use can also increase vulnerabilities, including instability of housing, high-risk sex, violence, and increased HIV risk (Pearce et al., 2015).

While additional empirical examinations are needed in all areas, understanding of trauma and its sequelae is enhanced by data on PTSD rates and ACE (adverse childhood events) scores. Burgeoning research on biological changes in response to trauma will also expand current knowledge. Not all people who are exposed to potentially traumatizing events develop psychological symptoms. Examinations of resilience in the face of trauma are crucial in fully understanding the range of responses.

Adverse childhood events

In the mid-1990s, researchers began to document the prevalence of childhood trauma and started to explore its implications for wellbeing in adulthood. The original CDC–Kaiser Permanente Childhood Experiences (ACE) Study collected over 17,000 confidential surveys in which respondents provided details of their childhood experiences, current health, and health behaviors. The study revealed that adverse childhood events are common, with almost two-thirds of respondents having one, and more than one in five having three or more.

ACE scores assess cumulative childhood stress. Adverse childhood events have implications for chronic disease, health-risk behaviors, and mental health problems. Higher scores are associated with a wide variety of risks, including alcohol misuse, pulmonary disease, illicit drug use, poor work performance, financial stress, domestic violence, sexually transmitted diseases, smoking, suicide attempts, sexual violence, and poor academic achievement (CDC, 2017). Military personnel with a history of adverse childhood events are at greater risk of developing PTSD after combat deployment (Arincorayan et al., 2017). In short, more adverse childhood events lead to a wide variety of problems in adulthood (Arincorayan et al., 2017).

Post-traumatic stress disorder

Post-traumatic stress disorder, a biological neuroadaptation, is one possible response to experiencing trauma (Ehlers, 2006). While initially this is an adaptive response to an extreme situation, lingering symptoms are maladaptive. Chronic hyperarousal is a key feature that can lead to secondary symptoms, such as anxiety, depression, emotional numbing, insomnia, and social withdrawal. PTSD lifetime prevalence estimates for the United States are in the range of 7–8 percent (Beals et al., 2013).

> PTSD requires an experience of intense fear, helplessness or horror during a traumatic event that threatened or produced physical injury or death (Criterion A), symptoms of reexperiencing (Criterion B), avoidance or dissociation (Criterion C), and hyperarousal (Criterion D), for a minimum of 1 month (Criterion E), producing social or occupational impairment (Criterion F).
>
> *(Bassett, Buchwald & Manson, 2014, p. 417)*

Internationally, rates of PTSD have been positively correlated with national political turmoil and negatively correlated with economic development (Beals et al., 2013). Indigenous populations are considered to be at greater risk of trauma and PTSD than other populations (Beals et al., 2013). The American Indian Service Utilization, Psychiatric Epidemiology, Risk and Protective Factors Project (AI-SUPERPTF) is the largest, most comprehensive study of Indigenous populations and trauma. It employed random sampling of enrolled members of two tribes, one in the Southwest and the other in the Northern Plains. All of the participants were living on or near reservations.

The AI-SUPERPTF examined PTSD prevalence using both single-event and three-event criteria (Beals et al., 2013). For single-event diagnosis, lifetime estimates of PTSD were 14.8 percent for female tribal members in the Southwest and 13.2 percent for Northern Plains women. Corresponding rates were 8.4 percent and 5.9 percent for men, respectively. Usually diagnostic interviews ask for the single worst event, but some ask for up to three events using a list of probable trauma.

In the AI-SUPERPTF study, using the three worst events criteria increased PTSD prevalence by 28 percent. This includes people who would not have been diagnosed using single-event criteria. Gender differences remained in the PTSD rates, regardless of event criteria: women with multiple qualifying traumas had dramatically higher lifetime PTSD estimates (Beals et al., 2013).

Common diagnostic categories such as PTSD are helpful in explaining some symptoms experienced by Native people but they do not adequately explain the impact of multiple traumatic events occurring across generations (Evans-Campbell, 2008). PTSD measures do not examine the impact of intergenerational transmission between individuals or communities, or the relationship between historical and contemporary trauma. Looking only at PTSD is limited and fails to reflect all of the complexities of many of the people who are exposed to trauma. Given these limitations, additional assessments are needed to understand the full impact of trauma for Indigenous clients. PTSD must be understood more broadly. Individuals from under-resourced communities often experience ongoing trauma concurrently with treatment. Protocols developed to treat clients who have suffered single traumatic events are inadequate for assisting clients with complex, ongoing trauma (McCrea, Guthrie & Bulanda, 2016).

The inadequate nature of trauma treatment protocols negatively affects Indigenous people. In Native American communities, trauma is cumulative and exacerbated by environmental factors, such as poverty (BigFoot & Schmidt, 2010). Native Americans rank highest on many ratings of violence and trauma (American Indian Law and Order Commission, 2015). They have multiple risk factors as well as high rates of PTSD. One out of every 30 Native youth age 14 or under has experienced trauma. This is more than double the rate for non-Native US youth and a blatant and painful example of Indigenous Peoples' increased vulnerability to trauma exposure (BigFoot & Schmidt, 2010). In another example, a study of 146 Native Americans found that PTSD has neurobiological consequences, including electroencephalogram findings of "hyperarousal, higher attentional levels to sad stimuli and slower processing of happy stimuli" (Ehlers et al., 2006, p. 125). In this study, 99 percent of the sample experienced at least one trauma, with the mean being five. Clearly, it is important to prevent trauma exposure in Native American communities in order to reduce PTSD and associated symptoms (Beals et al., 2013).

Epigenetics

The body can be changed by environmental forces throughout a lifetime. The study of epigenetics is illuminating how internal molecular pathways in the body can be altered as a result of external situations (Lock, 2015). Early life trauma can lead to persistent biological changes. For example, a study of adolescents who experienced physical abuse early in life found decreased peripheral levels of the thyroid hormone T3 (Machado et al., 2015).

Trauma can lead to changes in the brain and a variety of biological responses:

> The human stress response is triggered by trauma, fear, and other adverse conditions. It is regulated by the central nervous system (CNS), which activates the autonomic nervous system (ANS), the neuroendocrine system, and the immune system ... Exposure to extreme stress or trauma affects an individual's long-term capacity to modulate the ANS in response to subsequent stress. PTSD is associated with ANS dysfunction ... An individual with PTSD will respond to activation of the amygdala (immediate "fight or flight"

response) without being able to wait for the context provided by the cortex and hippocampus, thus moving into an emergency state of behavior where there is no emergency or real threat.

(Kelly et al., 2014, p. 414)

Environments, including the social environment, can have a shaping impact on human biology (Lock, 2015). Epigenetics theory proposes that genes carry memories of ancestral trauma and this influences how individuals react to contemporary trauma and stress (Pember, 2016). Historical trauma can lead to a psychobiological stress mechanism that influences neuroendocrine hyperactivity, autonomic and metabolic responses, and the immune system. This, in turn, can lead to diabetes, antisocial personality disorder, metabolic syndrome, substance abuse, and hypertension (Estrada, 2009). Significant adversity can lead to biological changes in stress response systems, the developing brain, the cardiovascular system, the immune system, and metabolic regulatory controls. These changes can result in lifelong impairments in physical health and mental health (Pember, 2016).

Epigenetic changes are not yet fully understood. Other research has shown that effects on gene function may be limited to short stretches of time (Lock, 2015). Intergenerational epigenetic changes vary significantly, meaning not all descendants are inevitably affected. More research is needed on the biological basis for intergenerational transmission of trauma. While studies have connected DNA methylation to intergenerational biological changes, it is possible that ribonucleic acid has an even more potent effect (Lock, 2015). Studies documenting biological changes in response to trauma can provide scientific evidence of the impact of historical trauma (Pember, 2016).

From the time of conception and throughout the lifespan of individuals, intrasomatic, cellular environments, and extrasomatic environments, physical and social, should be conceptualized as together bringing about transformation in material bodies. It remains an open question whether or not these interactions result in intergenerational transmission of effects. But sufficient evidence exists to argue that the body should not be conceptualized as a clearly bounded predetermined entity from birth.

(Lock, 2015, p. 177)

In order to comprehend the full impact of epigenetics, it is important to view them within historical, political, and ethnographic contexts while also considering their clinical implications (Lock, 2015). Epigenetic data could provide rigorous scientific evidence of the harm caused by discrimination. Governments and international bodies could then use this evidence to document and address human rights issues (Lock, 2015). Ultimately, societies must eliminate oppression and support human rights as a way to minimize trauma. It is important to examine issues of power and exploitation rather than seek new therapeutic techniques or medicine to help individuals and communities process trauma and adapt to oppression.

Resilience

There are also narratives of resilience, persistence, and strength that balance the psychologically driven deficit narratives of historical trauma that emphasize negative behavioral health impacts (Mohatt et al., 2014). When Indigenous elders from Southwestern tribes spoke of the impact of historical trauma in their communities, their accounts of this trauma were interwoven with descriptions of resilience and resilience strategies (Reinschmidt et al., 2016). Indigenous worldviews can frame how historical trauma is experienced. A holistic worldview in which mind, body, spirit, and context are interconnected translates to a framework where resilience and transcendence intertwine with risk and protective factors (Burnette & Figley, 2017).

Resilience is characterized by achieving positive outcomes in spite of significant adversity (Arincorayan et al., 2017; McCrea et al., 2016) or adaptive characteristics to recover from trauma (Iacoviello & Charney, 2014). Resilience can mitigate the onset of psychological, social, and behavioral problems associated with adverse childhood events (Arincorayan et al., 2017). Early research on resilience focused on individuals and their personal traits; only later did studies start to look at community characteristics or other aspects of social context (Reinschmidt et al., 2016). Both innate factors and the environmental context influence resilience, as does the availability of relationships with supportive adults (Arincorayan et al., 2017).

In most cases, trauma exposure does not lead to ongoing psychological distress. There is a range of potential responses, including resilience (Iacoviello & Charney, 2014). Often people demonstrate a remarkable ability to recover, and in some cases flourish, after trauma exposure. Trauma can lead to the development of new strengths, coping mechanisms, and insights (Goodman, 2013). Surviving difficult experiences can enhance an appreciation for life. It can also make an individual stronger and more thoughtful about their life choices. Coping resources have a mediating effect between trauma and mental wellbeing. Indeed, resilience is possible even in the face of extreme adversity (Maschi et al., 2014).

Psychosocial factors that contribute to resilience include optimism, cognitive flexibility, active coping skills, a strong support network, being attentive to physical wellbeing, and possession of a personal moral compass (Iacoviello & Charney, 2014). These factors can be cultivated as buffers against future traumatic events or bolstered by therapeutic interventions for trauma survivors. Enhancing them promotes resilience on individual and community levels.

Attachment theory posits the importance of human relationships in creating and enhancing resilience. There is increasing evidence that supportive relationships increase resilience and mitigate adverse childhood events. Resilience-enhancing relationships can include a variety of adults from primary caregivers to teachers, coaches, human service professionals, and spiritual leaders. Much resilience research focuses on children, but adults can also benefit from supportive relationships with people such as coworkers. A study of adverse childhood events and resilience in military personnel found that simple actions between and connections to peers became foundations for the resilience that is a crucial element in overcoming current and future adversity. For instance, bonds (a sense of community) between combat soldiers helped during deployment. Conversely, an absence of such bonds (lack of community) after the troops' return was linked to increased risk of PTSD (Arincorayan et al., 2017).

A deeper understanding of factors that contribute to resilience can inform efforts to alter social contexts and enhance resilience in communities. Ecological factors can promote or inhibit wellbeing. Environments that honor cultural differences and provide community support promote the wellbeing of people who have experienced trauma. Conversely, discriminatory environments inhibit healing from trauma (Goodman, 2013).

Treatment considerations

Trauma theory and treatment have been criticized for focusing on trauma as a past event with little recognition that many people continue to experience it. Trauma can be cumulative and ongoing, rather than a discrete, past event. Many clients experience multiple types of trauma as well as ongoing stressors. A study of low-income urban youth with enduring, concurrent, complex trauma found some elements of PTSD treatments were alienating. Traditional treatments, rather than helping, reduced engagement and aggravated symptoms. For example, requiring parental participation in youth treatment was unrealistic for families overburdened with multiple work and family responsibilities and led to dropping out. Also, discussing trauma—a central component of many treatments—may be more harmful than beneficial for youth immersed in unsafe environments (McCrea et al., 2016).

Discrimination and racism are sources of traumatic stress for both individuals and communities (Goodman, 2013). Historically, treatment models assumed that traumatic events were over before the treatment occurred. This model is not relevant for people suffering from poverty in violence-ridden communities who endure ongoing stressors. Traditional trauma treatment models must be revised to improve engagement and enhance outcomes for clients continuing to experience traumatic events (McCrea, et al., 2016).

Treatment must be culturally relevant and accessible. Cultural beliefs and norms about parenting, sexuality, and gender roles must be considered in the therapeutic process (BigFoot & Schmidt, 2010). The Transgenerational Trauma and Resilience Genogram was created as a tool to help human service providers apply an ecosystemic view of trauma and recognize family patterns. This culturally relevant tool was designed to aid in developing strengths-based interventions with attention to sociopolitical concerns that affect trauma and healing. Indeed, "cultural recovery may be integral to trauma recovery" (Goodman, 2013, p. 393). As such, it can be useful to consider how culturally grounded symbols like the Medicine Wheel dimensions of Mind, Body, Spirit, and Heart may interact with different aspects of resilience.

The Indigenous Peoples of the Americas Survey may inform clinical practice and research as it can be used to collect data in reservation and urban settings to explore the impact of collective trauma and lifespan exposure on behavioral health symptoms and to guide the development of culturally responsive interventions (Brave Heart et al., 2011). This Indigenous-specific instrument includes questions modified from the Harvard Trauma Questionnaire, a well-validated, frequently used assessment tool that was developed to assess trauma in Southeast Asian refugee populations.

Whitbeck and colleagues developed instruments to assess how often people thought about traumatic events and losses and their emotional responses to those losses. This research is part of a growing body of work generating empirical evidence that demonstrates a link between collective historical trauma and emotional sequelae compounded by contemporary trauma (Brave Heart et al., 2011).

The Connor–Davidson Resilience Scale (CD-RISC) is a 25-item self-report measure of resilience with good reliability and validity (Arincorayan et al., 2017; Iacoviello & Charney, 2014). It has been used with Indigenous elders in the United States and youth in Canada (Pearce et al., 2015), and can be used to evaluate resilience and guide clinicians in recognizing opportunities to support their clients.

Trauma-informed care

The concept of trauma-informed care (TIC) developed in the wake of a study of adverse childhood experiences conducted by the Centers for Disease Control and Prevention. Study results led to an increasing awareness that childhood trauma was both prevalent and had significant, lasting implications for physical health and mental health (Berliner & Kolko, 2016). Moreover, traumatic childhood experiences are frequently not isolated incidents. The cumulative burden of adversity increases the risk of many negative outcomes (Berliner & Kolko, 2016).

Trauma-informed care is distinct from trauma-specific interventions. It is not designed to treat the trauma itself but is grounded in the understanding that many service users have experienced trauma and that service delivery systems may exacerbate trauma symptoms (Kelly, 2014). A trauma-informed approach shifts assessment because it does not ask *what is wrong with a person* but *what happened to them*, thereby moving the blame away from the individual. Trauma-informed care is anchored in the principles of safety, trust, choice, collaboration, and empowerment. These principles are relevant to organizational structures and policies as well as work with individuals (Fallot & Harris, 2008). For example, agencies can implement policies and procedures to help clients feel safer and to promote collaboration and empowerment.

SAMSHA has taken the lead in promoting trauma-informed approaches. These approaches incorporate awareness of trauma and its impact throughout all aspects of services and the organizational context. Many federal and local governments and agencies are investing in training for TIC. While it is important to raise awareness about the prevalence of trauma and the need for trauma-informed care, more must be done to implement services grounded in these principles and to document the effectiveness of TIC (Berliner & Kolko, 2016).

Some critics question how trauma-informed care differs from simple good practice (Berliner & Kolko, 2016). Generally, people support the concept of TIC but uncertainty remains about how to operationalize it, including identification of necessary skills and strategies. The challenges of operationalizing the principles of trauma-informed care and the questions of how this is distinct from full implementation of quality care mirror the questions that have been raised about culturally competent service provision.

There is also concern that the current emphasis on trauma and TIC focus on psychological responses in ways that can pathologize the individual and fail to draw sufficient attention to ongoing violence, including structural violence. In response, some critics have called for the application of a decolonizing lens with explicit attention to historical and contemporary violence experienced by Indigenous Peoples. They emphasize that the primary focus must be on violence rather than prioritizing trauma and its psychological impacts. They fear a focus on trauma can obscure the conditions that support structural violence (Browne et al., 2016). As an alternative to TIC, Browne et al. (2016) propose an expanded model—trauma- and violence-informed care (TVIC)—that goes beyond eliciting trauma histories to foster a safe environment for clients based on an understanding of historical trauma, ongoing violence, and discrimination.

Supporting strengths and healing

The field of epigenetics may offer insight into how people develop resilience as well as negative responses to trauma (Pember, 2016). It is important to ensure that documenting the long-term impact of stressors does not become misused as a way to feed arguments about genetically based inferiority and eugenics. There must be a balanced understanding of the implications of historical trauma. While it is important to understand connections between trauma and various forms of health and wellbeing, it is equally important to avoid stigmatizing or employing only a deficit perspective. Like trauma, resilience can be transmitted across generations (Braga et al., 2012; Goodman, 2013).

Scholars note both the magnitude of risk factors and the danger of further stigmatizing Indigenous populations. The "deadly role historic and on-going trauma and violence plays … [makes Native Americans] the gold standard for disease in this country … We could be viewed as ground zero for Adverse Childhood Experiences" (Pember, 2016, p. 9). It is inappropriate to assume that all Native Americans are equally affected by historical trauma. Some scholars have expressed concern that the way that historical trauma theory has been applied glosses over various life experiences and promotes images of marginalized, traumatized Indians. Rather than speaking generally of Native Americans and historical trauma, it may be more appropriate to examine trauma experiences of specific Native communities or bands (Hartmann & Gone, 2014).

Effective ways of healing from historical trauma must emerge from within tribal communities, drawing on spirituality and traditions (Pember, 2016). More scholars are beginning to consider the importance of spirituality for healing. Spirituality and mindfulness may be noted as helpful but can be difficult to measure and validate in ways that create evidence-based practices. This limitation makes many culturally grounded treatments ineligible for federal funding (Pember, 2016).

Cultural revitalization on a macro as well as a micro level can be a remedy for historical trauma. This is a way to replenish what was lost with colonization (Hartmann & Gone, 2014). Decolonization and restorative processes are directly related to recovery from losses. Calls for decolonization add a political aspect to ideas about therapeutic healing from trauma. These address behavioral health disparities in ways that go beyond clinical interventions (Hartmann & Gone, 2014).

Healing can occur in many different ways. Acknowledging and treating psychological trauma and historical oppression are important, but structural change is integral to ongoing wellness (Hartmann & Gone, 2014). In addition to acknowledging different paths to healing, it is important to be attentive to the needs of different yet interconnected entities, such as individuals, families, communities, and nations, to heal.

Sustaining culture in spite of oppression is a powerful example of resilience. Indigenous Peoples have demonstrated tenacity, strength, and resilience in the face of colonization (Pearce et al., 2015). Culture continues to be intertwined with resilience. Familial connection to culture and language were strong predictors of resilience in urban Aboriginal drug users (Pearce et al., 2015).

Resilience is dynamic and can vary over time, due to a variety of factors. There may be times when an individual demonstrates significant resilience and other times when resilience seems to be depleted (Pearce et al., 2015). Understanding resilience in young Indigenous people must include an acknowledgement of historical and contemporary injustices that impede resilience balanced by culturally specific strengths that support it. Along these lines, research in Canada is beginning to move beyond individualistic, linear, and Western-based conceptualizations to explore how protective factors such as culture, language, and spirituality foster resilience (Pearce et al., 2015). For example, self-governance, tribal control of health and education services, and Indigenous language fluency have been associated with lower suicide rates in a study of 196 bands in British Columbia.

Self-care for helping professionals

It can be both rewarding and challenging for helping professionals to work with individuals and communities where trauma is prevalent. When working with these populations, helping professionals must find ways to cultivate their own sense of balance and nurture their own needs for wellness. In some ways this parallels the healing process for survivors of historical trauma. Mechanisms for promoting wellness differ from person to person. Each individual needs to develop a plan that makes sense for him or her and then use it, particularly when hearing stories of trauma. For example, artistic expression can be one of many effective ways to promote healing and let go of memories and narratives of trauma (Herman, 2010).

Placing a consistent emphasis on self-care is another important component of providing trauma-informed education for social workers and others entering the helping professions. This is particularly important in the context of teaching about intergenerational trauma. Professionals and students in the helping professions must learn ways to listen to the trauma of others without taking this as a burden on themselves. Learning about the numerous traumatic events experienced by Indigenous populations can lead to a trauma reaction in helping professionals who are trained to empathize with their clients. There are different ways in which helping professionals experience the suffering of others. They may react with numbness, remain oblivious, experience vicarious traumatization, or suffer compassion fatigue.

Of particular importance in human services education is the fact that many students learning about the intergenerational trauma experiences of Native Americans may come from backgrounds that included traumatic experiences. Educators must thoughtfully grapple with the implications of teaching this content in ways that are educationally sound and supportive of their students' needs. Students and professionals must learn to recognize how they may be triggered by or internalize stories of trauma and take steps to mitigate their impact.

Critiques and future directions

Theory about the impact of trauma on Native Americans has experienced significant development in the last two decades. Scholars have elaborated on nuanced distinctions among related ideas about historical trauma, intergenerational trauma, colonial trauma response, historical oppression, and related terms. These theoretical conceptualizations have received significant popular support from Native American communities and service providers (Hartmann & Gone, 2014).

The idea of historical trauma resonates with many Native Americans who find it a useful framework that reflects their life experiences. While empirical validation is still needed, the fact that this concept resonates so strongly with so many people whose experiences it seeks to explain suggests that it fills a significant gap (Evans-Campbell, 2008). Likewise, Indigenous helping professionals have embraced the theory, finding that it resonates with their own lived experiences and those of their Native clients.

Only recently have scholars begun to look at interventions for intergenerational trauma through the lens of evidence-based practice (Gone, 2009). Previously, theoretical development had been guided primarily by practice wisdom. While clinicians have identified intergenerational transmission of trauma in a wide variety of populations, some studies have failed to document similar findings (Braga et al., 2012). Indeed, there is still a significant amount of work to be done to identify appropriate ways to measure intergenerational trauma (Whitbeck et al., 2004).

Scholarship on historical trauma often includes limited explorations of resilience and strength. This deficit perspective is a limitation that can be easily remedied.

Indeed, the experiences of Indigenous Peoples are marked by stories of survival under extraordinarily difficult circumstances. As scholarship on historical trauma becomes more sophisticated, more exploration of strength and resilience is needed. Research should focus not only on trauma but also on healing. It is important to recognize that mental health issues caused by cultural losses are now being reversed, leading to renewed hope (Morgan & Freeman, 2009).

In reflecting critically on the literature on historical trauma it becomes clear that many sources of trauma are large-scale events that happened to whole communities or nations. On the other hand, many trauma interventions are conducted on an individual, clinical level. While individual interventions and healing are certainly needed, the primary use of individual-level interventions to redress large-scale trauma that happened to members of collectivist cultures may be something of a mismatch. There have, however, been grassroots efforts that promote macro-level healing in Indigenous communities. These projects can complement individual healing interventions and promote a sense of community wellness, resilience, and cultural strength that could not occur through micro-level interventions alone.

It is now commonly accepted that colonization, oppression, and policies promoting assimilation, both past and present, are the root causes of many health risks for Indigenous Peoples (Nutton & Fast, 2015). Conversely, decolonizing strategies, identity development, and culturally adapted interventions are presumed to buffer the impact of colonial oppression. It is notable that empirical investigations have progressed more slowly than theory development or acceptance of these ideas.

Acknowledging traumatic events and their lasting impact is seen as a prerequisite for progressing beyond dysfunctional, trauma-related coping mechanisms, such as substance misuse. Likewise, official recognition of genocide and trauma is part of the healing process, yet the United States was slow to sign up to the United Nations Declaration on the Rights of Indigenous Peoples (Brave Heart et al., 2011). This sort of lack of recognition may be one factor that has hindered development of empirical investigations of trauma and its impacts on Indigenous Peoples. While some empirical investigations have been conducted in this area, far more are needed.

Research is making progress in clarifying the impact that colonization, slavery, war, and genocide have on wellbeing. This research can inform how to address this type of exposure in the context of a presenting problem. While not all families exposed to trauma carry this burden through the generations, acknowledging the past can help others solidify resilience and look toward the future (Durham & Webb, 2014).

Significant opportunities exist for empirical examinations of the impact of trauma on Native Peoples. There are many areas that need further exploration, including biological, psychological, and social impacts of trauma on Indigenous individuals, families, and communities. While there is empirical evidence that intrusive thoughts of historical losses are linked with outcomes such as guilt, hopelessness, despair, anger, substance abuse, and depression, more data are needed to clarify connections between historical events and contemporary behaviors of Indigenous people (Walls & Whitbeck, 2012). It is also important to study treatment effectiveness and methods for enhancing resilience.

More research is needed on how current life stressors interface with historical trauma. These connections may be subtle, making it difficult to see a relationship between current reactions and historical trauma. Under these circumstances, emotional responses to seemingly small negative incidents may seem too intense, even to those directly involved (Evans-Campbell, 2008). Understanding connections between historical trauma and contemporary incidents can help contextualize and explain reactions to microaggressions.

Future research is needed to assess the range of responses to trauma as well as intertribal differences in experiences (Evans-Campbell, 2008). There is a need for greater description, assessment, and measurement of historical trauma. Once behaviors are identified, it is important to parse out what is dysfunctional and what is adaptive. For example, a certain amount of denial in the face of terror can be a reasonable coping strategy. More research is needed to develop and test interventions at the familial and community levels.

As research on historical trauma advances, it will be important to include more research on resilience and healing. It may be that experiencing historical trauma can strengthen community ties and heighten the importance of maintaining culture and traditions (Evans-Campbell, 2008). Another question for exploration is whether individuals develop resistance to current stressors like microaggressions based on previous exposure to trauma or whether these serve as triggers for trauma sequelae.

Urban relocation programs provide opportunities to examine the intergenerational impact of more recent events that many experienced as traumatic. Implementation of relocation programs began on a large scale in the 1950s. Unlike many earlier traumatic events, such as massacres, it is still possible to gather data from Native Americans born prior to implementation of this disruptive program for comparison with those born later to relocated families.

Historical trauma theory is often criticized for its focus on past trauma. This is seen as a significant limitation, particularly given the extensive continuing exposure to traumatic events experienced by Native Peoples today (Burnette, 2015; Burnette & Figley, 2017; Evans-Campbell, 2008; Mohatt et al., 2014). It is important to recognize that colonization is not simply a finite, historical traumatic event but rather a complex, ongoing set of processes and structures within contemporary US society (Hartmann & Gone, 2014). Scholars such as Burnette and Evans-Campbell have built on historical trauma theory and proposed theories such as historical oppression and colonial trauma response to provide a more comprehensive framework that includes history and contemporary interactions, thereby providing a remedy for what they view as a limitation in historical trauma theory.

In spite of frequent criticisms in this area, it should be noted that Brave Heart did acknowledge the impact of contemporary trauma in her development of historical trauma theory. She framed her development of historical trauma theory and historical trauma response as a context for understanding contemporary trauma exposure and reducing stigma about emotional distress (Brave Heart et al., 2011). The limitations of historical trauma theory may lie more in how it has been interpreted and applied (without consideration of contemporary trauma) rather than any inherent weakness in the theory itself.

Conclusion

This chapter has provided a brief overview of the development of trauma theory, including the concepts of post-traumatic stress disorder, adverse childhood events, and trauma-informed care. It has described the state of our knowledge and the need for additional research. There have been significant advances in trauma theory in the last century. While early theory development was spurred by attempts to understand the experiences of combat veterans, it has expanded to incorporate the experiences of many types of trauma survivors.

Clinicians working with survivors of the Jewish Holocaust identified inter-generational transmission of trauma, opening the door to explorations of trauma rooted in other atrocities, genocides, and colonization. Recent decades have seen a significant increase in the literature on historical trauma but much of this has been theoretical and conceptual. Significant research is needed to explore relationships between historical and contemporary trauma as well as relationships between individual and collective trauma. All these explorations must take into account the dynamics of resilience. Historical trauma and resilience are multifaceted, whereby the historical trauma and resilience of individuals are intertwined with those of families and communities (Reinschmidt et al., 2016).

2

A BRIEF HISTORY OF NATIVE AMERICANS

In order to understand contemporary Native American Peoples and issues it is important to understand historical events and policies. Understanding history informs an understanding of historical trauma as well as economic, health, and mental health disparities. Likewise, it sheds light on the substantial strength and resilience that led to the survival of Indigenous Peoples as contemporary nations and communities.

In spite of consistent intentions to de-indigenize all of Turtle Island (a.k.a. North America), US policies have had differential applications and impacts on various Native American Peoples. For example, since early contact between colonists and Native Americans was more pronounced in the Eastern United States, policies such as removals had a disproportionate impact on Eastern Indigenous Peoples. Some policies intended for all Native Americans, such as the Dawes Act (a.k.a. allotment, discussed below), were implemented on some reservations but rescinded before being applied to all. Likewise, termination policies began with some Native Nations but lost political favor before being applied to others. This chapter provides a general overview of key historical events and policies affecting Native Americans but it is important to understand that even policies with broad application, such as reservations, allotment, and the Indian Reorganization Act, had differential impacts on different tribal Nations, communities, and individuals.

Early encounters

Long before the arrival of people from other parts of the world, many diverse Indigenous groups inhabited the territory that has become the United States. These Indigenous populations had, and continue to have, a variety of social structures, including clans, societies, bands, tribes, and large intertribal confederacies. There is an unfounded stereotype that Indigenous Peoples of the Americas lived a primitive, changeless existence until European contact (Mann, 2005). In fact, by the time Columbus ventured into the Western Hemisphere, Indigenous relationships and trade routes had flourished in the Americas for more than 1500 years. Indigenous Peoples made significant modifications to the natural landscape, developed sophisticated understandings of science and mathematics, and built large urban centers with elaborate systems of governance and social relations. Before 1492, the Americas were a thriving, diverse place filled with tens of millions of people (Mann, 2005).

While many European colonists attributed their ability to colonize the Western Hemisphere to divine providence, the more likely explanation is extreme depopulation due to the ravages of disease, combined with more advanced weaponry. Indeed, smallpox had infected the hemisphere and decimated Indigenous populations before many Indigenous communities had even seen a European:

> When microbes arrived in the Western Hemisphere … they must have swept from the coastlines first visited by Europeans to inland areas first populated by Indians who had never seen a white person … Epidemics shot out like ghastly arrows from the limited areas they saw to every corner of the hemisphere, wreaking destruction in places that never appeared in the European historical record. The first whites to explore many parts of the Americas therefore would have encountered places that were *already* depopulated.
>
> *(Mann, 2005, p. 103; emphasis in original)*

While pre-contact population estimates remain controversial, the depopulation described by Mann, combined with estimates that 95 percent of the Indigenous population of the Americas died within the first 130 years of contact, leads to considerably higher population estimates than those proposed by early demographers. Today, it is generally believed that the population of the Western Hemisphere at the end of the fifteenth century (the time of the first encounters between Europeans and Indigenous Peoples) was about 150 million. About 40 percent of these Indigenous Peoples inhabited North America. At the time, the population of Europe was about 50 million (Dunbar-Ortiz, 2014).

Indigenous Peoples existed as distinct societies with a sense of territories and boundaries that separated them from their neighbors. Boundaries shifted as territories were gained or lost, alliances were made or dissolved, or nations joined with others to form confederacies. Indigenous societies maintained ways of remaining distinct from and incorporating others. For example, the Haudenosaunee (a.k.a. Iroquois) are a confederacy formed when five previously warring nations united after receiving the teachings of the Peacemaker. This amalgamation is depicted in the Hiawatha Wampum Belt, which also illustrates that other like-minded Indigenous Peoples are welcome to join. Subsequently, the Tuscarora Nation joined the Haudenosaunee Confederacy in 1722. Likewise, the Haudenosaunee Two Row Wampum Belt depicts the history of this confederacy's initial interactions with European newcomers and their determination that Indigenous and European Peoples had distinct ways of life that were equally valid, but non-intersecting.

Most Native Nations reacted to the European newcomers as potential allies and trading partners (Venables, 2004). As Europeans arrived in North America, they made treaties with the Indigenous Nations. These treaties recognized Indigenous sovereignty and documented a government-to-government relationship between European powers and Indigenous Nations. Treaties affirmed the land to be retained as well as documented payments and services promised in exchange for land cessions.

At least 395 treaties remain in force between Native Nations and the United States (Venables, 2004). In spite of numerous violations, they still carry legal weight. The obligations defined in these treaties bind non-Natives as well as tribal members, yet the United States has not fulfilled its responsibilities, even though these legal agreements are by far the cheapest land acquisitions in history (Venables, 2004). Although Indigenous Peoples once possessed all of the territory that has now become the United States, 98 percent of that land is no longer in Indigenous hands (Venables, 2004). In spite of extensive losses, Native Nations persisted and retained crucial elements of their cultures. Indeed, contemporary Indigenous Nations have been shaped by their resistance to colonialism (Dunbar-Ortiz, 2014).

The de-indigenization of Turtle Island

Some Indigenous Peoples of North America still refer to the continent as Turtle Island, based on the creation story of Skywoman, who fell from above to a world of water. She survived with the help of birds who caught her in mid-air, animals that dove deep in the water to find mud, and a turtle that allowed the mud and Skywoman onto its back, thus forming hospitable land for the woman and her descendants. Indigenous Peoples and colonists had fundamentally different value systems that led to diametrically opposed perspectives of colonization processes and the history of Turtle Island/North America.

The American continents have been systematically stripped of their Indigenous Peoples and heritage. This has been done in a variety of ways, fueled by values and philosophical perspectives that enabled the radical and violent shifts that are inherent in colonization. Annihilation and removal of Peoples, decimation of cultures, and seizure of lands and resources were all facets of de-indigenization.

Colonization and manifest destiny

Indigenous Peoples of the Americas and colonizing Europeans held very different worldviews. Native people viewed the world as populated by interdependent and equal beings, both humans and non-humans. In contrast, Europeans saw a divinely ordered hierarchy where only humans had souls (Venables, 2004). Indigenous worldviews allowed for fluid transitions between human and animal forms. There were few, if any, rigid, hierarchical distinctions between humans and other beings, sacred and secular, physical and spiritual. Stories tell of sacred beings like Cornmother who nourish people with their bodies, giving physical and spiritual sustenance, accompanied by traditions of people being made from corn (Kristianto, 2013).

The last five centuries of conquest in the Americas share a common theme: the replacement of one people by another. Indeed, the magnitude of the conquest of the Americas may very likely make it the most important conquest in all of human history. For five centuries after 1492, a territory greater than the Roman or any other empire was subdued with a brutality whose magnitude equaled the continents at stake. The initial wars of conquest ... brought wealth that helped Europe seize the economic leadership of the world and hold it into the twentieth century. The Europeans, with Africans and Asians pressed into the struggle, repopulated great parts of the American continents and imposed new political orders that in turn asserted their independence from Europe ... The conquest of the Americas stands as the greatest chain of military and social events in history.

(Venables, 2004, p. 2)

Colonization of the lands that became the United States is underpinned by two interrelated concept: the Doctrine of Discovery and manifest destiny. The Doctrine of Discovery was the principle, outlined in a series of fifteenth-century papal bulls, that European adventurers acquired title to land they *discovered* (Dunbar-Ortiz, 2014). This doctrine provided the legal justification for taking Indigenous territories, putting land in the hands of speculators, and ultimately transforming land previously held in common into private property (Dunbar-Ortiz, 2014).

After the founding of the United States, Thomas Jefferson sought to affirm that the rights granted to European powers under this doctrine could subsequently be passed to the United States. In 1823, the doctrine was solidified by the US Supreme Court in *Johnson v. McIntosh* (Dunbar-Ortiz, 2014). After the Louisiana Purchase, the United States became the first colonizer that did not recognize the Aboriginal title of the Indigenous Peoples of Louisiana (Klopotek, Lintinger & Barbry, 2008). The Doctrine of Discovery provides the foundation for contemporary federal laws and policies (Dunbar-Ortiz, 2014).

The concept of manifest destiny asserted that there was a moral obligation, perhaps divinely sanctioned, that accompanied the legal right to disposes Indigenous Peoples. A belief in manifest destiny is reflected in Woody Guthrie's classic song "This Land is Your Land" (Dunbar-Ortiz, 2014). The lyrics, which are intended to affirm equality among Americans, seem oblivious to the land's history of brutal dispossession and colonization. Becoming oblivious to violence and its institutionalization has lasting implications for subsequent generations.

Origin stories unify a sense of distinct identity or peoplehood while depicting core values and beliefs. Narratives of the founding of the United States tell the story of Puritans divinely ordained to take the land. These narratives, in turn, are reinforced by stories that depict the nobility of Columbus's voyages and the Doctrine of Discovery. They depict an empty land awaiting settlement (Dunbar-Ortiz, 2014).

To align with the philosophy that the colonists had a right or even a duty to populate this empty land, steps were taken to clear the land of Native Peoples. Colonization is a system that requires violence: "People do not hand over their land, resources, children, or futures without a fight, and that fight is met with violence. In employing the force necessary to accomplish its expansionist goals, a colonizing regime institutionalizes violence" (Dunbar-Ortiz, 2014, p. 8). In addition to more conventional forms of depopulation through combat, a growing understanding of disease as a potential weapon was employed by some colonizers. For example, Jeffrey Amherst, a British nobleman, wrote multiple letters documenting the distribution of blankets infected with smallpox to people in Native communities as a deliberate method of spreading disease (d'Errico, 2013).

Indigenous Peoples struggled to remain separate and distinct. Caught in the trajectory of the growing United States and viewed as an obstacle to its expansion, they resisted colonization and sought to retain their fundamental values. The desire to be left alone and maintain their ways of life was often a powerful motivation for signing treaties and moving away from settlements. On the other hand, ending the Native Nations' existence as distinct Peoples was a key objective of colonial powers (Dunbar-Ortiz, 2014).

The concept of manifest destiny spurred on many Europeans and subsequently Americans to overrun the continent. Some saw dispossession of Indigenous Peoples as justifiable and indeed a moral imperative. Warfare and conquest added to the trauma experienced by Native people. Many Indigenous communities were decimated by the spread of disease and warfare. Hostile and racist attitudes displayed by many Americans compounded the trauma. Indigenous Peoples were considered little more than vermin whose presence was an annoyance that could no longer be tolerated by the worthy and upstanding citizens of the United States. L. Frank Baum, author of the classic book *The Wizard of Oz*, expressed attitudes held by many Americans when he published newspaper editorials in 1890 and 1891 calling for the extermination of the Great Sioux Nation (Venables, 1990). His remarks were presented within weeks of the assassination of Chief Sitting Bull and the massacre of around 300 Lakota by the US 7th Cavalry at Wounded Knee.

The United States consolidated its power and the balance that had once been the norm in government-to-government relationships dramatically shifted. As the self-sufficiency of Native Nations was undermined by the loss of territory and resources, the federal government forcibly removed and isolated Native Americans, further undermining their self-reliance (BigFoot & Schmidt, 2010). The unremitting processes of colonization and racism continued to erode Indigenous resources, strength, and traditions by force, generating ongoing, daily trauma (Klopotek et al., 2008).

> US history, as well as inherited Indigenous trauma, cannot be understood without dealing with the genocide that the United States committed against Indigenous peoples. From the colonial period through the founding of the United States and continuing in the twenty-first century, this has entailed torture, terror, sexual abuse, massacres, systematic military occupations, and removals of Indigenous children to military-like boarding schools. The absence of even the slightest note of regret or tragedy in the annual celebration of the US independence betrays a deep disconnect in the consciousness of US Americans.
>
> *(Dunbar-Ortiz, 2014, p. 9)*

Clearing the land of Indigenous Peoples with social policies

As the growing United States sought more land and resources, policies were developed to deal with the remaining Indigenous Peoples. In the nineteenth century, this was done through a series of removals, establishing reservations, and taking land. This was echoed in the twentieth century with urban relocation programs. In addition to physically removing Native people, policies of the nineteenth and twentieth centuries created dependency and a wardship status, opening the door for ongoing exploitation. The theme of assimilation consistently underpinned social policies, serving as another way to de-indigenize the remaining Native population.

During the 1830s, many Native people were removed during the infamous Trail of Tears. Approximately 8000 of the 17,000 Cherokees who were forced to leave their territories in the Southeast died during this march. Likewise, the Creek and Seminole Nations suffered approximately 50 percent mortality when they were forcibly relocated to "Indian Territory" west of the Mississippi River. Many other Eastern tribes were decimated or completely wiped out prior to these relocation policies (Szlemko, Wood & Thurman, 2006). The 1863 Long Walk of the Dine' and Apache was another infamous removal during which 8000 people were incarcerated and about 2000 died at Fort Sumner, New Mexico (Dunbar-Ortiz, 2014). These are some of the most well-known removals, but the strategy was employed against many other Indigenous Peoples, too.

During removals, Indigenous Peoples were taken from their traditional territories and either imprisoned or forced to settle in new areas beyond the boundaries of the growing United States. At different times, various territories to the west of colonial settlements were used for removals, including what became the states of Wisconsin and Oklahoma. As Indigenous Peoples were forced from their own territories, they encroached on the territories of other Indigenous Peoples, sometimes sparking hostilities (Venables, 2004). Removals also happened within regions: for example, the Saginaw Chippewa were moved inland, away from the area that now bears their name in Michigan. Likewise, the Houma were pushed away from their traditional inland home in Louisiana and toward the Delta, and a reservation was established for the Nez Perce in Idaho, far from their homeland in the Wallowa Valley in what is now Oregon.

Removals were often disruptive. After each removal, Native people were "forced to rebuild their lives without resources. Most never returned to their homelands, and their communities were forever shattered. There were no Red Cross or crisis response teams to deal with the aftermath of Indian genocide" (Deschenie, 2006, p. 9). This was not an unavoidable natural disaster; rather, this was government policy and the decimation was intentional.

After the US Civil War and emancipation of African Americans, many Native Americans who remained in the Southeast moved into sharecropping roles. They often became trapped in subsistence living where they experienced paternalistic, controlling relationships with landlords, including violence like whipping. Violence is a learned behavior with ongoing implications. In some Southeastern tribes, the majority of today's older generation has experienced both boarding schools and sharecropping (Burnette, 2015). Much like African Americans, Native Americans experienced discrimination in the Jim Crow South.

As the settlers demanded more land, Indigenous Peoples lost ever more of their landholdings and territories dwindled to much smaller reservations. Initially, reservations were conceptualized as a way for Indigenous Nations to reserve some territory in exchange for services and federal protection from settlers. By the late nineteenth century, however, reservations came to be viewed as enclaves within states' boundaries, set aside by the United States as a charitable gesture (Dunbar-Ortiz, 2014).

The reservation system had a dual focus: it made large tracts of land available for American settlement and kept Indigenous Peoples in small areas where assimilation programs could be more easily implemented. In turn, assimilation had the potential to free up reservation land and dissolve the federal government's legal obligations if Native Americans were deemed no longer to exist as distinct Peoples. Indeed, by the mid-nineteenth century, there were many predictions of the vanishing Indian. Anthropologists, artists, writers, and photographers rushed to document Native people, as many Americans considered their demise to be imminent. However, the predicted demise did not happen quickly or completely, leading to the development of other assimilation policies, such as boarding schools (see below) and the allotment policy, also known as the Dawes Act.

The Dawes Act of 1877 sought to break up communal ownership of territory and allot parcels of land to the heads of nuclear families. These attacks on communal ways of life weakened and compromised cultural identity. After eligible tribal members received their parcels, additional land within reservation boundaries was deemed surplus and made available for non-Indigenous ownership. With the Dawes Act came requirements to verify Indigenous identity, but many Native Americans did not have documents to prove their ancestry. Such people were removed from their reservations and de-enrolled without compensation (Turner & Pope, 2009).

Allotment institutionalized the use of *blood quantum* as a measure of identity used by the federal government to determine Indigenous status (Schmidt, 2011). So called *full bloods* (Native people presumed to have no non-Native ancestry) were deemed less competent and in need of more restrictions on their allotted land. Even though the federal government promoted blood quantum as a marker of identity, this criterion was used selectively to advance federal policies, particularly when it came to how *mixed bloods* (people of Native and non-Native heritage) were to be treated. Mixed bloods received fewer land protections and were declared competent for the purpose of ceding land, but they were often not recognized as Indigenous for the purpose of receiving allotted land (Schmidt, 2011).

Although tribal governments are free to determine the criteria for citizenship in Native Nations, they have often adopted criteria based on blood quantum, mirroring the federal government's use of measures of presumed biological heritage. Under federal policies like the Dawes Act, external definitions of Native American heritage were often substituted for Indigenous measures. Indeed, for allotment purposes, federal commissions were sometimes established to determine who was legally a Native American (Ellinghaus, 2008). Strict blood quantum requirements limited the number of Native people, and fewer American Indians meant settlers faced fewer barriers to claiming land (Cavalieri, 2013). For instance, a large percentage of tribal members from the Five Civilized Tribes of Oklahoma were removed from census rolls at this time, affecting them as well as their descendants. Additionally, European and other Americans with no prior tribal connections were added to tribal rolls, making them eligible for treaty payments and allotted land (Turner & Pope, 2009).

By 1934, 118 reservations had undergone the allotment process (Schmidt, 2011). Proponents of the Dawes Act believed it would decrease poverty by encouraging farming and the development of a wage economy on reservations, but Native Americans receiving land distributions rarely achieved the predicted economic self-sufficiency (Turner & Pope, 2009). Desperate Native Americans sold their land allotments to buy food and supplies and were often swindled by land speculators. By the early 1920s, 80 percent of Oklahoma (a.k.a. Indian Territory) was in non-Native hands (Turner & Pope, 2009). Prior to allotment, Indigenous territories had already plummeted to 156 million acres, a small fraction of Turtle Island. When the Dawes Act was repealed in 1934, only about 50 million acres remained in Indigenous hands (Dunbar-Ortiz, 2014).

The economic status of Indigenous Peoples had become dire and heavily dependent on payments and services guaranteed by treaties. Colonial powers fostered economic dependency and developed ways to control Native Americans through Christian missionaries and alcohol (Dunbar-Ortiz, 2014). Throughout its history, the federal government reneged on treaty payments and continued to take land and undermine traditional methods of Indigenous self-sufficiency. The Supreme Court has held that Congress can abrogate a treaty unilaterally. This, however, is at odds with the United Nations Declaration on the Rights of Indigenous Peoples' emphasis on establishing a contemporary political relationship between Native Peoples and surrounding nation-states based on respect, trust, and political equality (Tsosie, 2012).

The taking of the sacred Black Hills is a particularly notorious example of unilateral action by the United States. This territory was reserved under the 1868 Treaty of Fort Laramie, then appropriated by the United States a few years later. The Lakota and Dakota Peoples have consistently asserted their claim to this land. Such land-grabs are human rights violations that can be remedied only with the return of the land to its original owners. Although the United States eventually recognized its wrongdoing and awarded monetary damages, this was done unilaterally and the financial reparations have never been accepted (Tsosie, 2012).

Re-examining the impact of federal policies

Under the leadership of Lewis Meriam, the Institute for Government Research undertook a national examination of the life conditions of Indigenous Peoples in the United States (Echo-Hawk, 2013; Venables, 2004). The Meriam Commission was a nine-member task force that included technical specialists in law, economic conditions, health, education, agriculture, family life, and urban communities, including one Native American member, Henry Roe Cloud, a member of the Omaha Nation and a Yale graduate. It studied living conditions on 85 reservations over the course of seven months. The resulting report, published in 1928, shocked public officials (Fixico, 2013).

While the Meriam Report continued to emphasize the importance of assimilation, it noted the Dawes Act had failed to assimilate Native people and resulted in extreme poverty. Consequently, it paved the way for policy change (Echo-Hawk, 2013; Fixico, 2013; Turner & Pope, 2009; Venables, 2004). In the wake of the Meriam Report, the federal government moved toward recognition of tribal distinctiveness, and acknowledged the need for improved educational and medical facilities as well as more regulation of and better-qualified Bureau of Indian Affairs (BIA) employees (Venables, 2004). It noted that corruption in the BIA had played a significant role in creating and exacerbating poverty among Indigenous Peoples.

Other studies at this time found that 55 percent of Native Americans had incomes below $200 per year, and 49 percent of those on allotted reservations had become landless. The living conditions of Indigenous Peoples continued to decline under the federal trust relationship. The federal government had assumed responsibility for ensuring the wellbeing of Native Americans as a result of legal decisions that defined them as domestic dependent Nations, akin to wards in need of protection. (See "Erosion of sovereignty," below, for the legal foundation of the federal trust responsibility.) It was assumed that this protected status would be a temporary step toward integration into the US mainstream. In spite of federal policies designed to promote assimilation, Native Americans had not become integrated within US society. Rather, tribal communities continued to exist as distinct entities in parallel to mainstream society (Fixico, 2013).

The Great Depression led to substantial policy reforms known as the New Deal. Likewise, policy makers developed the Indian Reorganization Act (IRA), colloquially known as the Indian New Deal. John Collier, head of the BIA, was the driving force behind the IRA. A former settlement house worker who had spent time in the pueblos, Collier revered Indigenous traditions, at least in the way that he interpreted them. He saw the IRA as a way to revitalize his vision of the "noble Indian" way of life.

The IRA, which was passed in 1934, was a significant piece of legislation that was controversial among Native Nations as well as many federal officials. Some US critics claimed that the Act no longer promoted the government goal of assimilation of Native Americans. Most notably, it stopped allotment completely and contained a provision that allowed Native Nations to opt in or out of the sections of the Act related to tribal governance. Many tribal members were confused about the implications of this. Tribes were often divided along heritage lines, with full bloods against the legislation and mixed bloods supporting it. Ultimately, 192 tribes accepted the IRA, with 161 of them adopting tribal constitutions by 1946. Meanwhile, 77 tribes rejected it (Fixico, 2013).

The IRA failed to solve all the problems noted in the Meriam Report. Reservations continued to struggle with the effects of colonization and federal dependency. One Plains medicine man insisted that ongoing problems on reservations were caused by systems of oppression that marginalized Native people and deliberately limited opportunity in an effort to push them off their land, which had the effect of fueling social problems and detaching community members from the traditional significance of the land. He also identified the legacy of the federal system as the cause of contemporary self-harm on reservations (Hartmann & Gone, 2014).

The IRA fostered self-governance but in a form that was palatable to the United States, based on federal guidelines. Essentially, it assimilated tribes into mainstream entities that were designed to be self-sufficient and economically independent. Once Native Americans integrated into the mainstream, federal responsibilities could be eliminated (Fixico, 2013). As Ramon Roubideaux, a Brule attorney, pointed out, "self-government by permission is not self-government at all" (quoted in Fixico, 2013, p. 88). Federal paternalism and perpetual wardship are inherently incompatible with sovereignty.

The complexities, contradictions, and ironies of federal Indian policy are highlighted by the Indian Reorganization Act—a law that provided an external mandate that could presumably dictate internal strength and sovereignty. But the latter is inherent and cannot be granted or legislated. Legislation that prohibits the federal government or other entities from infringing upon Indigenous sovereignty is all well and good; the federal government should be self-policing and penalize itself and its various incarnations, entities, and policies that promote dependency and wardship, thus undercutting sovereignty. However, Acts that attempt to *bestow* self-governance are no more logical than one of Frantz Kafka's novellas and no more credible than one of M.C. Escher's drawings.

Indigenous Peoples in both the United States and Canada are still legally considered wards or dependants of their respective federal governments. The sovereignty of Indigenous Nations is undermined, yet Native people in both countries have not been accorded full constitutional rights as citizens (Turner & Pope, 2009). This is an ongoing social justice issue. Federal governments still assert control over Indigenous lands and support exploitation of tribal lands for corporate profit on the basis that these lands are held by the federal government on behalf of Indigenous Peoples. Indigenous religious freedom is undermined and land held in trust for Indigenous Peoples is used for research and public recreation, or exploited for mineral extraction and the dumping of nuclear waste (Turner & Pope, 2009).

Helping professionals have played roles in creating policies and implementing programs that have undermined the wellbeing of Indigenous individuals and Nations. For example, social workers have been complicit in medical experimentation on Native people and promoting a eugenics agenda as part of social reform efforts. This has included using Children's Aid Society records to document so-called degeneracy and supporting a campaign to sterilize Abenaki Peoples (Johnston-Goodstar, 2013). Research has also been used as a tool of colonization and oppression (Bjorum, 2014).

Assimilation as cultural genocide

Forced assimilation is tantamount to cultural genocide (Dunbar-Ortiz, 2014; Schimmel, 2005). Article 8, part 1 of the United Nations Declaration on the Rights of Indigenous Peoples states, "Indigenous peoples and individuals have the right not to be subjected to forced assimilation or destruction of their culture." That right, however, is not respected under colonial regimes. Forced assimilation can take many forms, including prohibiting spiritual expression, usurping sovereignty, and disrupting intergenerational transmission of language and culture.

Spirituality is intimately intertwined with culture. In the United States, assimilation was often promoted through attacks on spirituality. John Collier noted, "the destruction of the native religions that yet lived was viewed by the Indian Bureau as a *political* necessity. The religions made the tribes strong, and made the individuals of the tribes immune to intimidation or corruption" (quoted in Venables, 2004, p. 289; emphasis in original).

Native Americans have never had equal protection for the free exercise of Indigenous religions (Tsosie, 2012). Indeed, explicit suppression of Native American spirituality was codified in 1883 with passage of the Indian Religious Crimes Code. This Act prohibited Indigenous ceremonies such as the Sundance and was passed with the specific intent of forcing assimilation (Venables, 2004). Indigenous bereavement practices were also banned (Brave Heart et al., 2011). Participation in traditional Indigenous ceremonies was punishable by imprisonment (Forbes-Boyte, 1999; O'Brien, 1991). Native Americans who gathered for Ghost Dance ceremonies at Wounded Knee Creek in 1890 were massacred. Their bodies, initially left frozen on the ground in a blizzard, were later dumped in a mass grave. Congress awarded 30 Medals of Honor to those who conducted the massacre (LaDuke, 2005; O'Brien, 1991). Likewise, hundreds of spiritual leaders were sent to the Hiawatha Asylum for Insane Indians for practicing their spiritual beliefs (LaDuke, 2005).

Controlling Indigenous spiritual expressions devastates cultural integrity (Weaver, 2011). Only incrementally have some Indigenous religious freedoms been restored under the 1978 American Indian Religious Freedom Act and subsequent amendments (O'Brien, 1991). However, some Indigenous practices, such as those related to traditional burials, are still prohibited (Brave Heart et al., 2011).

Canada also passed a series of laws that replaced traditional systems of governance, took control of finances, and outlawed traditional marriage and parenting practices (Turner & Pope, 2009). The country's Indian Act was implemented as an attack on nationhood. It usurped Indigenous sovereignty by promulgating rules and determinations of who is and who is not legally considered Indigenous. The original law, passed in 1857, allowed men to renounce their Indigenous status and ability to live on reserve lands so they could assimilate into general society. Women were given no such choice. Rather, a woman's status was determined by the choices made by her husband or father. An 1869 addition removed a Native woman's Indigenous status and place in her community if she married outside her tribe, even if her husband was also Indigenous. Children born to Indigenous women who married non-Indigenous men were not deemed Indigenous and therefore were ineligible for any rights guaranteed to Indigenous Peoples. The Indian Act remained in effect for more than a century (Amnesty International, 2004). As in the United States, reducing the number of people who were legally recognized as Indigenous in Canada meant that fewer people could assert claims to land and treaty rights.

Boarding schools: the ultimate tool of cultural destruction

As US policies shifted from warfare and containment of Native Americans to mechanisms for incorporating them within wider society, boarding schools became a primary method for assimilation. Other contexts with culturally distinct Indigenous populations, such as Canada, Australia, and Sweden, also implemented residential schools as a matter of federal policy.

The loss of children is the loss of the future. If children are taken from their families and communities and educated into a different value system and way of life, this threatens the continuation of Indigenous Peoples as distinct from wider society. The Indian Civilization Act of 1819 authorized instruction in reading, writing, arithmetic, and agriculture based on the belief that education would assimilate American Indians into the lower classes of US society, thus resolving the so-called "Indian problem" (Lajimodiere, 2012).

Boarding schools became the ultimate tool of cultural destruction. Colonial governments strategically focused on one of the most central and vulnerable facets of Indigenous communities—the children. Government and church-run boarding schools implemented a systematic process of colonization, religious conversion, and cultural genocide against Native people (Kristianto, 2013) from the late nineteenth until the mid-twentieth century. This education stripped away Indigenous languages, customs, traditions, and spirituality while simultaneously forcing assimilation into American and Christian value systems (Grayshield et al., 2015; Szlemko et al., 2006).

Civil War veteran Captain Richard H. Pratt is commonly known as the founder of the boarding school movement in the United States. In his own words:

> A great general has said that the only good Indian is a dead one, and that high sanction of his destruction has been an enormous factor in promoting Indian massacres. In a sense I agree with the sentiment, but only in this: that all the Indian there is in the race should be dead. Kill the Indian in him, and save the man.
>
> *(Quoted in History Matters, n.d.)*

Education was the vehicle used for cultural destruction, clearing the way to redeem and integrate the remaining cultureless shells.

Vacant cavalry barracks were granted to Pratt in Carlisle, Pennsylvania, in 1879 for use as an off-reservation boarding school (Lajimodiere, 2012). Another boarding school, Chemawa Industrial School, opened in Oregon the following year. Boarding schools employed a strict routine of bells, whistles, and marching based on a military model. Indigenous children were forced to attend church and speak English. The schools had a vocational emphasis and corporal punishment was widespread. Students often worked in the fields, growing food for their own consumption, or did carpentry work for the school. As one scholar reflected:

> While Wilkinson [founder of Chemawa] and Pratt [founder of Carlisle] were contemporaries and viewed by themselves, and others of their era, as heroes and enforcers of assimilationist policies and laws, I see them as having worked the tools of ethnic cleansing. The genocidal policies these men carried out were aimed at the destruction of the essential foundations of the lives of American Indian students. Their objective was the disintegration of the culture, language, spirituality, health, dignity, and even the lives of thousands of children attending Chemawa, Carlisle, and the many other on- and off-reservation boarding schools.
>
> *(Lajimodiere, 2012, p. 15)*

Industrial schools in Great Britain became the model for residential schools for First Nations Peoples in Canada. As in the United States, this was federal policy. The first residential schools in Canada opened in the mid-1870s (Dionne & Nixon, 2014) and banned Indigenous languages and customs. This was done to erode a sense of identity, thus driving a wedge between children and parents, with the ultimate goal of civilizing youth. The low-quality education in these schools focused on industrial trades for boys and domestic service for girls. The schools were run in collaboration with Christian churches until 1969, followed by a phase-out period that lasted until the mid-1980s, when they were run only by the federal government (Amnesty International, 2004). The last Canadian residential school closed in 1996 (Dionne & Nixon, 2014).

These schools had inhumane living conditions, chronic underfunding, and neglect. The school authorities beat the children, chained them to their beds, and denied them food. Individual members of staff participated in horrendous physical and sexual abuse (Amnesty International, 2004). School files documented extensive violence and dismal conditions that violated the norms of the day, yet these were ignored by both church and government officials.

Interviews with boarding school survivors revealed that they were stripped of their cultural identity, language, ceremonies, and traditions. Separation from parents and extended family led to feelings of loneliness, loss, worthlessness, and abandonment. Many of the students endured severe mental, physical, and sexual abuse as well as forced labor, hunger, and malnutrition. They continued to feel culturally disconnected when they returned home. Their experiences led to unresolved grief manifested as silence, mental health issues, relationship issues, and substance abuse (Warne & Lajimodiere, 2015). In Western belief systems, subjugation of the body is a logical way to save the soul. That logic underpinned the corporal punishment and physical abuse that were common throughout the boarding schools:

The obsession of the proponents of Christianity in America with the destruction of the body of native children to bring their souls to Christian salvation is
intriguing. There seems to be an acute hatred toward the human body on the
part of the perpetrators of violence in the boarding schools, i.e., the nuns and
the priests, across Christian denominations, which made them think that the
education of children could be performed using the instruments of violence ...
such as penetrating their tongues with sewing needles for speaking their native
languages, hitting the naked legs of runaway children using switches, as well as
punishments aimed at breaking their psyche such as having them lick milk on
all fours like animals in the presence of other children, having to wear "soiled
panties" on their heads for not cleaning themselves properly, and having to
consume the food that had been previously vomited.

(Kristianto, 2013, p. 42)

Boarding school staff inflicted this suffering without any accountability, yet their
actions would set in motion a chain of events that continues today. Many of the
children who experienced abuse were left with a sense of shame and self-hatred.
They came to believe that their own families, communities, cultures, and languages
were backward and demonic. They were denied positive parental role models and
passed on a legacy of violence and abuse to subsequent generations (Amnesty
International, 2004; Dionne & Nixon, 2014).

In Alberta, parents were threatened with prison if their children were not sent to
residential schools by a certain age (Dionne & Nixon, 2014). A study of residential
school survivors revealed that very young Native children had been abducted by
members of the clergy, Indian agents, and interpreters. The children often had no
idea what was happening and were denied contact with siblings at the same school
(Dionne & Nixon, 2014).

Boarding schools were places that undermined dignity and privacy. Children had
to shower with others. They were trained to respond to bells. They were told
what to wear. After being released from these institutions, they often had no idea
how to make their own choices. Residential school survivors have made connections between the schools and other institutional experiences. In both residential
schools and prisons, it is important to be alert and know how to "play the game."
For example, in the residential schools, children routinely gave their desserts to
other children in exchange for protection, a practice that was often replicated by
residential school survivors who were later incarcerated. Indeed, a study found that
some survivors were more comfortable with institutional living than life in the
outside world (Dionne & Nixon, 2014). For these individuals, the strict routines of
institutional living had become the only way of life that they knew (Dionne &
Nixon, 2014). Boarding schools left many survivors with a broken sense of self and
an impaired ability to envision a future (Kristianto, 2013).

The decades-long, massive removal of children from their communities led to
identity confusion, with boarding school survivors unable to fit into either their
home communities or the dominant society. In Canada, more than 140,000

Indigenous children were subjected to this educational policy, which was designed to suppress language and break connections to culture, families, and communities. In addition, more than 4000 children were recorded as dying in Canadian residential schools (Nutton & Fast, 2015).

There has often been a close connection between social reformers and Christian missionaries, with both playing roles in the assimilation of Indigenous Peoples (Johnston-Goodstar, 2013). Social workers have functioned as partners and proxies of the United States in the campaign for assimilation. Indeed, they have often had a role in implementing federal policies. As such, they have undermined Indigenous cultures and sovereignty (Johnston-Goodstar, 2013). The Child Welfare League of America worked with the BIA to place Native American children in non-Native homes, preferably far from their families and communities, as part of an assimilationist strategy. It is estimated that approximately half of all Native American people were raised away from their families and tribal contexts in the twentieth century (Cavalieri, 2013).

The National Boarding School Healing Project, sponsored by a coalition of Native agencies, works to document abuses that took place in the schools and their impact on families and communities, and demands justice from the federal government. Interviews conducted with survivors provide irrefutable evidence of countless human rights violations, including physical and sexual abuse, malnutrition, forced labor, religious and cultural suppression, and inadequate medical care. As in Canada, children died in these schools, sometimes through maltreatment and sometimes through suicide. Most of the survivors interviewed for the National Boarding School Healing Project had never told their children or grandchildren of their experiences (Lajimodiere, 2012). Trauma tends to fester when grief is silenced.

Although recent legislation was introduced with the intention of making reparations and promoting healing, the requirements have sometimes generated additional distress. For instance, residential school survivors were asked to disclose personal information about their experiences in the schools in order to receive financial compensation from the Canadian government. This requirement often led to resurfacing traumatic memories (Dionne & Nixon, 2014). Although compensation hearings were ostensibly private, sometimes survivors were asked to recount their experiences in front of their abusers. Their stories were judged by adjudicators who applied a compensation matrix based on the severity of the abuse and estimates of its emotional consequences. In this way, "cultural and human sacrifices are accounted for through a litigious system of monetary compensation for physical, sexual, and mental abuse" (Wiebe, 2016, p. 76). This is a long way from a trauma-informed approach that is designed to promote healing and reconciliation. Conversely, some boarding school survivors have found ways to recognize and shed the internalized oppression resulting from their experiences in the schools. Rather than continuing to carry the hurt, they have managed to forgive, let go of hatred, and move toward healing (Lajimodiere, 2012).

Erosion of sovereignty

Sovereignty was undermined and federal paternalism solidified with Supreme Court decisions known as the "Marshall trilogy." These cases formed the foundation of federal Indian law and defined tribal governments as *domestic dependent nations*. Marshall reasoned that Native Peoples maintained a separate political identity, illustrated by treaties signed with Great Britain and the United States and because they remained self-governing within their own territories. They were not, however, foreign nations as they existed within the boundaries of the United States. These legal decisions held that Native Peoples had a *right of occupancy* subject to extinguishment by the United States, which held sovereign title to the land through *discovery*. Marshall also noted that, because Native Americans did not have the same civilized status as Europeans, they were deemed wards of the federal government, thus giving the United States a duty to protect Native Americans from mistreatment by non-Natives (Tsosie, 2012).

These legal cases resulted in the doctrines of plenary power and federal trust responsibility. The latter confers a duty to protect while the former vests the federal government with the ability to regulate tribes, their lands, and their resources, regardless of Indigenous consent (Tsosie, 2012). Rather than possessing authority in their own lands, US legal doctrine has diminished Indigenous rights so that Native Americans are allowed to occupy their territories only at the discretion and whims of Congress. According to this line of thinking, Native Americans are the recipients of charity rather than vested with rights (Echo-Hawk, 2013). It should be noted that this dependent relationship, which is codified in US law, is at odds with subsequent international human rights doctrine that supports the rights of all Indigenous Peoples (Echo-Hawk, 2013; United Nations, 2008).

Sovereignty has also been consistently undermined for Indigenous Peoples in Canada. The 1884 Indian Advancement Act vested substantial authority in Indian agents as representatives of the federal government. These agents were given the authority to preside over band councils, and Indigenous people were required to seek their permission before leaving reserves (Wiebe, 2016).

In order for colonization and assimilation to be complete, the sovereignty of Native Nations must be undermined and ultimately obliterated. The history of Indigenous Peoples in the United States depicts a pattern of policies that dilute recognition of sovereignty, Indigenous assertions of nationhood, and inconsistent acknowledgement of the distinct legal status of Indigenous Nations and people. Key areas that shed light on the erosion of sovereignty are issues of federal recognition, relocation and termination programs, and the complicity of helping professions and professionals.

Federal recognition and its implications

Just as the federal government has attempted to define who is Indigenous, it exercises control over which Native Nations are officially recognized. The BIA has the authority to accept or reject petitions for federal recognition. Tribal recognition Bills have also moved through Congress, although the last tribes to gain federal recognition through this legislative process did so under the Clinton administration. At the time of writing, a Bill was seeking federal recognition for six Virginia tribes (Indianz.com, 2017).

Federal recognition is an acknowledgement by the US federal government that a tribe exists as a sovereign entity and therefore is entitled to a government-to-government relationship with the United States. Tribes can petition for recognition, which makes them eligible for a variety of federal services and funding. As of 2017, the US government recognized 567 Native Nations (*Federal Register*, 2017). In spite of federal recognition, however, the United States has increasingly encroached on the sovereignty of Native Nations. Tribal governments are not fully empowered to protect their land, resources, and members, thus infringing on their right of self-governance (Tsosie, 2012).

The rights of Indigenous Peoples without federal recognition are on an even more precarious footing. For example, non-federally recognized tribes are not entitled to repatriation of sacred objects and ancestral remains under the Native American Graves Protection and Repatriation Act. In addition, members of these tribes may face criminal prosecution for ceremonial use of peyote or for possessing sacred objects, like eagle feathers. This is because exemptions for Native Americans to use federally regulated items for religious purposes typically extend only to enrolled members of federally recognized tribes (Tsosie, 2012).

Some Indigenous Peoples within the United States have pursued a legal process seeking federal recognition. One historical example sheds light on this process. In 1938, a delegation of Tunica leaders traveled to Washington, DC, seeking federal recognition. Federal services had recently been received by the nearby Jena Choctaws and Coushattas. In addition, news of the Indian Reorganization Act may have encouraged the Tunica. Based on their application, Ruth Underhill, an anthropologist, was sent to conduct an evaluation of Tunica communities. Her visit lasted five days and the resulting report contains a host of historical, linguistic, and ethnological inaccuracies (Klopotek et al., 2008).

Underhill's criticisms included an accusation that Tunicas were a mixture of various Indigenous Peoples that had also mixed with Whites and African Americans. Characterization of their identity as ambiguous suggested that they might not be a legitimate Native American tribe worthy of federal assistance. Black ancestry among some Native tribes ultimately led the Office of Indian Affairs to eliminate services for all tribes in Louisiana by the 1940s (Klopotek et al., 2008).

Accusations of African heritage undermined claims to Indigenous status and therefore denied claims to land. According to the principle of hypodescent that governed social relations in much of the United States and particularly the South, one drop of *Black blood* defined an individual as African American, regardless of the rest of their heritage. The Tunicas were known locally as Redbones—Indigenous people with some African heritage.

> When they called Tunicas Redbones ... it was a means of disempowering Tunicas by erasing their indigenous legal and political status and highlighting their racial status. Black people or "colored" people did not have a collective right to the land under US law. Indian tribes did.
>
> *(Klopotek et al., 2008, p. 61)*

Some states recognize the existence of Indigenous Peoples that are not acknowledged by the federal government. State recognition may entitle these tribes to certain benefits and funding from state governments. As of October 2016, at least 63 tribes in 11 states were formally recognized as Native Peoples through state legislative action (Salazar, 2016).

Relocation and termination

The post-World War II urban relocation program was a large-scale government assimilation initiative that remains a source of trauma for many Native American adults today (Walls & Whitbeck, 2012). BIA-sponsored relocation legislation was designed to move Native Americans from reservations to urban centers for vocational training and integration into the mainstream economy. Assimilation has always been a way to reduce federal economic support for reservations. While the relocations were ostensibly voluntary, there was pressure for many Native people to participate. Relocation from small, tight-knit communities to cities was designed to undermine cultural values of sharing and intergenerational family connections (Walls & Whitbeck, 2012).

Relocation program jobs were often seasonal and poorly paid. Minimal training and job placement assistance were provided. Native Americans relocated to urban environments often struggled with adapting to their new cultural context. Indigenous cultural identity is rooted in place, which makes urban relocation particularly disruptive. Relocation experiences are linked to internalization of past cultural losses, amplifying a sense of dislocation and loss of land, community, and extended family (Walls & Whitbeck, 2012).

In Canada, the movement of Indigenous people to cities began organically. Later, this became a government policy that was promoted as an economic opportunity. The urban relocation policy focused on moving Native people to facilitate land development and centralize government administration of resources. Regardless of whether movement from reservations to urban settings was forced or voluntary, relocation became highly stressful and disruptive (Walls & Whitbeck, 2012).

Around the same time that relocation policies were being touted as a way to promote economic self-sufficiency for individuals, another US policy was designed to promote similar goals on a tribal level. The 1954 Termination and Relocation Act led to unilateral dissolution of Native Nations and encouraged assimilation through moving to designated urban areas (Szlemko et al., 2006). Like the relocation of individuals and families, termination policies did not succeed in promoting integration; rather, they resulted in the development of urban ghettos filled with Native people.

Termination legislation sought to eliminate the federal trust responsibility and all federal obligations to Native Americans (Fixico, 2013). The legislative language was phrased in a way that termination would free Native Americans from their burdens and make them just like everyone else in the United States. Reservations and all rights specific to Native Americans would be dissolved (Dunbar-Ortiz, 2014). A total of 109 termination cases were processed, beginning with the Menominee in 1961 (see Chapter 8 for further details). The termination and relocation policies both ended in 1973, as federal policies shifted their focus to self-determination (Fixico, 2013).

The global context

There are many commonalities shared by colonized peoples across the world. Just as Native Americans and Aboriginal Canadians experienced policies of assimilation, such as boarding schools, so did other Indigenous peoples, especially those who were surrounded by Anglo settler societies. In Australia, they speak of the "Stolen Generations" who were taken from their families. Like the US boarding school policy that sought to "kill the Indian and save the man," educational policies targeting Aboriginal Australians are an incarnation of assimilation as cultural genocide. As one scholar put it, in Australia, this was a way of "killing without murder" (Schimmel 2005).

Indigenous Peoples around the world have experienced trauma from colonial entities such as schools. This has led to ongoing mistrust of authorities, professionals, and the institutions they represent or are perceived to represent (Nicolai & Saus, 2013). The roles that social workers and other helping professionals have played in implementing federal policies have left a legacy of mistrust among Sami people. Helping professionals are often viewed as members of oppressive systems (Nicolai & Saus, 2013).

Beyond residential schools, various Indigenous populations around the world have been subjected to assimilationist policies implemented through child welfare systems. Like Native Americans, Sami have been subjected to child removal, placement in foster care or residential schools, and the criminalization of traditional religions and languages. These massive cultural losses and traumatic histories of colonization are associated with contemporary disparities (Nicolai & Saus, 2013).

Resilience is also a theme shared by Indigenous Peoples around the world. Native people from different regions speak to one another. They share their strength and healing as well as histories of colonization and trauma. As a result, Indigenous people are increasingly using international law to hold states accountable for historic and contemporary injustices (McMillan & Rigney, 2016).

Indigenous Peoples are finding ways to learn from others and borrow relevant strategies without wholeheartedly using someone else's experience to substitute for their own. The lived experiences of each Indigenous person are valuable and most relevant to their own situation. They can also gain strength from shared experiences. This is clearly articulated by Maori people, who have found ways to incorporate what they find meaningful from historical trauma theory and implement it as a companion to their own ways of knowing (Pihama et al., 2014).

Conclusion

It is important to understand history. It often frames contemporary realities. Native Americans, like other Indigenous Peoples around the world, continue to exist and display amazing resilience in the face of a variety of colonial assaults, both historical and contemporary. Indigenous Peoples transcend the ways in which federal bureaucrats and politicians try to define and confine them (Tsosie, 2012). Historical narratives depict significant trauma, yet close observers will also note recurring themes of resilience. Indigenous Peoples are survivors, in spite of many predictions of their demise.

We are not the same as our ancestors. We are changed by what they experienced. While our current incarnations have been forged by tragedy and atrocity, they are equally shaped by the strengths of those who have come before, our values, and the Great Mystery. Just as the buffalo puts her head down to walk through a blizzard knowing better weather is on the other side, Indigenous Peoples have weathered many storms and continue on our path for future generations.

3

CONTEMPORARY EXPERIENCES OF NATIVE AMERICANS

This chapter examines contemporary issues for Native Americans, beginning with an overview of the Native American population and a discussion of contemporary values and cultures. This is followed by an exploration of tensions between contemporary expressions of Indigenous nationhood and ongoing federal paternalism. The impact of multifaceted manifestations of racism is explored, as are activism, wellness, resilience, and healing. Contemporary experiences of Indigenous Peoples within the larger global context are also investigated. Beyond this general foundation, a more in-depth examination of specific issues is provided in subsequent chapters on child and family wellbeing, elders and veterans, education, health, and economic and community development.

Overview of contemporary Native Americans

The 2010 Census revealed that there were 5.2 million self-identified Native Americans living in the United States, constituting 1.7 percent of the total population (Norris, Vines & Hoeffel, 2012). Nearly half of these people (2.3 million) designated themselves as mixed heritage. Forty-one percent of the total lived in the West, while the South had the second-largest proportion, followed by the Midwest and the Northeast. Native Americans are a young and growing population, with every region in the United States experiencing a rise in their Indigenous population between 2000 and 2010. Fourteen percent of the Native American population resided in California, with Oklahoma boasting the second-largest figure, followed by Arizona, Texas, and New York State. New York City, Los Angeles, Phoenix, Oklahoma City, and Anchorage, Alaska, had the largest urban Indigenous populations, with 111,749, 54,235, 43,724, 36,572, and 36,062, respectively. Anchorage had the largest proportion of Indigenous people of any city at 12 percent. Only 20 percent of the total Native American population were living on reservations or Indigenous trust lands, although 31 percent of those who identified solely as Native American resided on tribal territories, compared to just 7 percent who identified as Native American with mixed heritage (Norris et al., 2012).

Many readers will be surprised to learn that 77 percent of the 4.6 million people who were living within what the federal government designates "American Indian areas" in 2010 did not identify as Indigenous (Norris et al., 2012). This is largely a result of federal policies such as allotment that led to the transfer of reservation land to non-Native owners.

The reservation with the largest Indigenous population was the Navajo Nation (169,321), followed by the Pine Ridge Reservation (16,906), and the Fort Apache Reservation (13,014). Among Alaska Native villages, Knik had the largest Native population (6,582), followed by Bethel (4,334) and Kenaitze (3,417). In terms of population, the Cherokee were the largest Native American Nation in the United States (819,105), followed by the Navajo (332,129), Choctaw (195,764), Menominee (175,494), and Chippewa (170,742). The Census also documented 332,129 people who identified as Mexican American Indian and 234,320 people who identified as Native American but listed no tribal affiliation (Norris et al., 2012).

Residing within a tribal territory, such as a reservation, or living in an urban area carries a wide range of connotations beyond a preference for a particular living context. In many ways, reservations have functioned as havens where culture and language receive more reinforcement than they do in urban contexts. Tribal territories are also sites of tribal governments and can maintain a level of self-determination that is impossible in other areas. While initially developed to confine and remove Native Americans from other lands, they afforded Indigenous Peoples a mechanism for keeping to themselves in ways that protected them from a societal context of violence and overt social inequality (Burnette, 2015). Reservation contexts also facilitated transmission of cultural knowledge and sometimes contained spiritually significant sacred places (Tucker, Wingate & O'Keefe, 2016). On the other hand, they can also be politically charged environments with limited economic and educational opportunities and a land base that is often too small to support tribal membership. Living on a reservation can remind residents of the unjust policies and laws that originally forced Native Americans onto these lands, thus reinforcing historical loss thinking (Tucker et al., 2016).

Urban areas can provide a variety of opportunities for education and employment beyond those available on tribal territories. These may entice additional Indigenous people to relocate, beyond those who participated in formal relocation programs. On the other hand, relocation has often led to bereavement and traumatic stress (Turner & Pope, 2009) as well as alienation and intergenerational poverty (Moghaddam, Momper & Fong, 2013). Substance misuse of relocated people is associated with substance misuse and depression in the next generation. This addiction can make second-generation urban dwellers less effective parents (Walls & Whitbeck, 2012). Their adolescents are at greater risk of developing depression and delinquency. Relocation is also a risk factor for intergenerational substance misuse (Walls & Whitbeck, 2012).

A study of urban Aboriginal street youth in Canada found that 92 percent had experienced some sort of maltreatment. In spite of this, most maintained significant resilience. Only emotional neglect was associated with decreased resilience. It may be that these youth can cope with just about anything, except for the failure of their caregivers to provide basic psychological and emotional nurturing and thus instill a sense of belonging. The effects of childhood emotional neglect extend well into adulthood (Pearce et al., 2015).

The experiences of urban Indigenous Peoples are multifaceted. While there are many negative effects, as noted above, cities were also places where Native people from many different backgrounds came into contact with one another and formed new pan-Indian communities. This became a source of empowerment, leading to significant activism and the creation of many urban Native American community centers and social service agencies (Means & Wolf, 1996).

In the cities, Native Americans encountered people from other tribes and other cultures. This often led to the formation of multi-tribal and multicultural families and communities (Weaver, 2012). This dynamic environment raises questions for Indigenous identity. It poses challenges for enrollment (establishing membership in a tribe), particularly for tribal groups who base enrollment on blood quantum measures. Many scholars view the latter as a deliberate attempt by the federal government to reduce the number of people who are legally designated as American Indian, ultimately leading to the statistical annihilation of whole Native Nations (Kiel, 2017). The adoption of blood quantum measures by tribes themselves is a reflection of internalized colonization. It amounts to a suicidal policy that will ultimately eliminate American Indians as distinct Peoples (Harjo, 2017; Wilkins & Wilkins, 2017).

Some Indigenous people have heritage from multiple tribes but insufficient heritage from any one tribe to meet the minimum requirements for enrollment. Others may have a mother from a tribe where enrollment is permitted only through patrilineal lineage and a father from a tribe with matrilineal descent, leaving them with full Native heritage yet ineligible for enrollment in either Native Nation (Kiel, 2017). Urban multicultural environments raise new questions as Indigenous Peoples grapple with what it means to be a Native American or a tribal member. Cultures are always changing and growing in ways that defy static stereotypes of identity.

Contemporary values and cultures

Indigenous cultures have changed over time but persist in the face of colonization and multiple efforts at assimilation. Therefore, they continue to provide a foundation for resilience in the face of trauma. One of the core values found across American Indian cultures is reflected in the Lakota phrase *mitakuye oyasin*—"we are all related." There is a sense of connection and relationship, accompanied by values of respect and responsibility. All beings are valued, including those that are not human. A sacredness is accorded to all living things, including entities that are rarely recognized as living by Western society, such as rocks, watercourses, and the earth. Within this cultural worldview everything is understood in terms of relationships (Nebelkopf et al., 2011).

People can fill many different roles. While these may be distinct, they are typically not perceived as hierarchical, with one role superior to another. This is reflected in a balance of gender roles and different responsibilities across the life cycle. There are different roles that contribute to the wellbeing of a community. These can include internal and external leadership roles as well as warriors and veterans. Indigenous cultures tend to be highly interconnected, including strong ties across generations. So, when community ties and intergenerational linkages are broken, this has significant consequences for subsequent generations (Walls & Whitbeck, 2012).

Indigenous societies have received traditional instructions about how to live in a good way. There are ways of keeping balance and maintaining wellness. Many Indigenous societies have experienced disruptions to their social norms and traditional ways. Virtually all Native American cultures have traditional beliefs and norms that prohibit interpersonal violence and substance abuse. Studies have documented higher rates of substance use among Indigenous people who do not identify with Indigenous values, and the lowest rates among those who feel comfortable with both Native and non-Native values (Szlemko, Wood & Thurman, 2006).

Traditional Indigenous values incorporate ways of mending disruptions and restoring balance. With cultural change can come adaptability and new ways of retaining and expressing core Indigenous values within new contexts. One epidemiological study in British Columbia demonstrated that culture and language have strong associations with resilience. The researchers found that cultural teachings, values, and traditional healing integrated with health services can support wellness in Native youth who use drugs (Pearce et al., 2015).

Traditional Indigenous identity is grounded within community. Resilience as conceptualized within a larger social context (rather than as an individual trait) fits within Indigenous understandings of interrelatedness. When the community and environment are resilient, this supports resilience and wellness in individuals:

> Distinct notions of personhood, where individuals are connected to the land and the environment, shape Indigenous ideas of individual resilience. Indigenous ideas of community resilience include revisioned collective histories that value Indigenous identity; the revitalization of language, culture, and spirituality; traditional activities; collective agency; and activism.
>
> *(Reinschmidt et al., 2016, p. 65)*

Indigenous nationhood and federal paternalism

There is ongoing tension between the self-determination inherent in the sovereignty of Indigenous Nations and federal paternalism. The Supreme Court has found that the federal government has the power to limit, modify, or eliminate tribal sovereignty. Others would argue that this is absurd and constitutes a human rights violation (Tsosie, 2012). This conundrum lies at the heart of Indigenous wellbeing. The unilateral exercise of federal plenary power violates international standards articulated in the United Nations Declaration on the Rights of Indigenous Peoples (United Nations, 2008). Tensions between Indigenous sovereignty and federal paternalism are rooted in history but also anchored in contemporary laws and policies. Social problems on reservations have historical roots but continue to be fed by contemporary, systemic oppression, particularly related to the federal government's failure to fulfill its treaty responsibilities (Hartmann & Gone, 2014).

The United States considers Native American tribes to be domestic dependent Nations (Tsosie, 2012). They are allowed to control their territory and membership and have the power to exclude non-members from tribal lands. On the other hand, the federal government controls recognition of tribes and defines what constitutes tribal territory. The jurisprudence that holds that Native Peoples remain distinct sovereign governments while simultaneously holding that the United States can unilaterally eliminate that sovereignty is a paradox that inhibits Indigenous self-determination (Tsosie, 2012). The United Nations Declaration on the Rights of Indigenous Peoples requires countries to work with Indigenous Peoples to establish free, prior, and informed consent before enacting anything that may affect them (Echo-Hawk, 2013; United Nations, 2008). Clearly, these US and UN principles are incompatible.

Beyond the dilemma of the United States' assertion that it has the power to eliminate Native Peoples is the question of federal recognition, introduced in Chapter 2. Federal recognition has continuing implications for access to funding and services. There are some tribal entities that the United States does not recognize as meeting its definition of "Indian tribe" and others that are currently seeking federal recognition.

> Today the question of which tribes are entitled to "federal acknowledgement" is governed by a byzantine federal administrative process which carefully sorts through the notion of "Indian identity" under a series of factors, including whether the group is recognized as an "American Indian entity" (by state or other tribal governments, by academics, or in publications), and whether the tribe has existed as a "distinct community" from historical times to the present. The federal acknowledgement process has been heavily criticized for its bureaucratic inefficiency and potential unfairness to tribes whose histories are not well documented by anthropologists and historians.
>
> *(Tsosie, 2012, pp. 939–940)*

The United States still grapples with its history of expansion, which led to massive dispossession of Native Americans. Many Native Peoples maintain strong spiritual and cultural ties to territories now designated as state or federal public lands, and they remain determined to protect the cultural and natural resources within these areas. In some cases, the United States treats Indigenous Peoples as stakeholders in the management of federal public lands, while on other occasions they negotiate co-management agreements to balance public use with tribal interests (Tsosie, 2012).

The Indian Citizenship Act of 1924 sought to increase the integration of Native Americans as individual citizens of the United States. Native Americans do not have a unified position on US citizenship: some still prefer separation and strongly assert their own Indigenous citizenship; others are strong advocates for integration and full participation in US society. Native Americans seeking inclusion have launched many lawsuits that demand Native American representation on state bodies that have an impact on tribes and their members, including school boards, transportation commissions, and redistricting planning groups seeking to ensure voting rights (Tsosie, 2012).

It is notable, however, that even within the United States all Indigenous Peoples are not treated equally. While the US federal government recognizes Native Hawaiians as Indigenous, they are not legally considered either a tribe or a domestic dependent nation (Taualii, 2017). On the centenary of the US overthrow of the Hawaiian government, President Clinton issued an apology to the Hawaiian people. In 2010, with President Obama's support, the US House of Representatives passed legislation that had been circulating for more than a decade in support of recognizing Hawaiian political authority, akin to federal recognition of American Indian tribes (Siler, 2012). However, this legislation was heavily contested and at the time of writing there was still no federal recognition of Native Hawaiians as a tribe or a sovereign government. Therefore, the Native Hawaiian sovereignty movement remains active (Lyte, 2017).

In the United States, many rights are guaranteed only to federally recognized or sometimes state-recognized tribes. On the other hand, the United Nations Declaration on the Rights of Indigenous Peoples speaks of the *inherent* human rights of all Indigenous Peoples. This may make it unjustifiable for the United States to treat some Indigenous groups (including Native Hawaiians) differently on the basis of their recognition status (Tsosie, 2012).

The legal status and governance structures of Indigenous Peoples in Alaska differ from those of Indigenous Peoples in the rest of the United States. Under the Alaska Native Claims Settlement Act, Native communities are designated as corporations that manage tribal resources using a business model. As corporations, they no longer possess the jurisdictional capacity and inherent sovereignty over their own territory that other Native Americans retain (Tsosie, 2012).

The United States' policies continue to perpetuate dependency and undermine sovereignty-based development initiatives. Some reservation dwellers are concerned that federal paternalism and a heavy regulatory environment discourages Native business ownership on reservations. The few stores are often owned and operated by non-Native people. This climate became entrenched after traditional forms of leadership and decision-making were replaced by an elected model of tribal governance mandated by the IRA (Hartmann & Gone, 2014). Under these circumstances, rather than being truly sovereign, tribal governments function as branches of the US government.

Leaders from many Native nations have identified the need for increased collaboration among federal agencies concerned with Indigenous wellbeing. Accordingly, tribes and various federal agencies established the National Tribal Behavioral Health Agenda, which was designed to promote coordination of services that focus on youth, culture, identity, and individual self-sufficiency. Services and policies in these areas are underpinned by an understanding of historical and intergenerational trauma (SAMHSA, 2017).

Article 5 of the United Nations Declaration on the Rights of Indigenous Peoples states that Indigenous Peoples can both participate in self-governance and be equal citizens of the national government. Native Americans can be full participants in both systems. This balance can be reflected in state–tribal agreements developed on matters of mutual concern, such as education, law enforcement, environmental regulation, and gaming compacts (Tsosie, 2012). This dual status must be recognized by non-Native people and entities. Along these lines, SAMHSA (2014) has produced tips for emergency responders that contextualize their status as outsiders within sovereign Nations and encourage them to work with tribal representatives to demonstrate respect for the culture and increase their credibility.

In spite of challenges, there continue to be examples of Indigenous Peoples functioning as self-governing Nations, at times lending support to the United States as well as surrounding states and communities. For example, in the wake of Hurricane Katrina, a tribal hotel in Marksville, Louisiana, became an evacuation center. Hospitality and generosity are central to Tunica traditions, so the Tunica–Biloxi council felt compelled to help all those affected by the disaster, regardless of whether they were members of the tribe. The tribal casino also became a designated Red Cross evacuation center. Tribal members devoted many volunteer hours, and hurricane relief efforts received significant financial support from the tribe (Klopotek, Lintinger & Barbry, 2008).

Shifting perspectives on the contemporary circumstances of Native Americans can play an important role in empowerment and addressing various disparities. It is important to move beyond a clinically based perspective of historical trauma that conceptualizes Native Americans primarily as patients in need of healing to a focus on nation building and Native Americans as empowered agents (Hartmann & Gone, 2014). Indeed, support for Indigenous nationhood as well as policy changes to eliminate federal paternalism and dependency can be important steps toward Indigenous revitalization and amelioration of many disparities. Empowerment through restoration of sovereignty would likely diminish symptoms of historical trauma, just as incursions on sovereignty led to trauma (Cavalieri, 2013). This, in turn, would enable tribal nations to continue to support the wellbeing of their non-Indigenous neighbors as well as tribal members.

The multifaceted manifestations of racism

Trauma is compounded by a sense of continuing injustice. Stereotypes and racism (including internalized oppression) can undermine the protective aspects of cultural identity. Bigotry, racism, and blatant hostility that continue to be expressed in statements such as "the only good Indian is a dead Indian" are chilling reminders that embracing Indigenous heritage is not always positively received. The psychological protective factors associated with a strong cultural identity can be muted by a climate of intolerance (Turner & Pope, 2009).

Native Americans live within a societal context where various forms of oppression are ever present. These can include blatant racism, discrimination, stereotyping, microaggressions, and environmental racism. These multiple layers of oppression contribute to ongoing stressors and experiences of trauma.

A Native American educator spoke of day-to-day indignities and the conscious trade-off between displaying cultural pride and opening the door to microaggressions and overt racism. In particular, he described the trade-offs to be considered in having license plates on his car issued by his reservation versus having state plates. Reservation plates can foster a sense of pride and belonging, but they can also be lightning rods for racism. While they are legal, they often draw negative attention, leading to police stops and even the impounding of vehicles. Some Native people opt out of having reservation plates out of fear and frustration—emotions that are far removed from the cultural pride and sense of sovereignty they were designed to foster (Peacock, 2011).

Native American youth can experience multiple challenges, including cumulative disadvantage, social exclusion, distrust, and shame in public schools where they comprise a minority. These youth may keep to themselves in schools and display a reluctance to venture into town. They may become withdrawn, fearful of mistreatment, and wary of speaking out or asking for help (Burnette, 2015).

Native Americans are frequently stigmatized and face extreme interpersonal and systemic discrimination (McQuaid et al., 2015). In a study of over 50,000 people, "Native American" was the only ethnic/racial category that was a predictor of reporting discrimination (Moghaddam et al., 2013). The effects of discrimination may diminish with support, but, equally, they can be exacerbated by negative or upsetting responses, such as blaming, distancing, and minimizing. Perceived discrimination is associated with increased historical loss thinking and directly related to symptoms of depression (Tucker et al., 2016). These, in turn, can lead to a sense of shame, self-hatred, and internalized oppression. Sometimes language or other cultural traditions are not passed on to children when they are perceived as disadvantages in succeeding in the mainstream world (Burnette, 2015).

In June 2017, the US Supreme Court ruled that racially offensive names cannot be censored, thus providing support for the NFL football team involved in a trademark case for continuing to use a name and promote merchandise that contain an anti-Native American racial slur (Swoyer, 2017). This decision affirms a social environment where racism and public use of racial slurs is deemed acceptable. This context of ongoing hostility has multiple consequences for the wellbeing of Native Americans, as perceived discrimination is associated with reduced access to preventive healthcare and delays in accessing services (Moghaddam et al., 2013).

Microaggressions are among the most persistent forms of discrimination experienced by Native Americans (Evans-Campbell, 2008) and continually reinforce feelings of being different and a lack of acceptance within mainstream society

(Myhra, 2011). Examples include asking if a person is a *real* Indian, doubting the authenticity of Indigenous people who do not conform to romanticized stereotypes, assertions that Native Americans only existed in the past and are not contemporary Peoples, and misappropriation of ceremonies and sacred objects. A 2003 study found two-thirds of respondents had been told they were "surprisingly articulate," more than three-quarters had been told they did not "look or act Indian," and one-third had received a request from an employer to change their appearance (Evans-Campbell, 2008). Such microaggressions are highly correlated with distress.

Microaggressions occur in a variety of contexts, including circumstances where Native Americans have the resources and skills to assist others. For example, after Hurricane Katrina, there was a significant need for teachers for displaced people throughout the Gulf region. When one tribal member with excellent credentials applied for a teaching job, her offer was rejected and she was told to seek employment at the casino (Klopotek et al., 2008). Microaggressions are fed by stereotypes including the false image of rich Indians who do not need to work because of the casinos. This can lead to a presumption that Native people either have no need for or should not seek jobs or support outside their own tribe. This bias is used to exclude Native Americans from employment opportunities, even though they are disproportionately affected by poverty (Klopotek et al., 2008).

One Native educator reflected on his childhood experiences and how these influence the way in which Native people think about themselves. He remembered walking with his grandfather as a young boy. His grandfather was humiliated to be called "Chief" but just looked down and did not respond. At the time, the young boy wanted to shrink, hide, and become invisible. This type of experience can turn to self-denigration and denial. It provides fuel for internalized oppression. The educator continued:

> I too have lived my life having to deal with the everyday denigration of ignorance and racism. When I was a young golf caddy, these same men also called me "Chief." Their children called me other names as well—redskin, wagon burner, "injun." Even the ones who adopted me as some kind of pet, whom I thought were my friends, called me an honest "injun." One Halloween a group of us reservation kids, too poor for masks or costumes, went to town to trick or treat, only to return with what we thought was a popcorn ball wrapped in tinfoil. There was a note inside: "Go home to the reservation." I wish I was there now.
>
> *(Peacock, 2011, p. 15)*

Like many others along the Gulf Coast of the United States, Indigenous Peoples suffered extensive damage from Hurricane Katrina. The Tunica–Biloxi lost the archives of their tribal history as well as other cultural items. Post-Katrina, tribal members faced multiple stereotypes based on their statuses as Native Americans, evacuees, and people of color (Klopotek et al., 2008) but also had access to unique resources from their tribe. The latter provided support to non-tribal evacuees too, but they were not immune to microagressions. In spite of their own losses and their efforts to assist others after the disaster, tribal members received the message, "That's what you get for living below sea level" (Klopotek et al., 2008).

Exploitation of the natural world

Exploitation of land is a continuing trauma for Indigenous Peoples. Many Native Americans have significant natural resources within their tribal territories but typically receive minimal compensation for extracted mineral wealth. They also experience significant pollution and environmental degradation. In large part, these are by-products of unsustainable development conducted by non-Native people. In one blatant example, parts of the Navajo Reservation are now unsafe for human habitation after radioactive material was left behind after uranium mining (Szlemko et al., 2006). The large uranium deposits on the reservation were exploited to fuel the Cold War and US advancement in the nuclear age. For decades, in the face of mounting evidence, state and federal regulatory bodies neglected to warn miners and community members of the devastating impact of uranium mining (Eichstaedt, 1994). Once rare birth defects are now common in some Navajo communities due to contaminated water supplies (Lewis et al., 2015).

While the United States and other societies grounded in Western ways of thinking typically conceptualize water, oil, minerals, and other parts of the natural environment as resources or commodities, Indigenous Peoples often view these same entities as relatives (Wildcat, 2009). These contrasting philosophies lead to diametrically opposed actions. Commodities exist to be exploited, consumed, or used with little thought for reciprocity, whereas relatives merit respect. Relationships are based on give and take, should be mutually beneficial and respectful, and we should be thankful for them.

When territories were taken from Indigenous Peoples, this was typically experienced as more than simply a loss of possessions. Loss of land carried a much deeper meaning. After the discovery of gold in the 1870s, the United States illegally seized the Black Hills from the Lakota, based on a desire to exploit this natural resource for financial gain. However, to the Lakota and other Indigenous Nations of the region, this area was the original source of the people and the buffalo—a sacred place inherent to survival. When the US Supreme Court eventually recognized the illegality of the seizure and offered monetary compensation, the Lakota consistently declined the proposed reparations on the basis that this wrong can be rectified only through the return of the Black Hills, a sustaining place that is central to Lakota identity and wellbeing (Ostler, 2010).

Indigenous Peoples have repeatedly experienced an inability to exercise control over their own territories in the face of colonization. This happened when miners invaded the Black Hills in violation of the 1868 Treaty of Fort Laramie (Ostler, 2010), when Tuscorosa land was taken for a hydroelectric power project in the early 1960s (Legal Information Institute, n.d.), and when more than half of the

Senecas' Allegany Reservation was flooded when the Army Corps of Engineers built the Kinzua Dam in the 1960s. In the latter example, while building the dam necessitated breaking a treaty, this was justified by the fact that finances for the project were included in the 1958 federal budget, indicating congressional approval (Haupton, 2015). Similar examples abound for Indigenous Peoples around the world. For instance, the United Nations Human Rights Commission condemned Canada's licensing of mineral extraction on Lubicon Cree lands in 1990 and 2006 (Turner & Pope, 2009).

For Indigenous Peoples, land is a source of strength and connection to culture. Deliberately disrupting this connection was used as a mechanism for forcing assimilation as well as making more land and natural resources available for settlers (Ostler, 2010). Ongoing violence against land, water, air, and other aspects of the natural world as well as disruption of the sacred relationships that Indigenous Peoples maintain with their territories continue to be experienced as attacks on Native Peoples and their identities.

In January 2017, four days after the inauguration of Donald Trump, completion of the Dakota Access Pipeline was authorized by presidential executive order with a mandate to expedite construction (University of Arizona Rogers College of Law, 2018). This was done in spite of the fact that this pipeline flows under a major water supply next to Standing Rock Reservation in an area guaranteed to the Lakota under the Treaty of Fort Laramie. A US District Court judge ruled that the fast-track approval was illegal since it did not consider a major component of the National Environmental Policy Act when it granted the easement under the Missouri River (*Indian Country Today*, 2017). This action is also in direct contravention of the United Nations Declaration on the Rights of Indigenous Peoples, which requires free, prior, and informed consent to be sought from affected Indigenous Peoples, particularly when water may be compromised (United Nations, 2008). This is yet another example of Indigenous people forced to bend to someone else's wishes while their attempts to assert their own rights and those of the environment go unheeded.

Peaceful demonstrations are a key method for advancing human rights, yet this form of activism is increasingly criminalized. Indigenous people who participate in peaceful demonstrations to defend land from resource extraction have been subject to both criminal prosecution and police violence. The encampments of Indigenous Peoples and allies that protested and attempted to halt the completion of the Dakota Access Pipeline were self-policing and non-violent. They received ongoing guidance from traditional elders and spiritual leaders. Yet, their resistance met with excessive force from state law enforcement and private security forces. Mass arrests were used to threaten, intimidate, and silence the activists. These violent actions displayed disregard for human rights and fundamental rights to free speech and assembly (University of Arizona Rogers College of Law, 2018). Unarmed protesters were confronted with paramilitary-style force (Devon, 2016; Stand with Standing Rock, 2016). The use of water cannons and police dogs against unarmed protesters, including praying women, was reminiscent of earlier acts of colonial violence perpetrated against Indigenous Peoples perceived to be standing in the way of what others defined as "progress."

Oil began flowing through the Dakota Access Pipeline on June 1, 2017. Similar pipelines have experienced leakage, including a 4200-barrel oil spill about 200 miles west of Standing Rock Reservation from the Belle Fourche Pipeline. This spill went undetected by electronic instrumentation but was noticed by a local landowner in December 2016. Additionally, more than 176,000 gallons of crude oil leaked, mostly into the Ash Coulee Creek, about 150 miles west of the Dakota Access Pipeline protests (Braine, 2016). At the time of writing, the US Army Corps of Engineers had missed a deadline for a new environmental analysis, but oil was still flowing through the pipeline (Bender, 2018). After becoming operational, the Dakota Access Pipeline leaked at least five times in the remainder of 2017 (University of Arizona Rogers College of Law, 2018). Indigenous Peoples continue to protest against the pipeline, but they now receive little media attention.

LaDuke (2005) speaks of recovering sacred relationships as a complex and multifaceted process that is essential for individual and community healing from the ravages of the past. In describing the sacred, she notes that spirituality is intimately intertwined with place. Spiritual relationships were violated when sacred mountains were seized as locations for observatories and lands were fouled by mineral extraction.

Another example is provided by the Anishinaabeg. Their lives are inextricably connected with their relative the sturgeon, but commercial overfishing and habitat destruction, resource exploitation, and pollution have led to the species' cataclysmic demise. In the 1990s, the Anishinaabeg reintroduced sturgeon from a Native-run hatchery in Canada. Traditional teachings from Anishinaabeg elders remind us that the strength of the fish population is directly connected to the strength of the human population. Tribal biologists and Native communities are working diligently to restore lost balance, including supporting traditional food sources, such as sturgeon for the Anishinaabeg and buffalo for Great Plains Peoples (LaDuke, 2005).

Even when traditional food sources remain available, environmental degradation poses significant problems. For example, sturgeon can live up to 150 years and absorb many toxins, including heavy metals and mercury. This process of bioaccumulation means that as the Anishinaabeg practice traditional ways of life, including fishing, toxins the fish have absorbed are transmitted to the people. Other Indigenous Peoples whose lives are closely intertwined with fish, such as the Mohawk, are similarly impacted by toxicity. Meanwhile, other sources of food and identity, such as wild rice, have also been contaminated and pass the toxins on to their human relatives (LaDuke, 2005).

Indigenous Peoples are disproportionately affected by climate change, yet environmental changes are largely caused by development and exploitation of resources by non-Indigenous people. This disproportionate impact, along with Indigenous Peoples' ongoing connections to the natural world, have led to their active efforts to limit climate change (LaDuke, 2005). Gulf Coast communities like the Houma Nation face chronic environmental changes. While outsiders often arrive to provide short-term relief after crises like hurricanes, trauma resulting from persistent, repeated loss of land due to climate change receives little attention. Coastal erosion has resulted in approximately 34 square miles of land loss each year over the past 50 years, and this seems likely to continue. Native Americans are among the most socially and physically vulnerable communities to environmental change (Billiot, 2017).

Activism, resilience, and healing

In spite of significant, ongoing trauma, Native Americans continue to find both traditional and novel ways to cultivate wellness and foster healing. A cultural resurgence is breaking the cyclical impact of historical trauma (Walls & Whitbeck, 2012). This resurgence is reconnecting generations and linking lives in positive ways to support the healthy growth of future generations.

There are many paths to healing and wellness. The varied contemporary circumstances of Native people make non-traditional healing and traditional healing effective for different people under different circumstances (Dionne & Nixon, 2014, p. 347). Oftentimes, a synthesis of traditional healing and Western therapeutic techniques can prove helpful.

A study of medicine men on the Great Plains revealed different conceptualizations of historical trauma. One medicine man saw historical trauma as a therapeutic discourse that reflects spiritual perspectives on distress and the need for healing. Another viewed discussions of historical trauma as a call for nation building, recognizing ongoing systemic oppression, and moving toward structural change (Hartmann & Gone, 2014). Both of these traditional healers emphasized resilience, healing, and positive change as companions that balance the deficit elements of historical trauma.

Elaborating on historical trauma, they spoke of contributing and protective factors. One cited lack of spiritual purification as a factor leading to historical trauma. Conversely, someone who had committed murder could participate in sweatlodge ceremonies to purge him- or herself and eliminate contamination. This ties in to traditional beliefs and protocols. Ceremony can function as a preventive mechanism for a variety of trauma sequelae, such as substance abuse, domestic violence, and suicide (Hartmann & Gone, 2014).

Various forms of traditional healing can promote wellness for contemporary Indigenous Peoples. Medicine people and other traditional healers can help Indigenous Peoples let go of negative self-images and internalized oppression (Grayshield et al., 2015). On a larger scale, community events such as the Wiping of the Tears ceremony, held in the Black Hills, have been used as interventions for historical trauma (Brave Heart et al., 2012).

A study of urban Aboriginal youth who use drugs confirmed that cultural teachings, values, and languages promote resilience in Indigenous people—a fact that these people have always known. Culture serves as a buffer against the devastation of colonization, and can protect Native people from severe health outcomes. Native people are survivors who have experienced multiple, intersecting adversities

(Pearce et al., 2015). Indeed, this is an important reminder that even under very difficult circumstances, such as homelessness and addiction, it is possible to find strength and resilience.

It is crucial that Indigenous Peoples struggling with various forms of adversity have access to culturally safe, trauma-informed interventions. Access to language and culture are particularly important pathways to enhancing resilience. This is true for individuals with a strong sense of cultural identity and those with limited cultural connections who may benefit from revitalization of their cultural identity to promote resilience (Pearce et al., 2015).

Culturally grounded resilience can also support macro-level change. For example, in Canada, the gendered aspects of the Indian Act made women particularly vulnerable to losing their status and ties to their home communities while making them more dependent on their spouses. This Act has also been linked to subsequent alienation and removal of children from Indigenous communities. Indigenous resilience and activism eventually led to changes in the Act, resulting in more than 130,000 people seeking to have their rights and status restored (Amnesty International, 2004).

Indigenous systems of helping still exist (to a greater or lesser extent) in various communities and can be meaningful for healing. Indigenous cultures and traditions have much to offer in terms of supporting contemporary wellness. Rather than Native American cultural teachings and practices being supplemental to behavioral healthcare, mainstream behavioral health systems must adapt so that they can effectively support Native healing practices:

> Before the United States existed, there were bodies of fundamental values, principles, and laws that Native people knew and survived on for many years. Many traditional healing ways were forcibly interrupted and western behavioral health treatments were introduced. Thus, given the process of colonization that occurred, the solution cannot be conceived of as the integration of two equal systems of care. Instead, it must involve primacy being given to traditional teachings and an overall emphasis on the restoration of harmony.
>
> *(Goodkind et al., 2010, p. 391)*

Indigenous people experience multiple stressors and traumas that are not adequately addressed by behavioral health systems. These problems can be ameliorated by increasing reimbursement for traditional healers, funding infrastructure that connects primary care and behavioral health in a holistic manner, and emphasizing practice-based evidence over evidence-based practice. Systems must consider the context and recognize current realities and the multiple stressors facing Native people. It is important to fund programs that bridge prevention and treatment and offer alternative licensing for experienced Native American providers to facilitate reimbursement (Goodkind et al., 2010).

As Canada phased out residential schools, Indigenous survivors began to speak out about their experiences and started to demand justice. Some residential school staff were prosecuted in the 1990s for abusing students. Following a 1996 Royal

Commission on Aboriginal Peoples report, the federal government established a $350 million fund to support healing programs for survivors and their families. In spite of this funding and an apology from the federal government, critics remain concerned that no public inquiry has been launched, resources continue to be dwarfed by need, and these remedies do not adequately address the magnitude of the trauma resulting from multigenerational loss of culture and identity or the legacy of intergenerational abuse suffered in the schools (Amnesty International, 2004).

Indigenous communities are developing their own healing paradigms for survivors of abuse in residential schools (Dionne & Nixon, 2014). Striving for wellness can include a mixture of traditional and mainstream healing practices, including holistic approaches that involve family, friends, and community members, so survivors do not feel isolated. It is important to pursue healing at all levels, including language and spiritual reclamation. Telling their stories allows residential school survivors to be acknowledged, let go of oppression, and begin healing (Dionne & Nixon, 2014).

There are many types of traditional healing. Different tribes and communities have their own traditions and ceremonies. Traditional forms of healing, including sweatlodge and pipe ceremonies, have sometimes been combined with psychological interventions, such as transpersonal psychology (Prussia, 2018). These methods seek a deeper healing of spirit and soul based on the beliefs that human nature is spiritual, consciousness is multidimensional, and there is an ongoing search for wholeness and awareness (Dionne & Nixon, 2014).

Helping professionals and the need for change

As noted in Chapter 2, helping professionals have often implemented biased policies and promoted assimilation. Most behavioral health interventions do not adequately address distress and dysfunction resulting from colonization (Nebelkopf et al., 2011). Additionally, the growing emphasis on evidence-based practice continues to disadvantage Native communities and agencies by pressuring them to implement interventions validated with non-Native populations that may be counterproductive in Indigenous contexts (Nebelkopf et al., 2011). Community-based and tribal organizations often have limited resources and do not have the capacity to implement the gold standard of rigorous experimental conditions required to develop evidence-based practices:

> There may be an inherent bias against Native American cultural communities expressed by making it a requirement to use EBPs [evidence-based practices] to get funding. EBPs are not tested in cultural communities so their results cannot be applied with the expectation of success. Mandated use of EBPs discriminates against community-defined best practices that are rooted in culture. Communities facing larger disparities in health care need interventions that focus on the community, not the single individual. This bias has found its

way into the behavioral health field and mirrors many of the racist assumptions that prevailed in the past, such as that improvement of quality of life means being deprogrammed from one's cultural identity.

(Nebelkopf et al., 2011, p. 266)

As an alternative, Indigenous Peoples and other communities of color have called for practice-based evidence. This can be defined as treatment approaches derived from, used with, and known to be effective by local communities. There is consensus or practice-based evidence that these interventions meet the therapeutic and healing needs of individuals, families, and communities (Nebelkopf et al., 2011). Community-defined evidence is reminiscent of the Native American push for self-determination. In this case, Indigenous Peoples strive for recognition and acceptance that we know what works for us.

Significant concerns have also been raised about research and its utility in informing best practices with Native people and communities. Often, when data are collected, Native Americans may not be included in analyses due to their small numbers. This can be perceived as dismissive and an excuse not to include Native Americans in discussions of best practices. This type of invisibility further perpetuates disparities and allows funders, policy makers, and society in general to continue to ignore the needs of Native Americans (Goodkind et al., 2010).

Although SAMHSA had historically welcomed cultural models, by the mid-2000s it was linking funding to evidence-based practices. This shift limited community-based and culturally based programs' ability to secure funding (Nebelkopf et al., 2011). Few Native American-specific interventions are listed in the *National Registry of Effective Programs and Practices* or verified as evidence-based practices. The handful that are include the suicide prevention curriculum, American Indian Life Skills Development/ Zuni Life Skills Development, and a substance abuse prevention program—the Red Cliff Wellness School Curriculum (Nebelkopf et al., 2011).

Helping professionals have the potential to be key allies in promoting wellness among Indigenous people. By drawing on local knowledge and culture, it is possible to ground social work practice in ways that make it relevant, authentic, and culturally appropriate (Nicolai & Saus, 2013). For example, cognitive behavioral approaches are often amenable to integration with traditional healing practices (BigFoot & Funderburk, 2011).

Social work education must prepare future social workers to be trauma-informed and responsive to Indigenous clients and communities. Johnston-Goodstar and colleagues provide examples of activities to teach social work students about microaggressions (Johnston-Goodstar, Piescher & LaLiberte, 2016). Their work is based on the premise that Native community members have unique, collective knowledge. The histories of local tribes are often representative of larger policies and trends, so they provide ideal learning opportunities for students in the helping professions. Educators can use creative techniques, such as treaty-mapping exercises, to engage students with Indigenous content.

The global context

The contemporary circumstances of Native Americans bear substantial similarities to Indigenous Peoples in other parts of the world. For example, like their counterparts in the United States, First Nations Peoples in Canada experience more childhood adversity than other citizens, compounded by high levels of discrimination as adults (McQuaid et al., 2015). In 1999, the Canadian government identified the state of affairs of Indigenous people as its most pressing human rights concern (Amnesty International, 2004).

As in the United States, there are federally recognized Indigenous Peoples in Canada and throughout the rest of the world (Lawrence, 2013) as well as Indigenous groups who remain unrecognized. Struggles for recognition and issues of identity are still commonplace among Indigenous Peoples around the world. For example, the question of who should be classified as Indigenous is a crucial aspect of both internal and federal-level discussions in Canada. The basic categories of First Nations, Inuit, and Metis are complicated by issues of urban and reserve, status and non-status people, those covered by treaties and those who are not, and various combinations of these categories (Patrick, 2013).

In recent decades, Indigenous people in Costa Rica, previously ignored by the federal government or assumed to be annihilated by colonization, have sought tribal recognition and restoration of a land base (Stocker, 2013). Likewise, Caribs in Trinidad assert their indigeneity, challenging narratives of their extinction and loss of identity through miscegenation (Forte, 2013). Since the 1990s, many Indigenous communities in Brazil have achieved recognition, land, and a high degree of autonomy and self-determination (Warren, 2013).

Violence against Indigenous women is a significant concern in many parts of the world. In 2004, Amnesty International made the following recommendations:

1. acknowledge the seriousness of the problems;
2. support research on the extent and causes of violence against Indigenous women;
3. take immediate action to protect the women at greatest risk;
4. provide training and resources for police to make prevention a priority;
5. address social and economic factors that perpetuate extreme vulnerabilities to violence; and
6. end marginalization of Indigenous women.*(Amnesty International, 2004)*

Indigenous women's vulnerability has received far more attention in Canada than the United States.

After more than 25 years of discussions, negotiations, and debates, the United Nations General Assembly finally passed its Declaration on the Rights of Indigenous Peoples (UNDRIP). This document affirms Indigenous Peoples' rights to self-determination and the maintenance of distinct cultural and political status. At the time of its passage, the United States, Canada, Australia, and New Zealand all voted against UNDRIP, but each subsequently reversed its position (Tsosie, 2012). UNDRIP is a statement of principles rather than an enforceable treaty, but it articulates benchmarks for just relationships between Indigenous Peoples and the nation-states that surround them (Tsosie, 2012, p. 925). This ground-breaking international human rights document takes an important stance that goes beyond US laws and policies in supporting the human rights and wellbeing of Indigenous Peoples. The United States and other countries would do well to follow its guidance and modify their laws and policies accordingly in order to support human rights, minimize oppression, and advance the wellbeing of Indigenous Peoples. Unfortunately, though, many positive developments generate a backlash. The United Nations Human Rights Office (n.d.) reports increasing intimidation of and reprisals against people who engage with the UN on various human rights issues.

Conclusion

The contemporary circumstances of Native Americans, as well as other Indigenous Peoples around the world, are inextricably linked with their histories. Colonization, far from being simply a historical process, has many insidious, contemporary manifestations that provide the structural framework for a multitude of disparities. Contemporary Native Americans are a young, growing, and increasingly urban population. In spite of ongoing racism, federal paternalism, and health and economic disparities, many continue to derive sustenance and empowerment from traditional value systems adapted for contemporary circumstances. Native Peoples around the world grapple with what it means to be Indigenous in contemporary, often multicultural contexts. This includes both internal and external criteria and ideas about embracing and asserting identity.

Tribal governments continue to operate and assert sovereignty, albeit in highly constricted legal environments. Indigenous communities seek creative ways to partner with state and federal bodies to respond to contemporary circumstances in our shared world. Social workers and other helping professionals must rise to the occasion and partner with Indigenous Peoples, both individuals and communities, to provide the responsive and respectful services that are needed to help Native Americans define their own needs and priorities. How this may be achieved with specific clients, such as children, families, elders, and communities, will be explored in subsequent chapters.

4

OUR HOPES FOR THE FUTURE

The wellbeing of Indigenous children and families

Children and families are at the heart of Indigenous communities and Nations. Indigenous societies are typically grounded in a network of distinct yet balanced roles that support the wellbeing of the Nations and their members. All roles are necessary and valued, and children are sacred within this interwoven network. They are the future of Indigenous Nations.

The roles and responsibilities of families and communities are intimately intertwined with the wellbeing of youth. This chapter examines the challenges and strengths of Native American children and families, including the impact of trauma and resilience on their wellbeing. Edwin Gonzalez-Santin and Dr. Priscilla Day were asked to share their perspectives, knowledge, and insights on this subject as both have decades of experience working in tribal communities with a particular focus on children and families. Many of the needs and strengths of Native American children and families, as well as many helping practices, both successful and unsuccessful, are not fully documented in the scholarly literature. Therefore, insights from experts who have worked closely with tribes and committed their careers to this area can illuminate important issues that otherwise might go unnoticed.

Edwin Gonzalez-Santin has served as Director of the Office of American Indian Projects at Arizona State University School of Social Work since 1984. He has conducted extensive evaluation work for the Navajo Nation Division of Social Services, the Salt River Pima-Maricopa Indian Community, and the Gila River Tribe. He serves as a consultant for social services for the Hopi, Gila River Indian Community, Navajo Nation, and Fort McDowell Indian community on issues related to child abuse, foster care, and case management. He also serves on various inter-tribal and national bodies, such as the Inter-Tribal Council of Arizona Health and Social Service Working Group, the National Fathers and Families Coalition of America, and the National Advisory Committee to FRIENDS National Center for Community-based Child Abuse Prevention. Throughout his career, his work has focused on evaluating American Indian child welfare and behavioral health programs, with particular emphasis on the intersections between child welfare and behavioral health.

Gonzalez-Santin sought out specific educational opportunities that would prepare him for work in tribal communities. As a social work student, he encountered service providers who were ready to give up on a young American Indian student. He volunteered to work with the student, and guaranteed that he would pass his classes. Through this work, Gonzalez-Santin recognized how systemic and environmental issues contributed to barriers that affected Native youth and families. These challenges mirrored his own experiences and led him to commit his life to enhancing the wellbeing of American Indians.

Dr. Priscilla Day is an Anishinaabe tribal member from Leech Lake Reservation and a tenured full professor in the Department of Social Work at the University of Duluth, where she has worked since 1993. Her research focuses on American Indian family preservation and she serves as Director of the Center for Regional and Tribal Child Welfare Studies, whose mission is "to advance the wellbeing of children by strengthening families and communities through social work education, research, and outreach in the region." In addition, she is an advisory board member and consultant for the Children's Bureau Capacity Building Center for Tribes, a mother of three, and a grandmother of nine. She brings both a professional and a personal perspective to her commentary on the wellbeing of Indigenous children and families as a professional who has worked with tribal communities for decades and someone with lived experiences as a tribal, family, and community member.

Day worked with a reservation-based sexual assault program prior to attending college. This gave her an opportunity to learn more about reservation communities and tribes that she had not encountered while growing up on her reservation. After completing her master's degree in social work, she became the Director of Mental Health for her tribe before entering academia.

The wellbeing of children and families is the cornerstone of many issues impacting Indigenous Peoples. There is a synergistic, multidirectional relationship between various aspects of Indigenous wellness. For example, the radiating impact of trauma affects health as well as gender roles, family structures, the roles of elders, and the ability to nurture youth. While this chapter focuses on children and families, it is understood that issues such as substance misuse, economic wellbeing, and education are intricately intertwined with the wellbeing of families and their members.

Traditional Native American families

Day reflected on the commonalities and differences across Indigenous groups. While there are tribal variations, there are common beliefs about family, community, and certain values. In particular, helping professionals must understand extended family networks and the importance of spirituality and culture. Historical trauma and oppression have had a lasting impact on families and communities, as is apparent in the prevalence of many social issues and health challenges.

Traditional Native American communities have never been characterized by Western models of the nuclear family, in which one father and one mother bear responsibility for raising children (Ball, 2010). By contrast, Indigenous families are typically immersed in their communities, with various community members playing significant roles in supporting both parents and children. While, to many people, the term parent implies one or two adults with exclusive responsibilities for the safety and guidance of their children, in Native American families multiple significant adults often assume caregiving roles. For instance, elders have responsibility for passing on cultural norms and traditions to later generations:

> Caregivers' responsibility was to cultivate the positive nature of the child, to touch the child with honor and respect. Because a child was considered a gift from the Creator, caretakers had the responsibility to return to the Creator a person who respected him/herself and others. Children, parents, and grandparents were secure in their relationships within the family. Children learned respect for their parents from the way they were valued and respected by their own parents, and by the respect shown to elders.
>
> *(BigFoot & Funderburk, 2011, p. 312)*

Traditional child-rearing is characterized by indirect guidance and modeling. Examples were often offered in the form of storytelling, which taught children about expected behaviors and self-control (BigFoot & Funderburk, 2011). Expectations were clear and reinforced through a combination of non-interference and ignoring. Adolescents and adults alike could be shunned or removed from the community for serious inappropriate behavior (BigFoot & Funderburk, 2011).

As collectivist societies, Native American communities are built on extensive interconnections among many people. Rather than individualistic societies where independence is highly valued, Native American cultures prioritize interdependence. There are often reciprocal relationships across age groups, including strong bonds between elders and youth. Multigenerational households are common, and elders continue to play valued roles in both their families and their communities.

Traditionally, Native American families and communities had balanced, distinct gender roles. Men and women held complementary responsibilities. This egalitarian balance was often characterized by women owning the family home and having responsibility for issues relating to internal community life, including local gathering and food provision, while men had external responsibilities, such as hunting and protecting the community. Women were also often the keepers and teachers of health and wellness practices. However, many of these traditional roles were undermined by colonization (Brown, 2016).

Gender is not inherently determined by biology; rather, it is a social construction of masculine and feminine (Sheppard & Mayo, 2013). As such, it is not surprising that different societies have different expectations for male and female roles. As an example, boarding schools socialized Native American men into farming as a suitable vocation on the basis of Western notions of appropriate male roles. By contrast, some Native societies, such as those of the Great Plains, typically viewed farming and tending gardens as women's work, since these were internal community functions.

While the dominant US society typically recognizes male and female gender categories and associates these with particular social roles, traditions like those of the Dine' (a.k.a. Navajo) recognize fluidity and the existence of more than two genders (Sheppard & Mayo, 2013). Gender identity and expression are viewed in terms of a continuum rather than confined to inflexible, binary definitions. Different expressions of sexuality were typically respected and seen to fit within families and communities. Therefore, the ways in which Native Americans have traditionally conceptualized gender and sexuality differ from the Western worldview anchored in heteronormative assumptions (Sheppard & Mayo, 2013). Someone born with an equal balance of male and female may be considered *two spirit*. This term may be used for someone who does not identify solely as male or female or for someone who is LGBTQ. Traditionally, two spirit people were valued, did not have their identity questioned, and were not rejected because of that identity. Indeed, some two spirit people undertook important ceremonial roles on behalf of their communities.

Disrupted families

The disruption of family ties has a lingering impact. In boarding schools, contact with grandparents was impeded, which inhibited cultural transmission, sometimes leading to a loss of cultural knowledge and practices (Byers, 2010). This disconnect was perpetuated by extensive child removals into the child welfare system. American Indians were often labeled unfit parents for using shared child-rearing practices, such as leaving a child with a relative for an extended period of time. The majority of out-of-home placements were justified on the basis of this practice (Byers, 2010). Helping professionals have often failed to recognize—or at times have deliberately ignored or undermined—the strong roles of the traditional extended family. In April 2001, the Child Welfare League of America apologized for its role in the Indian Adoption Project, an initiative that took many Native American children from their families and placed them in non-Native homes (Byers, 2010).

The intentional destruction of Indigenous families and cultures by the US government is at the root of various dysfunctions and disparities that are evident in Native American communities today. Families are the foundation for wellness, so disruption of them has a ripple effect. Family stories of historical trauma shape how Native youth think about their own adversity and resilience (Mohatt et al., 2014). Ethnic cleansing and government policies of forced assimilation deliberately destroyed protective intergenerational linkages. Physical and emotional separation of children from their families produced generations with no parenting guidance or role models (Ball, 2010; Walls & Whitbeck, 2012).

The boarding schools system has had a lasting disruptive impact. Cultural destruction was conceptualized as a means to incorporate American Indians into mainstream society. In addition to learning vocational skills, Indigenous youth absorbed the learned behavior of physical, sexual, and emotional abuse that was perpetrated against them in the schools, then carried it back to their own communities. Intergenerational trauma from the boarding schools is so pervasive that contemporary young people who never attended one of these institutions still feel the effects (Ball, 2010; Hedrick, 2016). As one author noted, "our people are hurt, many of our men are not present, and our roles as men have been stolen, leaving us incomplete and feeling unnecessary" (Hedrick, 2016, p. 49).

The disruption of traditional gender roles

Many assimilation policies targeted Native American families. Traditional families transmitted Indigenous values and their composition did not mirror the nuclear models that were considered the norm in US society. This made them primary targets for change. Egalitarian gender roles and fluid gender identities were perceived as deviant and nonconforming. These roles were undermined and conformity to Western standards was enforced as the ideal. Understanding how traditional Native American families were specifically and deliberately targeted for change (both in values and composition) by various policies of assimilation is central to understanding the ongoing effects of trauma for Native American families and children.

Historically, settlers viewed Native Americans as savages, while people who expressed gender nonconformity or same-sex sexuality were dubbed sick, insane, or criminal (Balestrery, 2012). Some contemporary Native people continue to espouse traditional beliefs about gender fluidity and sexuality, but others have become more acculturated to the rigid binary standards that are more typical of Western belief systems. This may be accompanied by the adoption of Western prejudices in a process of psychological colonization (Balestrery, 2012). Bias against Native Americans combined with bias against gender fluidity can produce a form of compounded colonization, which may be conceptualized as a form of intersecting oppressions rooted in history.

Boarding schools imposed Western-based gender norms that undermined egalitarian values. Men traditionally served as protectors of the people and the land, but destruction of their traditional gender roles has led some boys and young men to embrace gang culture (Brave Heart et al., 2012). Boarding schools disconnected Indigenous people from their traditional roles and cultures. Consequently, Indigenous men who become fathers often have no positive models for fulfilling this role (Ball, 2010).

Colonization also undermined many female-centered social arrangements that promoted respect for women and balance in family relationships. Patriarchal colonialism—a synergistic combination of colonialism, sexism, and racism—provides an additional layer of structural inequality and interlocking oppressions that serve as risk factors for interpersonal violence in the lives of Indigenous women (Burnette, 2016). Disruption of traditional gender roles in tribal communities included incorporation of misogynistic attitudes, behaviors, and practices that led to oppression, denigration, and violence against women (Chenault, 2011).

Devaluing the lives of Native women, entrenched racism, marginalization, and an environment that is often dominated by poverty and a lack of resources create a context of vulnerability. This context has led to many Native women disappearing or being murdered. For instance, more than 1000 Indigenous women were murdered in Canada between 1980 and 2012, while many others are missing (Bourgeois, 2018). The small size of Canada's Indigenous population and the low national violent crime rate make this number (which is probably a significant underestimate) even more appalling. Governmental indifference exacerbates vulnerabilities (Amnesty International, 2009). Indeed, it may be said that the colonial state enables and perpetuates violence against Indigenous women (Bourgeois, 2018).

There are connections between contemporary violence in the lives of many Indigenous women and historical policies that undermined women's roles. In Canada, this is linked to both the boarding school system and many women's loss of their Indigenous status under the Indian Act. Everything is connected. Indigenous women interviewed by Amnesty International described how the loss of culture, community, and self-esteem led to increasing desperation (Amnesty International, 2004). The crisis of missing and murdered Indigenous women is a direct result of colonization, patriarchy, and racism (Bourgeois, 2018).

The Stolen Sisters movement acknowledges the many Native women who have disappeared. Sometimes their bodies are found, but many families never learn what happened to their wives, daughters, mothers, and sisters (Amnesty International, 2004; 2009). Without any sort of closure, families and communities are left wondering, which adds another layer of trauma.

Violence and substance misuse

The various traumas experienced by Indigenous Peoples have had a significant and lasting impact on Native American families. Trauma has disrupted traditional family structures, undermined gender roles, fostered violence, and led to other issues, such as substance use problems and premature death, which damage family systems and impede caregiving roles. Intergenerational emotional neglect stemming from the boarding schools is a significant element of historical trauma. Native youth may use drugs and alcohol as maladaptive coping mechanisms to numb the pain of this intergenerational legacy (Pearce et al., 2015).

Native youth (ages 15–24) have the highest youth suicide rates in the United States: 34 per 100,000 compared to 11 per 100,000 overall. These behavioral health disparities can be attributed to:

1. disproportionate exposure to violence, trauma, and traumatic loss;
2. historic and contemporary oppression, racism, and discrimination;
3. inadequate funding for services;
4. disregard for effective Indigenous practices;
5. overemphasis on evidence-based practices;
6. lack of cultural competence; and
7. various barriers to care.*(Goodkind et al., 2010)*

Internalized oppression is one of the most insidious effects of colonization and trauma. Some Indigenous people have internalized negative perceptions of themselves, their cultures, and all aspects of indigeneity. As a result, they perpetuate discrimination based on a variety of factors, such as skin color, enrollment status, and sexuality (Brave Heart et al., 2012). Recognizing and remediating the impact of internalized oppression must occur in tandem with system-level changes. Both of these are necessary to realize positive change.

Internalized oppression leads to oppressing both the self and others. This often manifests in vicious and dysfunctional tribal politics as well as high rates of crime, violence, and addiction. Internalized racism feeds into mental illness, self-harm, and suicide as well as other types of disintegration of both individuals and communities. Indigenous Peoples must recognize and address internalized oppression and racism or risk implosion and extinction (Peacock, 2011).

Rates of violence are higher for Native American women than any other group of women in the United States (Burnette, 2016). Native women traditionally turned to their families for support, but family divisions and parental impairments, including intergenerational patterns of impaired bonding, alcohol misuse, and absent or deceased parental figures, limit available support (Burnette, 2016). Historical oppression has been internalized in the lives of many Native families, thus increasing women's vulnerability to violence. Centuries of oppression have created a toxic social context that has led some people to normalize and feel resigned to violence in their own families and communities (Burnette, 2016; Kipp, 2004). This toxic environment not only desensitizes people to violence but can silence women's voices and perpetuate the intergenerational cycle of violence (Burnette, 2016).

A study of Southeastern Indigenous women who experienced domestic violence learned that most of them had also been victimized as children. This study linked current family dysfunction and violence to colonial processes and an internalization of violence as acceptable. These patterns of dysfunction have been transmitted across generations, and participants in the study made specific connections between contemporary alcohol use and colonization (Burnette, 2016).

> Abuse is a part of our tribal communities. It is not a part that we want to acknowledge, not even a part we will always admit to, but drug and alcohol, physical, sexual, and spiritual abuse are, in some cases, more a part of our community than tradition and culture. Native youth in our communities feel

the impact of drugs and alcohol from family members. Domestic violence and sexual abuse are prevalent in our communities, but rarely reported and usually hushed. In some communities there has not been a ceremony for generations. Most, if not all, of this abuse has been facilitated by intergenerational trauma.

(Hedrick, 2016, p. 49)

A qualitative study of multigenerational families found that multiple exposures to lifetime trauma are linked to early onset of substance misuse. Older adults were noted to have experienced more than twice as much sexual abuse, more physical abuse, and more mental health issues and discrimination compared to those in the next generation (Myhra & Wieling, 2014). The sexual abuse experienced by the older generation was typically perpetrated by family members, mothers' boyfriends, and neighbors. For their children, sexual abuse most often occurred at the hands of peers or babysitters who were also minors (Myhra & Wieling, 2014). Those in the parent group often did not report the abuse due to shame or fear of skepticism and disbelief.

Neglect was common in both generations, and this was often related to substance misuse. Accidents were related to lack of parental supervision and the parents' own substance misuse, especially in the older generation. Many tragic and untimely deaths of family members and close friends occurred due to substance misuse, accidents, and suicide (Myhra & Wieling, 2014). Participants spoke of the challenges of unstable housing and unsafe neighborhoods as well as exposure to drugs and alcohol, in both urban areas and reservations. Risk factors for violence were often related to poverty and lack of opportunities.

Girls are more likely than boys to experience sexual abuse (Stevens et al., 2015). A study of adolescents in substance misuse treatment also found girls had higher levels of traumatic stress. Women in substance abuse treatment and the child welfare system similarly reported higher rates of both physical and sexual abuse (Stevens et al., 2015).

Greater trauma is associated with more substance misuse, so it is unsurprising that people in treatment for the latter report the former (Stevens et al., 2015). There are complex and reinforcing connections between trauma and addiction. Trauma may lead to substance use in the hope of numbing feelings and memories. In turn, substance use may lead to addiction and consequent impaired decision making, declining motor skills, and poor functioning (Stevens et al., 2015). These impairments may then generate additional trauma due to accidents, domestic violence, or neglectful parenting.

Native adolescents in residential facilities for substance misuse report an average of 4.1 lifetime traumas, with the most common being the threat of injury or witnessing injury. Trauma is pervasive among this population, with sexual trauma being particularly stigmatizing (Deters et al., 2006). Psychological and physical trauma forms part of everyday life for many Native youth.

Two spirit people report more childhood trauma in their families, including physical abuse. They also report more psychological symptoms, alcohol and other drug use, and more service utilization (Balsam et al., 2004). In addition, they experience higher rates of assault than non-Native LGBTQ people. In contemporary society, the multiple layers of oppressed status frequently lead to stress, trauma, and substance misuse. Conversely, many people also have a multilayered resilience framework that supports them in responding to many challenges (Elm et al., 2016).

Loss and American Indian families

There is a theme of loss interwoven throughout many Native American families and communities. This includes loss of traditional family structures, values, and roles. It also includes the loss of people who would have traditionally played key roles in sustaining families and communities. More than half of the women in a study on interpersonal violence had a parent die before they reached adulthood (Burnette, 2016).

Ultimately, the loss of children in Native American families and communities is equated with the loss of future prospects and an ability to exist as culturally distinct Peoples.

American Indians continue to experience various forms of loss disproportionately. For example, a family member may be mentally or emotionally unavailable due to substance misuse. Other losses result when a family member is taken away, as happened under the boarding schools system and when children are removed and taken into the child welfare system. Additional loss is evident when a family member is lost to suicide or to death from health disparities, or when they go missing for unknown reasons. It is more difficult to understand the impact of ambiguous loss than loss through death. The former, when a family member has left but return often remains possible (such as parental incarceration or removal of a child into protective custody), is associated with negative childhood effects that can include rage, behavioral problems, substance misuse, and PTSD (Stevens et al., 2015).

The loss of relatives has a staggering, disproportionate impact on Native families because of the relatively high child mortality rate and low life expectancy of the Native American population (Stevens et al., 2015). A sample of Native American, Latina, and White substance-abusing mothers explored different types of family loss. These included loss through death (of a parent, child, or partner), stillborn children, removal of children by social service agencies, and incarceration (of self or a family member). Native Americans were more likely to have been involved with Child Protective Services as children but were also less likely to be abandoned by a parent. They suffered disproportionate family loss, particularly death of a father. This was the case for 50 percent of the Native Americans, 19.6 percent of the Latinas, and 31.8 percent of the Whites in the study. Death of a partner was suffered by 28.3 percent, 7.1 percent, and 12.7 percent, respectively (Stevens et al., 2015).

Men are absent in many Native families and communities. This absence may be due to any one of multiple causes, including incarceration, alcohol and drugs, or death. Many Native American families are affected by the incarceration of one or more of their members. In part, this is because Native Americans tend to be sentenced more harshly than White, African American, and Latino offenders in US federal courts, with young Native American males receiving especially harsh sentences (Franklin, 2013). This has led to disproportionate incarceration of Native parents. Maternal incarceration has forced many Native American grandmothers to raise their grandchildren (Byers, 2010). While grandmothers traditionally played significant roles in child-rearing, this was done within a supportive network rather than on their own.

Native youth are also affected by disproportionate incarceration. There is a significant relationship between racial discrimination and the criminal justice system. Among incarcerated youth, Native Americans and other males of color are more likely to feel labeled as criminals than their White counterparts. White privilege fosters more lenient sentencing, second chances from law enforcement, decriminalized behavior, and greater opportunities for bail for White juvenile offenders (Feinstein, 2015). For Native youth, labeling theory informs how negative perceptions can become self-fulfilling prophecies. When they are labeled as criminals, they begin to see themselves as criminals and subsequently begin to act as criminals (Feinstein, 2015). The emphasis on skin color in US society means that youth of color who engage in deviant behavior are more likely to be given a criminal label than their White peers. Assumptions about the association between skin color and deviant behavior influence the perceptions and actions of teachers, neighbors, police, and prosecutors, leading to increased likelihood of arrest and contact with the criminal justice system, creating a self-fulfilling prophecy (Feinstein, 2015).

Interventions with American Indian children and families

It is important to be aware that families often face multiple challenges. Native families involved with the child welfare system due to substance misuse often struggle with untreated trauma exposure. These families typically experience multiple problems, including intergenerational substance misuse and violence that affects multiple family members. These high-need families are among the most vulnerable in the child welfare system. Helping professionals must be conscious of connections between ongoing discrimination against Native people, current child welfare involvement, and the history of genocidal policies designed to destroy Native families (Lucero & Bussey, 2015). High levels of trauma, unresolved grief and undiagnosed or untreated mental health concerns are the root causes of many substance abuse issues.

Helping professionals must recognize the challenges faced by American Indian families and not overburden them with unrealistic goals in the process of serving them. Families who become involved in the child welfare system are often mandated to engage with multiple services in order to fulfill the requirements of their family service plans. This can place substantial burdens on the families' time, energy, and finances, making success unlikely (Lucero & Bussey, 2015). On the surface, parental engagement may seem a reasonable and important expectation, but parents' ability to engage with the child welfare system is often severely undermined by the issues that brought them into the system in the first place. Families may have lifestyles that are chaotic, which makes it hard for them to meet basic needs, like housing and food. A parent who is overwhelmed and immersed in struggles such as addiction may be severely hampered in terms of their ability to connect, function, and make progress on service plan goals to meet the child welfare system's expectations. In turn, failure to progress can have devastating consequences, such as termination of parental rights (Lucero & Bussey, 2015).

Gonzalez-Santin stressed that helping professionals must appreciate the importance of the history, policies, and value systems of American Indian people. Native Americans and mainstream helping systems may have different perspectives on wellbeing and safety. For example, mainstream approaches to child welfare tend to be child-centered, whereas Indigenous cultures view children's wellbeing within the context of the family and cultural continuity. Differing worldviews contribute to differing perspectives on safety. Helping professionals must be open to inquiry and learn about the cultural context to avoid misinterpreting what is happening in American Indian families. Gonzalez-Santin also mentioned strengths, including the importance of clans, songs, and traditional worldviews that have allowed many Indigenous Peoples to transcend myriad challenges. Throughout his interview, he repeatedly and emphatically highlighted the importance of relationships, the strength of families, and the destructive intent of many social policies.

Relationships are core components of Native American families, communities, and cultures. Family relationships and community roles are key elements in Indigenous worldviews and serve as protective factors that support the resilience of Native people (Hill, 2006). Personal relationships are also crucial for service providers. Actively listening, providing concrete assistance, and displaying empathy are important means to build relationships. Gonzalez-Santin decried the lip service that agencies often give to Indigenous communities and clients, such as naming buildings after Native leaders, while failing to establish real connections with tribal communities. They expect Native people to come to them for services rather than reach out to tribal communities and offer services where the people live. They fail to recognize how agencies and service providers perpetuate barriers when prospective clients have limited time, energy, and transportation options to access services. Both Gonzalez-Santin and Day emphasized that establishing and nurturing relationships are essential to engaging and serving Native youth and families.

Along with the importance of establishing relationships, helping professionals must recognize the strength of Indigenous families, which serve as the foundation for Native people. Helping professionals must understand how families are defined within tribal contexts, not just according to Western standards. This can include extended family members and people who are considered family through clan or even non-biological connections. Gonzalez-Santin and Day both noted the importance of working within family relationships to engage American Indian people successfully.

Enhancing wellness and resilience

Wellness can exist at many different but interconnected levels. True wellness can be attained only when all system levels are aligned, including wellness for individuals, families, communities, and societies. This must include a social and policy environment that nurtures wellbeing as well as adequate funding to support programs and initiatives for Native children and families. Likewise, there are many different ways to enhance wellness and support resilience for American Indian children and families.

An understanding of trauma among Native Americans must be balanced with a counter-narrative of resilience (Grayshield et al., 2015). There is a need to identify mediators between stressors (like trauma) and poor outcomes (like depression) in order to guide prevention and intervention efforts (McQuaid et al., 2015). It is important to examine positive aspects of Indigenous experiences that can be passed intergenerationally, not just trauma. These include language, ceremonies, positive parenting, culture, and a strong sense of identity and belonging.

A study of intergenerational family trauma found that stories of healing, forgiveness, and hope balance the many struggles in the people's lives (Myhra & Wieling, 2014). While the younger generation displayed elevated levels of trauma compared to the general population, they were exposed to less trauma than their parents' generation. This speaks to the parents' efforts to protect their children from their own negative experiences and struggles. Healing also requires addressing internalized oppression. Raising awareness of historical trauma diminishes shame and can free people from internalizing blame (Brave Heart et al., 2012).

Various risk and protective factors combine to produce a likelihood of resilience. These consist of multiple independent factors on individual, familial, and societal levels (Stevens et al., 2015). A heightened sense of spirituality and an emphasis on community both facilitate resilience in Native Americans, more so than individual traits. Promoting a return to traditional practices can provide healing from historical trauma and help Native families to recognize and let go of internalized oppression (Grayshield et al., 2015).

A study of Native American fathers found that they consistently spoke of *circles of care* to depict how families are embedded within collectivist communities and the intertwined relationships among family members that provide a caring network for children (Ball, 2010). Although fathers are sometimes absent, Indigenous fatherhood must not be understood from a deficit perspective. Historical trauma and contemporary challenges, such as poverty, have disenfranchised Indigenous men from their traditional caregiving roles, yet vestiges of these important functions remain and they can be rekindled and integrated into culturally grounded, contemporary iterations of Indigenous fatherhood and families.

Enhancing wellness for Native American children and families must be done within a context of promoting wellness on the community level. Healthy communities are needed to sustain healthy families. Helping efforts initiated by tribes or Native organizations are ideally positioned to advance wellness, given that the latter is inextricably linked with culture among American Indians (Grayshield et al., 2015). Healing Native families and communities is also linked to promoting self-determination, as it is important to restore what has been lost or undermined.

The White Bison Center has developed a "wellbriety" movement that combines wellness and sobriety to offer support to individuals and communities. In 2009, members of this movement undertook a 7000-mile "Journey of Forgiveness" carrying a sacred hoop of 100 eagle feathers to raise awareness of human rights violations and intergenerational trauma stemming from the boarding schools system. They visited 24 boarding school sites and recorded elders' stories, having offered a safe environment for boarding school survivors to tell their stories. "Elders had placed into the hoop the four gifts of healing, hope, unity, and the power to forgive the unforgivable … The elders told us we would not be free from this trauma unless we could forgive the unforgivable" (Lajimodiere, 2012, p. 14).

Evidence-based practice and practice-based evidence

It can be challenging to identify the best ways to support the wellness of Indigenous children and families. Recent years have seen an increasing emphasis on evidence-based practice, particularly from funding sources. While this concept may seem reasonable, it has often been applied without scrutiny or critical thinking. Indeed, Native American researchers and helping professionals have questioned what constitutes evidence, given fundamentally different worldviews, and note the need to bridge the gap between Western science and Indigenous knowledge (Nebelkopf et al., 2011). Most interventions labeled as evidence-based or best practices have been developed with non-Native populations and have not been evaluated for their effectiveness with Native Americans.

A few models of Native American interventions are accepted as evidence-based practices, including manuals for Native adaptations of motivational interviewing, parent–child interaction therapy, and trauma-focused cognitive behavioral therapy (Nebelkopf et al., 2011). The Indian Country Child Trauma Center developed a Native American adaptation of an evidence-based cognitive behavioral intervention for treating trauma in children named "Honoring Children, Mending the Circle." This is a blend of traditional teachings and cognitive behavioral methods (BigFoot & Schmidt, 2010).

There are many more examples of *practice*-based evidence—interventions developed with Native populations that have documented effectiveness. There is a strength and power to be found in reclaiming culture and language that in turn promotes resilience (Myhra, 2011). Mending family relationships can help individuals achieve and maintain sobriety. Family connections can be important, even when family members have been apart for years. There is a need for providers to help the home become a safe place where all family members can heal, thus enabling families to stay together. Family connections provide a source of motivation and support for substance misuse recovery. Healing families can be an appropriate treatment goal that supports the wellbeing of individual members (Myhra, 2011).

Rebalancing gender roles

Even in communities where interpersonal violence is pervasive, there is a resurgence of women's power and leadership. There are tight-knit family support networks where grandmothers and female relatives offer support. Although traditional gender roles have been undermined, cultural values of female-centeredness are often still present and can be supported by cultural programs and helping professionals who recognize and draw on these protective values (Burnette, 2015).

There is a need for healing in Native communities. This includes recovering strong roles for Native men to restore the balance that was undermined by colonization (Hedrick, 2016). Indigenous men experience significant health disparities, often related to their participation in risky behaviors. Interventions to restore wellbeing and the traditional roles of boys and men can restore hope and minimize their participation in high-risk behaviors, such as drug use. Reclaiming strong male roles such as *wicasa was'aka* ("strong men") for the Lakota may facilitate wellness in Native communities (Brave Heart et al., 2012).

Native men are able to tap into traditional strengths and roles to promote healing for themselves and their families. For example, a Native American men's gathering was held in California to break the cycle of trauma. The participants recognized that men needed help to heal themselves and stop violence against women. It was important to have a safe context for them to begin acknowledging and healing from trauma (Hedrick, 2016). A quote shared at the gathering resonated with participants: "Wellness is not owned, it's leased and the rent is due every day." During this gathering, the men noted:

> We set the tone that we were there to heal. There would be no pulled punches, no subject would be avoided or ignored. To heal we must take responsibility for our abusive actions and admit to abuse inflicted upon us. Many men are guilty of abandoning our children, families, culture, and communities. Many of us are guilty of not pointing that out to one another and standing up for the women in our lives.
>
> *(Hedrick, 2016, p. 50)*

There are other examples of Indigenous men reclaiming traditional roles in ways that promote healing. For example, some Lakota tribal police and Gulf War veterans volunteered at Ground Zero after the 9/11 terrorist attacks in New York City. They saw this work as part of a traditional identity as *akicita*—"protectors of the people." They made connections between historical trauma, ongoing trauma exposure, experiences at Ground Zero, and their work as first responders on the reservation. By embracing the traditional *akicita* role in contemporary times, they protect and serve the Lakota and the rest of humanity. They are positive role models for boys struggling to navigate what it means to be Indigenous males serving and protecting their communities within a context of historical and contemporary trauma (Brave Heart et al., 2012).

Policies

It is also crucial to understand the intentional destruction that targeted American Indian families. Gonzalez-Santin described the ongoing efforts to *capture* Native children. It is impossible to have a nation without children, so the removal of tribal children is an existential threat to the Native Nations. It is testament to the inherent strengths of tribal people that they have survived the onslaught of policies designed to destroy Native families and a social environment where they are bombarded with negative, stereotypical, and racist images. Gonzalez-Santin noted the impact of unfunded mandates where the federal government continues to under-resource required services, at best characterized as benign neglect but more accurately as calculated omission.

While the federal government may make statements in support of tribal self-determination and the importance of Indigenous families, its ongoing intent to destroy tribal families is affirmed through these unfunded mandates. Gonzalez-Santin described the federal government as "consistently inconsistent; giving with one hand and taking away with the other," thus reinforcing mistrust. Some Native people succumb to these overwhelming pressures and become mired in addictions and other dysfunctional behaviors, but the majority maintain sobriety and resilience.

Gonzalez-Santin noted this is a dangerous time when unfavorable legal decisions, federal inconsistency, and a lack of funding continue to threaten the wellbeing of American Indian children and families. On the other hand, tribes are investing in their communities by sending more people into higher education, thus increasing their social capital and ability to use established systems to their advantage. Day similarly emphasized the destructive nature of policies of assimilation that have led to a sense of powerlessness that continues to fuel violence, poverty, addiction, and mental health problems. She emphasized that tribal sovereignty is constantly under attack.

Policy has a shaping influence on the social environment and context for Native American children and families. Earlier chapters have illustrated how some policies can have traumatic impacts, and they continue to facilitate unwarranted disruption of parenting and intergenerational attachment. In the future, policies must do more to promote healing among Native families.

Structural changes are needed in the criminal justice system, including revising policies and practices that undermine parenting. Current policy allows women in Arizona to be incarcerated in facilities that are well over 200 miles from their children. This makes visitation and the maintenance of familial ties extraordinarily difficult, which in turn exacerbates intergenerational family loss and trauma for both mothers and children. By contrast, policies that maintain connection and communication enhance the mother–child bond and foster resilience for both (Stevens et al., 2015).

The unmet treatment needs of women with addictions are high and hamper family reunification efforts. Child welfare workers may experience pressure to terminate parental rights under the Adoption and Safe Families Act. There is a need for comprehensive structural reform to be more responsive to the circumstances and needs of American Indian families (Stevens et al., 2015). The best efforts of child welfare professionals will continue to be hampered until adequate systems are in place to address pressing needs, such as poverty and addiction.

Child and family welfare

It is possible to re-envision child welfare services in ways that support family connections and collaborative efforts between various entities concerned with the wellbeing of Native American families and children. It is imperative to move away from unilateral, heavy-handed interventions that circumvent sovereignty and the rights of Native Nations and communities. Service providers can access specific guidance on interventions and policies from the National Indian Child Welfare Association (www.nicwa.org), an organization that offers training institutes, conferences, an online course, and advocacy on issues related to American Indian child and family wellbeing.

The ongoing effects of colonization must be acknowledged and addressed. For example, a state–tribal child welfare collaboration in Maine found they could not make real progress until past and present experiences of Wabanaki people were acknowledged (Bjorum, 2014). This recognition led to a mandate to launch a Maine Wabanaki–State Child Welfare Truth and Reconciliation Commission in 2012. The historical trauma perpetuated by child welfare systems can be acknowledged through such efforts.

Similarly, noncompliance with the Indian Child Welfare Act (ICWA) must be both acknowledged and addressed. The organized governmental effort to remove Native children from their families and communities that began in the late nineteenth century is reflected in current efforts to undermine this Act (Dotremon, 2013). This federal law is designed to foster cultural continuity for Native American children but there has always been concern about limited funding, training, and enforcement of its provisions.

Different states have different interpretations of the ICWA. While some monitor ICWA compliance, there is no nationwide federal monitoring system and substantive change is slow in coming (Bjorum, 2014). There is often confusion and disagreement about how to proceed when an "Indian child" (as defined under the terms of ICWA) is given up for adoption by a non-Native custodial parent (Dotremon, 2013). Significant controversy also surrounds differential applications based on interpretations of what constitutes an "existing Indian family." South Carolina, Alaska, Arizona, Colorado, Idaho, Illinois, Kansas, Michigan, Montana, New Jersey, New York, North Dakota, Oregon, and Utah apply the ICWA even when a child has not lived in the same household with American Indian parents, but this is not the case in other states. Inconsistency in the implementation of this federal mandate across the states leads to substantial confusion and patchy services for Native children and families (Dotremon, 2013).

Day identified how adoption agencies have used targeted efforts to undermine the ICWA. She viewed this as an attack on tribal sovereignty. In particular, she pointed to the Baby Veronica case, in which a Cherokee father lost his child to an adoptive White family with the assistance of a system that worked to keep her with non-relatives. The baby's non-Native biological mother consented to the adoption, but this was later contested by the Cherokee Nation and the child's biological father. When the South Carolina Supreme Court upheld the ICWA and ruled the child must be removed from her non-Indian adoptive parents, this led to considerable outrage in the media about the disrupted adoption. Of course, there were many interested parties in this precedent-setting case, ranging from adoption groups to tribes. The father had been notified of the adoption when his baby was four months old, at which point he had contested it. The Cherokee Nation then argued that the placement preferences articulated in the ICWA are intricately related to sovereignty and their continued existence as a tribe (Dotremon, 2013), but their argument was ultimately unsuccessful.

Boarding schools deliberately separated children from their American Indian families and cultures and are now recognized as perpetrating cultural genocide. This legacy continues as the ICWA is either ignored or interpreted so narrowly as to be inapplicable to American Indian children and families.

Resilience, hope, and best practices

As noted by Gonzalez-Santin, more American Indian people are obtaining advanced degrees and using their knowledge for the benefit of their people. There is now a better understanding of how to identify and access funding and training, resulting in greater ability to implement enhanced services. This has a slow, subtle impact on tribal communities. Gonzalez-Santin pointed out that there has been a great deal of positive change over the last three decades. Communities have adapted and developed hybrid models of service, such as Lake County in California, which has shaped programming with the input of elders. There has been a rise in Indigenous leadership, including engaged tribal workers who understand their own communities. There are also strong partnerships with non-Indigenous allies to provide high-quality services for American Indian youth and families. There is a level of empowerment. When your voice is heard, you can share your stories. In turn, this leads to an acknowledgement of trauma and its role in creating substance misuse and other problems.

Gonzalez-Santin noted that best practices are grounded in an ability to listen. Helping professionals need to understand the events that shaped individuals, elicit information from them, and ask appropriate questions. He highlighted an "ah ha moment" when American Indians recognized that the original ACEs study (see Chapter 1) and trauma-informed care movement, initially discussed by White scholars, held tremendous relevance for Indigenous communities that have experienced trauma continuously since their first encounters with early explorers. He identified a new generation of American Indian scholars who can use their knowledge about trauma to examine the past and change the future of Native children and families.

Day emphasized the incredible resilience of Native people. Stories of historical resilience balance the narratives of historical trauma. There is power in the way that American Indian children and families have persisted and reached for healing from trauma. It is important that we tell these stories, too. Indeed, there are many stories of strength and resilience, including one that Day shared about her own family:

> My grandmother was taken from her mother when she was four years old, not because of abuse but because she was Native. She was placed in a boarding school where no one spoke her first language, Ojibwe, and she was physically abused for using her only language. She credits her aunt for helping her. Her aunt was nice and knew English. My grandma always said she would have had it a lot worse if her aunt weren't there. Still, she was only four and was beaten and kept away from her family. She was one of the most upbeat and positive people I have ever known. She loved her family and everyone she met. She embodies resilience in spite of horrendous circumstances.

Day also identified an exemplary White Earth Nation program—MOMS (Maternal Outreach and Mitigation Services). This is a culturally specific holistic treatment program for pregnant women who are suffering from opioid addiction. It is run by tribal people who treat the participants as family members, both loving them and ensuring they remain accountable. Every participant who has completed the program has either kept or regained custody of their children. Day noted that the program interrupts the cycle of trauma. In it, service providers recognize that addiction can require a medical response, similar to diabetics requiring insulin. Participants are treated as people who have experienced trauma and use drugs as coping mechanisms. MOMS offers support to the whole person, with attention given to their physical, mental, and emotional safety. It provides boundaries with lots of support and never gives up on participants. Even if someone needs to leave the program for a while, they are welcomed back when they are ready to try again.

Another example of a model program is Honoring Children–Making Relatives. This intervention is designed to improve the parenting skills of Native American parents who are struggling with either personal deficits or children with problematic behaviors (BigFoot & Funderburk, 2011). It draws on traditional models of incorporating an array of supportive people into a nurturing child-rearing network. Members of the network listen, watch, support, and nurture children as the center of the circle, thus supporting both parents and children (BigFoot & Funderburk, 2011). The researchers who developed the project adapted empirically based treatment options to make them culturally congruent for Indigenous people.

RezRIDERS is a youth intervention program that was developed to disseminate health and prevention messages within high-risk peer groups in reservation environments. It targets Native youth who are at risk of depression and substance abuse. Extreme sports are used to engage the youth, promote positive peer groups and adult networks, and shift risk-taking behaviors to controlled program settings while promoting culturally grounded protective factors. This culturally tailored intervention was developed from community-based participatory research and can be modified to meet the needs of different tribal communities. It fosters strengths such as leadership, pride, and stewardship of the sacred water cycle (Brave Heart et al., 2012; Sarche et al., 2017).

Trauma-informed and culturally responsive services

Application of the principles of trauma-informed care is crucial in serving Indigenous children and families, given the history of oppression, including boarding schools and contemporary child removal. There are many reasons why Native families may not trust systems or feel safe within them. Helping professionals have often implemented policies and acted on behalf of systems that have caused trauma. Human service workers may not be seen as providing meaningful support and essential advocacy.

To provide trauma-informed services, helping professionals must recognize the pervasiveness of trauma in the lives of Native Americans and plan interventions and delivery systems accordingly. A trauma-informed approach minimizes stigma and the deficit perspective that is inherent in many explorations of health and social disparities. This is done by recognizing the detrimental impact of trauma on individuals and communities. Trauma-informed care requires attentiveness to its five principles of safety, trustworthiness, choice, collaboration, and empowerment in all aspects of service provision. Perhaps this is most important on a societal level: it is crucial to interrupt ongoing trauma and this requires large-scale changes. Ultimately, the colonial context that perpetuates oppression must be dismantled. Simultaneously, with systemic change, it is important to recognize and remediate trauma. Applying the principles of trauma-informed care minimizes the risk of compounding trauma or intensifying trauma symptoms.

Trauma-informed care must be integrated into the service environment and interventions. The agency's setting and procedures must help clients feel physically, emotionally, and culturally safe (Lucero & Bussey, 2015). Helping professionals must be aware and respectful of cultural norms. For example, the Indigenous value of silence may inhibit a Native person from disclosing trauma (Nicolai & Saus, 2013). Agencies must establish a comfortable and safe environment that recognizes American Indian beliefs and cultural expressions, such as the value of silence, so that those who need help feel safe enough to request it. A culturally responsive approach includes creating an agency environment where workers understand Indigenous cultural worldviews and values, especially those of local populations, understand both historical and contemporary issues of Native Peoples, hear and accept how clients express different levels of cultural connection and identity, and demonstrate a willingness to include traditional ways of helping (Lucero & Bussey, 2015).

Service providers must employ a trauma-informed lens to facilitate understanding of family needs. This can include intensive, proactive case management for high-need families using a brief screening tool for trauma exposure. Caseworkers can learn to identify trauma symptoms, make appropriate referrals to specialists who are skilled in working with Native clients, and offer an agency context that is focused on safety and trustworthiness.

There must be a commitment from the agency to foster a culturally responsive environment and support workers' training needs for trauma-informed services to be realized. Practice-informed evidence is an important mechanism for ongoing evaluation and to develop best practices for Native families (Lucero & Bussey, 2015). Trauma-informed, culturally responsive intensive case management can be effective in helping urban Natives Americans struggling with substance misuse and child welfare issues (Lucero & Bussey, 2015).

It is important to move beyond Western models of interventions to address trauma and loss effectively for Native American clients. One way to achieve this is to offer culturally grounded women's healing centers that provide culture-driven, trauma-informed interventions with community and social support. Such healing centers are based on a holistic model that focuses on wellness through an integration of body, mind, spirit, and emotion (Stevens et al., 2015). Traditional healing and teachings provide the basis for an effective synthesis for culturally driven interventions.

Helping professionals: be part of the solution, not part of the problem

Helping professionals can play important roles in changing the systems that have caused so much damage to American Indian children and families. Advocating for social justice can influence policies and alter systems. This begins with helping professionals' reflections on their own standpoints, biases, attitudes, and the need for change.

Child welfare removals and cross-cultural adoptions have historically been based on the underlying premise that most Native children would be better off growing up non-Native. This narrative is grounded in a power differential whereby the dominant society is able to define standards and express its beliefs about Native families, while an Indigenous counter-narrative about children, families, and communities goes unheard. The result is disproportionally higher numbers of American Indian children in the child welfare system (Bjorum, 2014). That dominant narrative must be challenged not only by Native people but by allies, both within and outside of service delivery systems.

It is important to recognize not only how human service workers have contributed to problems in the past but how they continue to do so. Some American Indian clients may feel a need to educate non-Native human service workers about their culture and the contemporary realities for Native people. They are afraid they will be stereotyped. Workers may not believe their urban clients are Native or minimize the importance of culture because they live in a city. These factors all present barriers to American Indians accessing services (Lucero & Bussey, 2015). The burden for promoting awareness and cross-cultural understanding should be on the human service provider, not the client.

A study of state and tribal child welfare workers revealed differences in how they perceived and approached their work. Tribally based child welfare workers felt that their state counterparts failed to understand the impact of removing children from Native communities. One study participant described a vast difference in the level of investment between state and tribal child welfare workers, with the former viewing clients as cases, while the latter thought of them as their own children, part of their survival. It is crucial to keep Native children connected to their tribes, especially when there are so few Native Americans. Tribal child welfare workers understood that the whole community hurts when a child is removed, and felt that state workers prioritized mandates, rules, regulations, and guidelines over people (Bjorum, 2014).

Human service workers have key roles to play that go beyond direct service provision. For instance, advocacy is essential. Helping professionals can influence laws and policies that are detrimental to Native children and families, and advocate for passage and implementation of more progressive policies that support Indigenous wellbeing. They can develop appropriate trauma-informed, culturally responsive services and push for adequate funding for initiatives that serve American Indians. Most importantly, they can help change the social environment and create a socially just context for everyone, thus minimizing ongoing oppression and trauma exposure.

Indigenous populations around the world have faced and continue to experience disproportionate child removals and attacks on culturally based family configurations and values. This has occurred not only on individual levels but as part of state-sanctioned policies anchored in the belief that the destruction of Indigenous families is key to assimilation and integration within wider society. Far too often, helping professionals have been the means to implement these regressive policies.

Higher education can play an important role in preparing helping professionals to serve American Indian children and families effectively. In fall 2018 a historic agreement was signed between the Navajo Nation, the Navajo Division of Social Services, the Department of Family Services, the Arizona State University School of Social Work, and the Office of American Indian Projects to support the education and training of social service workers. Russell Begaye, President of the Navajo Nation, touted this partnership as a way to protect Navajo children. The program, funded under Title IV-E of the Social Security Act, is the first of its kind to establish a collaboration between a university and a federally recognized tribal partner (Navajo Nation & Office of the President and Vice President, 2018). This collaboration may serve as a model to enhance capacity to serve American Indian children and families.

Conclusion

Trauma-informed care employs a perspective that asks "What happened to you?" rather than "What's wrong with you?" This chapter has provided an overview of what has happened and continues to happen to undermine American Indian children and families. It is important to move away from the deficit perspective that has frequently characterized views of Native families and children. This perspective has fueled assimilationist policies and attempts to destroy Native families and cultures, leading to overwhelming trauma and self-fulfilling disparities. We must examine the impact of policies and service systems, including how they have perpetuated trauma. Informed by this analysis, it is imperative to make thoughtful choices about interventions, service delivery systems, and policies that support American Indian Nations and communities, ultimately to enhance the wellbeing of American Indian children and families.

The subject-matter experts noted both challenges and positive aspects to working with American Indian children and families. Gonzalez-Santin found it particularly rewarding to have an opportunity to work with and see positive changes in people whom others had abandoned. However, he warned of continuing attacks on American Indian families, including subtle incursions, such as federal requirements to implement service models that are unsuitable for Indigenous Peoples. To be effective, all programs must be based on tribal, not external, norms. He reminds us that American Indian families are at the heart of cultural preservation.

Likewise, Day's message conveyed both hope and caution as she reflected on the internal work that American Indian people must do. We must acknowledge how we have internalized oppression based on the trauma experienced by our ancestors. We must recognize how this manifests in our actions. Likewise, we must draw on our ancestors' resilience and survival skills. Remediating internalized oppression is necessary to break the cycle of trauma.

Both experts identified the importance of extended families and knowledge about culture as informing culturally relevant helping services. Perhaps most notable is the emphasis that both placed on the continuing threat to Indigenous children and families present in the contemporary social and policy environment. Policies have had a destructive impact on American Indian families, and this impact has created a significant, ongoing, hostile context for American Indian children and families. Helping professionals must use their skills to alter this destructive environment if they are to have a significant, positive influence on Native families.

American Indian children and families continue to demonstrate resilience in the face of ongoing challenges. Far too frequently, social policies and human service workers have undermined rather than facilitated the wellbeing of Native children and families. Applying a culturally responsive, trauma-informed framework will allow service providers to partner with American Indian families and help them thrive, drawing on the strengths of cultural traditions while accessing appropriate and meaningful services, as needed.

5

HOLDERS OF KNOWLEDGE AND PROTECTORS OF COMMUNITIES

The wellbeing of elders and veterans

This chapter reviews contemporary circumstances for Native American elders, beginning with a review of their role in traditional Indigenous societies and a demographic overview. It explores the challenges faced by Native American elders as well as their strengths and resilience. Particular attention is given to veterans. Model programs and trauma-informed interventions are also reviewed.

Elderhood can be defined in different ways, based on age, life experience, or a combination of both. While mainstream programs often use the age of 65 as the starting point for elder status, that is not necessarily the case in tribal communities. Elder status is typically based on esteem for experience and community contributions, so it is not necessarily synonymous with a particular age. Additionally, with the lower life expectancy for Native Americans, people under 65 may be considered elders in some contexts (Shure & Goins, 2017). This chapter examines the life circumstances of older Native Americans, paying particular attention to elder status based on community perceptions and roles. It draws on the expertise of Dr. Suzanne Cross and Dr. Jordan Lewis. Input from these subject-matter experts informs a discussion of what helping professionals need to know about Native elders. Based on their extensive experience, they give their perspectives on the major issues facing these elders. In addition to challenges, they share stories of resilience and best practices for serving Indigenous elders.

Cross is a citizen of the Saginaw Chippewa Tribe of Michigan, a social worker, a gerontologist, and Associate Professor Emeritus at Michigan State University School of Social Work, where much of her scholarship has focused on American Indian grandparents. She received the Council on Social Work Education Senior Scholar Award, chaired that organization's Native American Task Force, and received the Mit Joyner Gerontology Award in 2012 for her work with American Indian elders. Now an elder herself, she is a traditional dancer as well as a beadwork and shawl artisan. Her artistic creations have been exhibited at multiple sites, including the Washington State History Museum and the Comprehensive Cancer Center at the University of Michigan. In addition to her professional and artistic accomplishments, she and her husband have served as foster parents for American Indian children.

Cross was raised in a traditionally grounded way that valued elders as teachers, healers, caregivers, and culture keepers. Her parents frequently brought her to community meetings and gatherings that included opportunities to be with and listen to elders. Although she was encouraged to play with other children, she always felt comfortable with elders. They welcomed her and included her in their conversations. She learned traditional crafts as well as life lessons. She has always been surrounded and nurtured by elders. They taught her how to love and care for others, grieve losses, create art, and, most of all, how to be an American Indian woman and now an elder herself.

Lewis, an Aleut/Unangan from the Native village of Naknek, is Director of the National Resource Center for Alaska Native Elders and an associate professor in the WWAMI School of Medical Education, University of Alaska, Anchorage. Trained as a cross-cultural community psychologist, social worker, and gerontologist, he partners with tribal communities to explore cultural understandings of successful aging, dementia, and intergenerational programming in tribal communities, as well as collecting stories to improve program and service delivery in long-term care settings. In 2009, he received the National Rural Aging and Public Health Research Award from the American Public Health Association. The following year, he won the Dennis Demmert Appreciation and Recognition Award from the University of Alaska, Fairbanks.

Lewis's mother valued spending time with elders, so, as a youth, he spent each day visiting and helping different elders. As a social work student he did an internship in a long-term care facility where he was confronted with the very different way Western society perceived elders. He questioned why mainstream society feared aging and wanted to reverse the aging process. The values instilled in him since childhood blended with his professional aspirations, leading him toward the field of gerontology, but his coursework contained few Indigenous perspectives. Lewis believed that all older adults should be respected and honored, regardless of background. His passions led him to focus on policy issues and he completed a Native health fellowship in Washington, DC, that included research into long-term care and home-based services. He then returned to Alaska, where his Ph.D. focused on serving his own elders and bringing the voices of Indigenous elders into the scholarly literature.

Elders in Indigenous societies

In Indigenous societies, elderhood is a significant life stage imbued with respect and valued community roles. As Lewis noted, many Indigenous people look forward to becoming an elder. Indigenous societies offer a counter-narrative to Western perspectives of aging as a time of increasing decrepitude and decreasing value (Grande, 2018). Cross noted that she often forgets how mainstream society perceives elders differently than urban and reservation tribal communities. She is often asked to speak or act because of her status as an elder, while those who are asked to speak in mainstream society often receive the request on the basis of formal credentials or titles. She noted the kindness and respect that Native people have for elders and shared a story:

> A young boy about eight years old came running up to his dad and said, "Can I have a dollar?" His father asked him why he needed it. He responded, "I need to buy George a bottle of water." George is an elder who is a veteran and a dancer. How kind of this young child to show his care for this elder.

The physical and mental changes that often accompany aging are perceived differently in different cultural contexts. Indigenous teachings often depict elderhood as a time of moving back toward the Creator and reconnecting with the spiritual realm. This reconnection is considered normal and provides alternative perspectives on what mainstream society may consider irrational behavior or even dementia-related conditions. Indeed, cognitive travel beyond daily reality is normal and valued (Grande, 2018).

Elders are highly valued in Indigenous societies around the world. Cross related that they contribute significantly to the stability and strength of tribal nations as wisdom keepers and storytellers. They may appear to be quiet and unassuming, but when needed will speak out for the benefit of their people. Elders traditionally had meaningful involvement in the lives of their grandchildren and other youth in the community (Cross, Day & Byers, 2010), and they continue to do so to a greater or lesser extent, depending upon the family or community.

Elders are recognized in their communities and families for their wisdom, cultural knowledge, and accumulated life experience. Their advice is often sought and they play key roles in sustaining their families and communities. They receive honor and respect for serving as role models, embodying Indigenous traditions, engaging in healthy behaviors, and teaching others. They have faced many life- and culture-changing experiences but need not be viewed from a deficit perspective. Rather, they possess tremendous resilience (Lewis, 2016).

Traditionally, elders possessed and transmitted intergenerational knowledge. Dedication to continuity while adapting to historical and cultural change speaks to cultural resilience (Byers, 2010). Indigenous elders took on many roles, including as caregivers, role models, and ceremonial leaders. As knowledge holders, they understand how best to offer ethical, culturally competent services to address historical trauma (Grayshield et al., 2015).

Institutions seeking to re-indigenize or ground themselves in traditional values are increasingly seeking the guidance of elders. For example, some social agencies and universities have instituted Councils of Elders to shape policies and guide services. Elders may serve as advisors, co-teachers, co-researchers (Momper, Dennis & Mueller-Williams, 2017), and/or consultants prior to research (Dennis & Brewer,

2017). For example, in one project elders facilitated groups and developed an interview guide prior to project implementation. They were able to draw on their own perspectives and experiences to engage research participants and develop a meaningful research instrument (Kahn, 2016).

Demographics of Native American elders

Native Americans age 65 and older are a growing population. In 2012, they accounted for approximately 0.6 percent of the US population aged 65 and over. In 2050, this figure is projected to rise to 1.2 percent. Native Hawaiians and other Pacific Islanders were 0.1 percent in 2012, which is projected to rise to 0.3 percent by 2050. Elders of more advanced age are also a growing population. Native Americans aged 65–84 currently comprise 0.7 percent of that age group in the US population, which is projected to rise to 1.3 percent by 2050. The Native Hawaiian and Pacific Islanders population in this age range was 0.1 percent, which is projected to triple by 2050. Native American elders aged 85 and older are currently 0.4 percent of the total US population in this age group, which is projected to rise to 1 percent by 2050. Native Hawaiians and Pacific Islanders are currently 0.1 of the total US population for this age group, which is projected to double by 2050 (all percentages from Ortman, Velkoff & Hogan, 2014). In sum, the number of Native Americans aged 65 and older is expected at least to triple between by 2050. The number aged 85 and older is expected to increase more than sevenfold (Schure & Goins, 2017). These predicted population increases, combined with the lifelong disparities experienced by Native Americans, mean that it is becoming increasingly urgent to understand and address elders' needs.

While the number of Indigenous elders is increasing, their average life expectancy continues to lag three to four years behind that of the general population. Indigenous elders are also significantly more likely to experience chest pain, obesity, shortness of breath, foot problems, depression, vision and hearing problems, and impairment in more than one of the activities of daily living (ADLs) than their White counterparts (Braun & LaCounte, 2015). Historical trauma, social determinants of health, and access to care explain these ongoing health disparities (Braun & LaCounte, 2015).

Veterans

Native Americans have higher rates of military service than any other ethnic group in the United States (Kaufmann et al., 2014; Shreve, 2017). Even before they had citizenship rights, thousands volunteered for military service in World War I (Neumann, 2017). During that war, an estimated 10,000 Native people served in the US Army and 2,000 in the US Navy. Many others served in the National Guard (Neumann, 2017).

Native Americans assisted the US military and colonial forces from the very beginning, often serving as key allies who controlled the balance of power between warring European powers. This early service is generally poorly documented, although there are some notable exceptions. For example, Ely Parker, a Seneca from New York State, served as a Union officer, eventually rising to the rank of brigadier general and military secretary to General Grant in the US Civil War. He wrote the terms of surrender for the Confederacy at Appomattox Courthouse, but was subsequently denied the right to practice law in New York State because he was Native American and therefore not legally recognized as a citizen (Campbell, 2000).

Veterans hold an esteemed status in traditional Indigenous societies, where they are respected and honored for their role in protecting the people. With colonization, many other traditional Indigenous roles were undermined or eroded, but military service was an exception. Traditional protector roles that warriors filled in Indigenous societies often transitioned to service in US, Canadian, or other militaries. After their military service, Indigenous veterans returned to their home communities and were held in high esteem, much as they were prior to colonization. They continue to provide strong leadership in their communities to this day (Kaufman et al., 2016).

Interviews and focus groups with Native veterans and their family members affirm that they continue to be valued and are often publicly honored in Indigenous communities, a distinction they appreciate is uncommon for other groups (Kaufman et al., 2016). Combat veterans often witness extraordinary acts of violence, death, and destruction in a short span of time. Undergoing so many experiences, some of them exceptionally painful, may lead to *age acceleration*, generating a degree of wisdom that is typically only associated with advanced age. In that respect, Indigenous societies often view elders and warriors as worthy of esteem and respect for all they have seen and endured, often in support of the wellbeing of their communities (Holm, 2017). Native veterans are publicly acknowledged at dinners, pow wows, and community events. They are given gifts, called to eat before others, and verbally acknowledged. People often stand to acclaim them, frequently with honor songs.

There is a powerful social contract between warriors and their communities that involves mutual responsibilities. Native Americans typically view veterans as relatives who have taken on the role of serving and protecting their community. Indigenous societies prepare their warriors for battle and also carry a responsibility for their reintegration upon return. There are ceremonial ways for Native American communities to cleanse returning veterans that can be helpful for other trauma survivors, too (Holm, 2017). One veteran contextualized veterans' position in Native communities by paraphrasing Sitting Bull:

> Warriors are not what you think of as warriors. The warrior is not someone who fights, because no one has the right to take another life. The warrior, for us, is one who sacrifices himself for the good of others. His task is to care for the elderly, the defenseless, those who cannot provide for themselves, and above all, the children, the future of humanity.
>
> *(Quoted in Kaufman et al., 2016, p. 69)*

The Vietnam War was unpopular in the United States and many returning veterans faced challenges including a lack of acknowledgement for their service. The context was different for Native American veterans. Many Native Americans opposed participation in the war because, although they were subject to the draft, the US government continued to violate treaties and failed to acknowledge Indigenous sovereignty and human rights. In spite of these significant objections, many Native veterans saw their service in the context of their own cultural values rather than their political views (Holm, 2017).

During wartime, Native Americans were disproportionately deployed on the front lines or in high-combat areas, which obviously increased their exposure to psychological trauma. Understandably, then, these veterans have higher rates of PTSD, depression, and substance misuse than their non-Native counterparts (Kaufmann et al., 2014). It is likely that untreated depression or PTSD leads to self-medication and substance misuse. Given the highly interconnected nature of Indigenous societies, this affects not only the veterans themselves but also their families and communities.

Native people served in many capacities in the military, including as messengers and telephone operators, using Indigenous languages. The Lakota were among the first "code talkers" in the US military in World War I (Neumann, 2017). Code talkers used their Indigenous languages to transmit messages that could not be understood by any enemy troops who might be listening. Their oath of silence meant much of their service was unknown to their families and remained unrecognized until very recently, often posthumously. Their work in 1917–1918 set the stage for expansion of the code talking program in World War II. The program was declassified in 1968 but was largely unpublicized until 2001. At that time, the few remaining Navajo code talkers finally received Congressional Gold Medals, almost 60 years after the creation of the military code based on their language. Navajo was used as the basis for secret communication during World War II because it is a complex oral language with no written equivalent. The code was never broken by the Japanese and was ultimately credited with saving countless lives (Lindsay, 2016).

Many tribal colleges and universities (TCUs) make a point of honoring and recognizing veterans. They also frequently offer specialized programming and services to help them transition to civilian life and college (Shreve, 2017). Higher education is undoubtedly enriched by the presence of these veteran students. In planning its new campus, Red Lake Nation College designed a memorial to list the names of all the tribal members who had ever served in the military. It included a stand for tobacco offerings, benches for elders, and a fire pit for honorings (King, 2017). The United Tribes Technical College similarly honored Native veterans from North Dakota who had served in World War I with a memorial on its campus (Neumann, 2017), while Haskell Indian Nations University erected yet another memorial to mark the centenary of that conflict (Shreve, 2017). Teaching about historical trauma can help veteran students process both survivor's guilt and identity issues (Shreve, 2017), while TCUs also help Indigenous veterans maintain a visible place in academia.

Community esteem for Native veterans contrasts sharply with their reports of their treatment by mainstream organizations such as the Veterans Administration (VA; Kaufman et al., 2016). While relationships between Native people and VA offices are better in some communities than others, many Native veterans have faced prejudice, discrimination, and stereotyping when trying to access benefits. Indeed, in spite of high rates of military service, Native Americans are the most underserved segment of the veteran population. Only 55 percent of these veterans make use of VA services (Kaufman et al., 2016), with stigma, limited awareness of benefits, and distance to care frequently cited as reasons for lack of engagement (Kaufmann et al., 2014). Reservation-based veterans often have difficulties negotiating the VA system, do not have adequate transportation, and do not receive culturally competent care. Their families are typically their primary caregivers, but they operate without adequate support, information, financial means, or other resources.

Similar to other Native Americans, veterans experience significant disparities compared with their non-Native peers. A study of rural and reservation elderly veterans receiving home-based primary care found that those who were Indian Health Service (IHS) clients tended to be younger and sicker than other veterans. Native American veterans also have higher rates of disability, despite being younger than their non-Native counterparts (Kramer et al., 2018). A community sample of 252 Native American veterans from both urban and rural areas showed correlations between combat and PTSD and other anxiety disorders as well as mood disorders, although not substance misuse (Westermeyer & Canive, 2013). In fact, in this study, substance misuse was inversely associated with PTSD, a finding that contradicted most other research in this area.

Challenges

As Cross emphasized, there is both significant diversity and similarities across Native Nations. Some Native elders continue to live within supportive traditional contexts while others do not. Many contemporary elders face a number of significant challenges, including some of the highest rates of chronic health conditions in the country (Conte, Schure & Goins, 2015). They therefore experience more functional limitations than other elders and have higher rates of depressive symptomatology than their non-Native peers (Schure & Goins, 2017).

Cross noted that many elders do not seek healthcare because they cannot afford it due to limited income or lack of transportation. Native Americans aged 65 and older are also less likely to have health insurance than other elders (Towne, Lee Smith & Ory, 2014). As a result, they may use traditional healing methods or homeopathic treatments. Additionally, they accept illness as an inevitable aspect of the aging process. Each individual was born with a number of days in their hand. In other words, no one knows how long their life will be. This is natural and should be accepted.

Lewis emphasized that while Indigenous cultures traditionally embrace aging as a normal stage of life, today's elders often face a variety of barriers to healthy aging. Their wellbeing can be affected by a combination of age, social determinants of health, and environmental infrastructure limitations, such as a lack of IHS services in urban areas where the majority of Native people reside (Towne et al., 2014). Issues that affect younger community members, such as poverty, lack of transportation, limited education, discrimination, and health issues, persist throughout life.

As mentioned, Native veterans experience disparities in both health and access to care. They have less education, homeownership, and employment than other veterans. Barriers to care include lack of transportation, a shortage of appropriate diagnostic and specialty healthcare, and difficulties securing appointments. They have greater mental health needs and are four times as likely as White veterans to report unmet health needs (Noe et al., 2014). They also report dissatisfaction with VA services and a preference for mental health services from traditional healers. Access to appropriate housing is another significant issue for many veterans (Kaufman et al., 2016).

Trauma

Lewis noted that unresolved trauma can be a serious issue for Native elders. Likewise, Cross emphasized that it is important for helping professionals to understand how historical trauma, including population decimation, has affected family relations, child-rearing, and elders' coping skills. Centuries of colonial influence have disrupted Indigenous communities and distorted roles for a variety of people, including elders.

The traditional roles and esteem accorded to elders remain intact in some communities, although they have diminished in others. In particular, colonization posed challenges to the status of female elders. Historically, as the US government gained power, its representatives refused to negotiate with elders and women leaders, thus undermining traditional Indigenous values and imposing the Western worldview that young men should speak for their communities. Indigenous societies were indoctrinated with patriarchal and youth-focused values to the detriment of the authority of all elders, and especially female elders (Byers, 2010).

A study of 233 Native Americans over the age of 50 found that adverse childhood events can have profound effects across the lifespan (Roh et al., 2015). In another study, Southwest elders lamented the loss of culture, language, traditions, and family life. Many of these losses were linked to their experiences in boarding schools. They expressed a yearning for the past, admiration for the strengths of their ancestors, and a desire to learn from those who have gone, while attributing contemporary adversity to past injustice and trauma (Reinschmidt et al., 2016).

Today's elders were heavily affected by the boarding school system. As Cross noted, there is substantial information about abuses that occurred in these schools, but little understanding of the guilt that survivors continue to feel. Older children in the boarding schools often experienced guilt over their inability to protect younger siblings or peers from abuse. At times, older students were even forced to discipline younger children in order to avoid being disciplined themselves. This left a heavy burden of guilt for those who were coerced to abuse others.

Cross noted that the cultural losses people who are now elders experienced in the boarding schools affect subsequent generations. Elders express concern that they were unable to raise their children effectively because of the institutional care that they received. They may carry feelings of abandonment by their own parents and suspect that they were inadequate parents who were unable to express affection because they did not receive it themselves.

According to Cross, elders who attended boarding schools often feel isolated in a crowd and may have difficulty relating to others in a positive way. They are often afraid to touch a child with affection, both because they have not experienced this themselves and because children in boarding schools were often touched inappropriately. Elders who survived the boarding schools need someone to listen to them and touch them in ways that are positive, affirming, and safe.

Cross also cautioned that we should not lose sight of the different experiences that Native people had in the boarding schools. Drawing comparisons between experiences, and especially attempting to determine whose experiences were more traumatic, is unhelpful. Cross recounted several discussions about the negative impact of boarding schools during which survivors focused on comparing their experiences and presumed levels of loss and suffering. These comparisons invariably caused participants to shut down and inhibited healing.

Many individuals have chosen not to speak openly about the trauma they experienced, although Lewis noted that elders with dementia may no longer refrain from sharing these memories. Indeed, their thought processes may dwell on a particular memory for an extended period of time. Under these circumstances, family members may be suddenly confronted with traumatic experiences from their elder's past about which they were previously unaware.

Physical health

Native elders have less access to health services and poorer health outcomes than non-Native elders. For example, they have less access to and utilization of cancer-screening services than their non-Native peers. This is true across the United States, even after adjusting for income and education. Native American elders have lower rates for mammograms and colonoscopies and must travel longer distances for testing. Indeed, Native women over the age of 50 have the lowest screening rates among *all* women in the country. In addition, there is a severe gap in available services (Towne et al., 2014). It seems certain that these disparities will only increase as the Native population continues to grow.

Elders may be at particular risk of adverse health outcomes associated with inactivity. A study of physical activity among Native American adults found only 27 percent met recommended levels, according to self-reports (Sawchuk et al., 2017). Objective measures of physical activity were even worse, reporting that only 9 percent met recommended levels. Barriers to physical activity vary considerably depending on age, gender, tribe, and neighborhood features, but include limited willpower, lack of childcare, inadequate time, and poor access to exercise facilities or even safe walking areas (Sawchuk et al., 2017).

Environmental circumstances can also pose health risks. In the Western United States, rocks and soil contain naturally occurring moderate to high levels of inorganic arsenic—a neurotoxin. This can affect the well water on which many rural Native communities depend, placing them at high risk of long-term arsenic exposure (Carroll et al., 2017). Data collected from the Strong Heart Study with 13 Western Native American tribes and communities documented associations between arsenic and cancer mortality, cardiovascular disease, diabetes, and albuminuria (Carroll et al., 2017). A subsequent study investigated the effects of long-term, low-dose exposure to inorganic arsenic on the neuropsychological functioning of Native American elders aged 64–95. Measurements were taken 20 years after baseline data on neuropsychological functioning were collected and revealed that this sort of exposure affects fine motor functioning and processing speed, but not other neuropsychological functioning. Arsenic concentrations were highest in the Southwest, moderate in the Northern Plains, and lowest in the Central Plains. Elders' cumulative neurological damage may inhibit their memory and capacity for intergenerational transmission of language and cultural knowledge, ultimately threatening cultural continuity for Indigenous communities (Carroll et al., 2017).

Mental health

A study of one tribe in the Southeast (Schure & Goins, 2017) found that 13.24 percent of the population were suffering from clinically significant depression, but the condition was most prevalent (19.9 percent) among the 50–64 age group. Lower rates were reported for older cohorts: 8.2 percent of those aged 65–74 were clinically depressed, while the rate for those over 75 was 12.1 percent. Respondents with some college education or a college degree were less likely to be depressed than those with a high-school diploma or less (7.9 percent against 15.7 percent). Depression did not vary by either gender or marital status.

Depression in Native American older adults is associated with suicide and mortality disparities (Burnette et al., 2017). One study of Native Americans aged over 50 found that childhood neglect and household dysfunction were associated with depression. Living alone and elders' negative perceptions of their own health also predicted depressive symptoms. Social support moderated these symptoms (Burnette et al., 2017). It is noteworthy that childhood abuse did not predict depression for older Native Americans, whereas childhood neglect and household dysfunction did. This may be due to the centrality of connectedness and family in Native cultures. Family and community ties may buffer the impact of abuse (Roh et al., 2015).

A study examining the differences between Native elders and their non-Native counterparts (Burnette et al., 2017) found the former had a mean Adverse Childhood Events (ACE) score of 2.55—significantly higher than the mean score 0.83 for non-Native elders. The Native elders were also significantly higher on the subscales for childhood abuse, childhood neglect, and childhood household dysfunction (mean scores of 0.68, 0.32, and 1.59, respectively) compared to non-Native elders (mean scores of 0.27, 0.14, and 0.42, respectively). Culturally specific outcomes may lead to a nuanced differential effect of ACE dimensions on depressive symptoms (Burnette et al., 2017). Given their significantly higher ACE scores, Native elders were predicted to have significantly higher depressive symptoms, but this was not the case. Instead, Native and non-Native elders had comparable rates of depressive symptoms and social support, indicating substantial resilience among the former cohort. In spite of a lifetime of disparities that accumulate in old age, the dimensions of ACE differentially affected Native and non-Native elders, suggesting culturally distinct risk and protective factors (Burnette et al., 2017; see also Roh et al., 2015).

Indigenous elders are less likely to live alone than their non-Indigenous counterparts. While 43 percent of White elders live alone, only 37.1 percent of Native American and a mere 26.7 percent of Native Hawaiian and Pacific Islander elders do (Braun & LaCounte, 2015). Living alone is a risk factor for depression in Native elders, but this was not found to be the case for non-Native elders. This difference may be accounted for by cultural norms. Elders are well integrated in traditional Indigenous societies, and this social connectedness may buffer depression. On the other hand, an elder who falls outside this cultural expectation may feel isolation particularly keenly (Burnette et al., 2017).

Changing families

As people age, they may require care from others. Historically, Indigenous elders were cared for by family and extended family members. In contemporary times, extended family networks may be fragmented, which often leaves individual women with the responsibility for caring for elders. This shift in responsibility from a network to an individual can result in significant social, economic, and personal health stressors on caregivers, which in turn can affect their quality of life and ultimately the wellbeing of elders and the community as a whole (Ryser, Korn & Berridge, 2014).

Lewis noted that this changing family structure diminishes opportunities for youth to engage with elders and learn how to live as healthy Native people. Sometimes young adults relocate to cities, presenting elders with the difficult choice of moving with them or staying behind in their familiar cultural context. When Native people move to urban settings without elders they may become a missing generation without the cultural knowledge they would have learned from close proximity. In these situations, elders are also diminished and lose the opportunity to pass on their knowledge and assume traditional roles as teachers. This may impact their mental wellbeing.

Changing values can also lead to what Lewis termed a "generative mismatch" between what elders want to share and what youth are interested in hearing. Youth may be focused on contemporary technology—an area in which elders usually have little experience—and this can constrain their traditional ability to impart knowledge. Under these circumstances, elders may wonder whether youth will be fully prepared to assume the role of elders when it is their turn.

Grief and loss

Elders may deal with layers of loss that have accumulated across their lifetimes. Grief and loss often begin in childhood (Dennis, 2014). Cross also noted that the sterilization of Native American women, which was common practice in the 1960s and 1970s, may continue to be traumatic for these individuals, who are now elders. Statistically, bereavement, which is associated with negative physical, social, and emotional consequences as well as increased use of medical services, occurs more frequently and at a younger age for Native Americans. One study exploring the relationship between loss and health in Lakota elders (Dennis, 2014) found that multiple losses of loved ones and community members were common. Many of these elders grew up in a socio-economic context with few resources, and many families were affected by frequent illnesses culminating in death. Elders often reported siblings who died in their youth when few health services were available on reservations.

Parental deaths were also common in this community, occurred suddenly, and typically led to a period of instability. The bereaved children were often sent to boarding schools, resulting in the loss of a familiar cultural context, identity and place, and connection to extended family members. Others lost connections to family and community when they were sent to tuberculosis hospitals—a regular occurrence in many communities. Elders reported experiencing confusion and grief from these multiple losses that framed their childhoods.

Throughout their adulthood, the elders continued to experience many health issues as well as accidental deaths of family and community members, which are common in many Native communities. Health disparities lead to shorter life spans. Elders often suffered the death of children as well as spouses. As young widows, women were often obliged to fill multiple, significant responsibilities. Multiple losses are compounded by such multiple responsibilities, taking a heavy toll. Cumulative losses and grief often result in emotional struggles for elderly women who strive to raise children and grandchildren in a resource-poor environment.

During the course of her research project, Dennis (2014) noted multiple incidents that led to injury or death. It was clear that the elders took the loss of each child personally, feeling a heavy weight of collective responsibility for all community members. They frequently discussed the many deaths in their community, attended the funerals and wakes, and helped one another cope with feelings of helplessness and loss.

The repercussions of addictions

Both Cross and Lewis emphasized that substance misuse and its many repercussions have a deep impact on elders, both when they misuse substances themselves and when others in their families and communities do so. In fact, struggles with addiction may interfere with adults' ability to acquire the knowledge and experience necessary to personify the esteemed role of elder (Lewis & Allen, 2017). Addiction may compromise parents' ability to raise their children, thus compelling some elders to take on full-time caregiving roles for their grandchildren or other young community members. Cross noted that adult offspring sometimes exploit their elders' willingness to provide childcare and may leave children from earlier relationships with them in order to start a new relationship or family.

She also noted that the financial drain caused by addiction can lead some parents to traffic their children, sell possessions, including those of spiritual or cultural significance, and financially victimize elders. People struggling with addiction may pressure elders for money or steal from them, particularly around the time when per capita tribal money is distributed. Cross felt that elders are often reluctant to report this sort of victimization because of a wish to protect "my child, the one I raised."

Strengths and resilience

Resilience is a multidimensional construct characterized by the ability to adapt in the face of adversity. It is associated with successful aging, despite challenges. Native American elders face persistent health and economic disparities, yet they are resilient and demonstrate considerable strength on behalf of their families and communities. Cross and Lewis both emphasized that these elders possess a wealth of knowledge, and there is inherent strength and resilience in knowing your own culture, roots, and how to teach others. This foundational knowledge and strength enables Native people to assert themselves and correct inaccuracies, stereotypes, and misconceptions.

Traditionally, gender and age converged to create an esteemed status for grandmothers that was grounded in the role they played as mothers. Women's ability to nurture a baby parallels the earth's sustainment of life. Nurturing life is celebrated in Indigenous cultures, so unique sources of wisdom are acknowledged and honored in Native grandmothers (Byers, 2010).

The current cohort of elders have navigated their way through both mainstream society and their own Indigenous culture. They are prepared and willing to teach the skills that are necessary to remain Indigenous in the contemporary, multicultural world. While there are many challenges in this world, Indigenous communities, families, and particularly elders have the answers that will resolve most of them. As Lewis stated, they just need to be asked.

Maintaining a positive outlook

Lewis pointed out that becoming an elder is a demonstration of hope and resilience in and of itself. He reported that 98 percent of the elders he has encountered are optimistic that tomorrow will be a better day and youth will become the people they need to be. He has seen incredible strength in many communities, both urban and remote.

Cross highlighted humor and laughter as key aspects of elders' resilience and wellbeing. She noted that this is one way in which they engage with each other and younger family members, and offered an example of the prevalence of laughter:

> My husband, who is non-Native, once asked me: "Why do Indians giggle?" I said rather strongly: "We don't giggle!" Then, we were at the pow wow and we walked by some teens who were full of quiet laughter and giggling, but I thought, "They are teens, and teens tend to giggle." Then, we walked by a small group of elders and one had told a story, and they all began to laugh quietly, which I again perceived to be giggling. I thought of different times and events in my life when the elders did the most "giggling" after they had shared stories of their experience.

Cross described how Native elders can maintain a positive outlook even through significant adversity. She noted how one of her mother's friends always seemed to get on with life in a matter-of-fact way and not let anything bother her. She always seemed happy, leaving Cross to speculate about the key to her happiness. This particular elder maintained a positive spirit through financial woes, her daughter's job loss, and even the deaths of her husband, a close friend, and other community members. In spite of these multiple challenges and losses, she always kept the same positive outlook. Cross commented, "I like being around her spirit." She noted that many elders demonstrate this sort of remarkable resilience and an ability to move beyond seemingly devastating experiences: "I see healing occur when they have turned to their cultures; they become more alive and experience happiness. Their personalities appear more complete and relaxed. From my perspective, they are home." We can all learn from the calm way in which many elders proceed through the ups and downs of life.

Elders can serve as role models. They are living examples who demonstrate how to survive adversity. In turn, they can pass on resilience through intergenerational teaching, either formally or informally. Storytelling is a traditional resilience strategy that connected contemporary elders to their grandparents. It can continue to serve as a way to connect contemporary youth to their culture, history, and community (Reinschmidt et al., 2016).

Lewis perceived significant strength and resilience in stories of recovery from addiction. Native Americans have high rates of abstinence, with many achieving sobriety or never drinking in the first place, but we seldom hear those stories. Their motivation for sobriety is often the birth of a grandchild or preparation to fulfill the responsibilities that are expected of an elder. Many make a conscious decision to become healthy. One study of Alaskan Natives over the age of 50 (Lewis & Allen, 2017) found that they abstained from alcohol or quit drinking because of and with support from their spirituality and family. Their own understanding of what it means to be an elder and a positive role model encouraged them to assume Indigenous cultural roles and activities within and on behalf of their families and community. They wanted to share traditional values, history, and spirituality, as well as what they had learned in their own lives by engaging in culturally grounded activities with youth. Fulfilling these traditional roles as elders and teachers encouraged them to maintain their own sobriety and enhanced the wellbeing of the whole community. Leading and teaching future generations leaves a positive legacy for the future. This teaching often includes stories of personal challenges and resilience.

Belonging and interconnection

Connections with others and social engagement facilitate better health and cognitive wellbeing among Native elders (Nelson et al., 2013). The Native Elder Care study (Conte et al., 2015), which was conducted with 505 community-dwelling members of one Southeastern tribe over the age of 55, found high levels of social support for the oldest generation (over 75). This was likely the result of strong cultural values of caring for elders and community cooperation. The study highlights the close relationship between health and social support in elders. Social support is associated with positive health indicators, such as less depression and chronic pain. Improving social support may also mitigate negative health outcomes.

Native American cultural traditions often emphasize shared responsibility across generations. Contemporary Indigenous people have a responsibility to plan for future generations, just as their ancestors took steps to ensure cultural continuity and the survival of today's generation. The ability to pass on traditions, values, and ways of knowing is grounded in what has been learned from those who have come before us and will ultimately benefit those who will come after us. To fulfill the responsibility of passing on a culture, individuals must first experience a sense of belonging. Elders' ability to share and mentor others affirms belonging and their connections with both ancestors and future generations (Lewis & Allen, 2017).

Lewis & Allen (2017) propose a specific Indigenous model of cultural generativity focused on collective wellbeing. Rather than focusing on an individual legacy, this model is centered on activities that benefit the whole family, community, and culture. This is done through activities such as teaching traditional values, beliefs, and subsistence practices. In this way, history, culture, and language are preserved for future generations, ensuring continuity of Indigenous values and ways of life. When elders feel they have a meaningful role to play in their families and community, they often gain the motivation to achieve and maintain sobriety. In this way, both elders and their communities benefit.

Reciprocity is intertwined with Indigenous cultural values of connectedness and interdependence. When practiced among community members, it supports the wellbeing of each and the community as a whole. This is readily apparent when looking at elder wellbeing. The traditional value of interconnectedness is embedded in Indigenous cultures and also serves as the foundation for wellness programming. The resilience of Native American and Native Hawaiian elders can be supported through culture, youth activities, and education (Kahn et al., 2016). Throughout their lives, elders have used culturally grounded strategies to overcome adversity. These strategies can be transmitted to youth to help them build their own resilience.

Elders as caregivers

Elders often find themselves in caregiving roles that are affirming yet simultaneously pose significant challenges to their own wellbeing (Dennis & Brewer, 2017). By guiding and supporting youth, Native American elders embody traditional roles in contemporary times. Exploring the multifaceted experiences of elders as caregivers provides insight into how challenges and resilience are often interwoven. Raising grandchildren may involve living in a multigenerational household with shared responsibilities, and elders can benefit from close interactions with their grandchildren (Cross et al., 2010). Many elders believe that children bring happiness, and they are viewed as the future of the tribe. Indigenous worldviews emphasize the importance of family and keeping people together.

Participating in child-rearing with other adult family members can be affirming for elders. Indigenous elders also often feel entitled to be supported and respected in their older adulthood. This can lead to balanced, mutually beneficial family roles and relationships (Dennis & Brewer, 2017). Contemporary elders often reflect on the importance of their own grandparents, particularly grandmothers, during their childhoods. They want to pass on similar values and experiences to their own grandchildren (Dennis & Brewer, 2017).

Traditionally, grandparents provided childcare and helped raise their grandchildren within a supportive social environment. Parents and other community members were present and supported both the children and the grandparents. This may or may not be the reality for today's grandparents. In particular, high incarceration rates of Native women in states like Oklahoma may lead to elders raising children without parental support. Grandparents', and in particular grandmothers', significant involvement in childcare and child-rearing has been consistently identified across studies (Byers, 2010).

Grandparents can serve as cultural conservators who are able to transmit traditions, rather than just fill in due to crises, parental neglect, or abandonment. Elders can offer strength to youth, but they may suffer emotional and/or physical consequences (Byers, 2010). When one granddaughter disclosed being teased for the color of her skin, her grandfather stated:

> I had to look away. As she spoke, I wept silently on the inside and did not want her to see me as weak and powerless, or furious knowing that she, too, will have to carry the burden of racism into her generation.
>
> (Quoted in Peacock, 2011, p. 16)

Sometimes elders, far from being dependent and passive, are our most powerful and articulate advocates.

Elders who serve as caregivers often experience both positive and negative effects. A qualitative study of 25 reservation-based Lakota elders explored their experiences as caregiving grandparents. While caregiving can take an emotional and spiritual toll on such elders, it can also be fulfilling for them to devote their time, love, and compassion in ways that provide family support and stability to children who otherwise might receive none (Dennis & Brewer, 2017). The experiences of caregivers are multidimensional. In spite of adversity, they need not be framed by a deficit perspective.

The challenges of grandparent caregivers

As Cross noted, the Indian Child Welfare Act advocates keeping Native children within their familial and cultural contexts. This provides a legal framework for grandparents as well as other family members to care for children when parents are unable to do so, although Native grandparents who raise their grandchildren still face a host of challenges and inequalities. For instance, caring for grandchildren can become a financial burden. Compared to Native peers who do not live with their grandchildren, grandparent carers are more likely to be older, single women, disabled, less educated, and have less income (Byers, 2010).

Grandparents may be physically or emotionally overburdened with caregiving roles yet often remain reluctant to seek support or services. These elders may have ongoing fears and mistrust that prevent them from seeking services based on their own experiences in boarding schools or fear that they will be deemed too old to parent. Distrust of social agencies and legal bureaucracies may also discourage them from initiating formal custody arrangements. A study of 31 caregiver grandparents found 20 had no legal authorization to care for their grandchildren (Cross et al., 2010).

On average, Native elders are three times more likely to be the sole carers of their grandchildren than non-Native elders (Cross et al., 2010), although the prevalence of grandparent caregiving varies across the tribes. This family model is particularly high in Oklahoma due to this state having the highest number of incarcerated females, which leaves many families without residential mothers. In the state, 64.3 percent of all Cherokee grandparents and 58.9 percent of all Muskogee Creek grandparents were raising their grandchildren at the end of the 2000s, compared to 42 percent for all Native grandparents (Byers, 2010).

Like the mainstream population, Native grandparents may become carers when parents are unavailable due to factors such as substance misuse, incarceration, mental health issues, or death. Alternatively, given the limited educational and economic opportunities on reservations, parents may seek employment elsewhere and leave their children with grandparents to enable them to maintain tribal connections (Dennis & Brewer, 2017). A study of caregiving grandparents found that many chose to raise children again specifically because they feared their removal from the household and the loss of traditional values and cultural norms. They may also choose to raise their grandchildren to avoid separating siblings or because of the risk of abuse in the child welfare system. In particular, they reference the historical trauma resulting from the boarding schools and want to avoid out-of-home care for their family members if at all possible (Cross et al., 2010).

Economic and health vulnerabilities can be pressing issues for grandparents who care for their grandchildren. They can experience a variety of stressors, including inadequate finances, housing, food, clothing, and medical care. Also, while initially they may view caregiving as temporary, complex and sometimes intractable family issues may necessitate long-term commitment to the role (Cross et al., 2010).

The role of trauma in caregiving

The earlier traumatic experiences of elders are often reawakened when they take on caregiving roles. Some grandchildren were intentionally given to the grandparents while others were abandoned or removed from unstable homes, and these children often carry their own unresolved emotional issues. This can rekindle elders' own feelings of abandonment, trauma, and anger. Beyond caring for immediate relatives, they may give various types of support to the community's grandchildren, many of whom may be unsupervised or hungry.

One Lakota elder described trying to raise her grandson, who was abandoned outside in the winter and only survived by huddling with dogs for warmth. The grandson's abandonment led him to struggle with anger, while his grandmother was also anguished, concerned, and flooded with memories and feelings about her own experiences in boarding school. Therefore, she could relate to her grandson's anger and frustration. Limited resources on reservations often make it difficult for both elders and youth to heal from such experiences (Dennis & Brewer, 2017).

Interventions

Interventions that support the wellbeing of elders can be either formal or informal. They may be done in the context of families or under tribal or other governmental auspices. Indigenous elders' needs can exceed Indigenous-specific resources, so they often receive care in mainstream settings. These contact zones between Indigenous and non-Indigenous people can be sites of contested power that can feel disempowering as mainstream services often reflect legacies of oppression. Native elders may not feel comfortable seeking services in mainstream settings where they fear discrimination. Likewise, mainstream service providers may be keenly aware of past inequities and fear that Native elders will be hostile and judgemental (Balestrery, 2016).

Multicultural service settings in Alaska can reflect historical trauma and the colonial legacy of service sites. For some Native elders, anxiety can be triggered in social service agencies where they encounter non-Native people. Generations of pain can lead to charged emotions, such as guilt and fear (Balestrery, 2016). Indigenous elders and non-Native service providers can panic when in the presence of the other. The elders are often conscious they may trigger panic in the service providers and take responsibility for lessening tension in the interaction. There is prejudice and wounding on both sides, with each feeling dehumanized and stereotyping the other. There can be a clash of values between Western and Indigenous ways of helping. Social agencies can be contested sites that include discrepancies between individual and community foci. The wellbeing of individuals, land, and community are still integral and intertwined with a subsistence lifestyle in Alaska. Healing this legacy must involve everyone (Balestrery, 2016).

Engagement and assessment

Cross and Lewis both emphasized that elders possess a wealth of knowledge. This cohort has been largely successful in negotiating both Native and non-Native society, so they demonstrate the strength of adaptation. Helping professionals need to do more to engage with and learn from them. However, Lewis cautioned that social workers must understand that elders' needs vary from individual to individual and community to community. To engage them and provide the most assistance, human service professionals must be patient, listen, and learn to be present. Some assessment tools have been tested for their utility with Indigenous elders. For example, the full and abbreviated versions of the Center for Epidemiologic Studies' Depression Scale have excellent internal reliability and concurrent validity with Native American elders (Schure & Goins, 2017).

When working with American Indian elders, helping professionals must be comfortable asking questions and learning from mistakes. Lewis noted that elders are good at "calling you out" and pointing out when a helping professional makes assumptions or mistakes. This can provide opportunities to display cultural humility and be open to learning. He emphasized that helping professionals must recognize resilience, strength, and success stories. Elders remind us they are doing many things right, and we must not view their life situations from a deficit perspective. The answers to many problems lie in the community, and community members usually know how best to address concerns.

Clear communication is an important component of engaging and working with clients. When clients and helping professionals come from different backgrounds, it is imperative to minimize potential misunderstandings. It is essential to check for understanding when communicating health risks to Native American elders (LaVallie et al., 2012). Understanding health information and providing informed consent are crucial.

Lack of trust in healthcare providers and organizations likely contributes to health disparities. A study of elders at Cherokee Nation health clinics (Simonds et al., 2014) found that 95 percent trusted their individual provider but only 46 percent trusted their healthcare institution. Elders who endorsed a strong Indigenous cultural identity had the least trust in the institution. People who trust are more amenable to medical advice and more likely to adhere to treatment recommendations.

Caregiving and social support

Little attention is paid to the needs of those who care for elders. These may be family members or people employed through county or tribal programs. The American Indian Caregiver Health Study (Ryser et al., 2014) found the average

age of caregivers was 50. These caregivers had significant physical and psycho-logical health concerns, including chronic stress and pain, depression, digestive problems, hyperlipidemia, and adrenal exhaustion. They also had high rates of trauma exposure, were on the verge of burnout, and some were at risk of sudden death from heart rate variability. Of course, these health challenges affect their ability to help elders.

Family is at the heart of elder wellbeing, providing a foundation that goes beyond formal interventions. Strengthening existing social and family supports is central to preventing and treating depression in Native elders (Roh et al., 2015). Companion programs can be a strategy to enhance social support and health ben-efits for isolated elders (Conte et al., 2015). Some programs use senior volunteers, which benefits both the volunteer and the service recipient. As noted earlier, intergenerational programs can enhance social support for elders, provide mentor-ship, and support cultural traditions among youth and others (Kahn et al., 2016).

Elders and youth may have fewer opportunities to connect with each other in urban settings, but the growing disconnect across generations can be remedied with intergenerational interventions (Kahn et al., 2016). Libraries can play an important role in offering opportunities for intergenerational support. For instance, they can host storytelling events to encourage interactions across the generations and allow elders to become role models for reading (Ford & Hughes, 2017).

Understanding protective factors such as social support can help develop viable health-promoting interventions, thus reducing health disparities (Conte et al., 2015). A study of 185 non-institutionalized elders over the age of 55 found high levels of resilience were associated with fewer depressive symptoms and less chronic pain as well as improved mental and physical health (Schure, Odden & Goins, 2013).

Empowerment and supporting resilience

Resilience is exemplified in the lives of American Indian, Alaska Native, and Native Hawaiian elders. Elders have survived, and even thrived, despite adversity (Kahn et al., 2016). Resilience strategies are linked to cultural teachings and values. Elders' life stories hold rich lessons and traditional knowledge that can foster cul-tural identity and life skills for future generations.

As Lewis noted, more elders are finding their voices and speaking out. An Aleut elder emphasized that we must "stop dealing with the symptoms and deal with the root causes, and the root cause is here [pointing to the heart], its separation, its disconnection that's creating all the sickness" (quoted in Balestrery, 2016, p. 311). Helping professionals can use an empowerment and a strengths-based framework to draw on the knowledge and empower Indigenous elders in ways that affirm and strengthen their sense of purpose and identity.

Engaging and empowering Alaskan Native elders to fulfill community roles based on their own preferences can be a trauma-informed way to enhance their health and wellbeing. By serving as teachers and mentors, elders can demonstrate how to age well—with dignity and pride. They may teach language and

Indigenous arts, volunteer, or serve in leadership positions. Elders' community engagement and desire to help others are often grounded in their sense of spirituality (Lewis, 2017). As they actively engage with other community members, they share valuable knowledge, stories, and healing practices in ways that foster language and cultural revitalization. Elders are now moving beyond being quiet observers to become advocates, leaders, and culture bearers for their families and communities (Kahn et al., 2016; Lewis, 2016).

A research project in the Southwest (Reinschmidt et al., 2016) found many urban elders felt youth did not understand and appreciate the impact of historical trauma. They believed educating Native youth was crucial to ending intergenerational transmission of historical trauma. Elders have also used talking circles to teach youth about alcohol and associated problems (Momper et al., 2017). Storytelling can rejuvenate traditional methods of teaching. In one example, elders began to convey their own stories unexpectedly during a research project. These stories described pathways to healthy living and contained prevention messages about substance misuse (Momper et al., 2017).

Social workers and other helping professionals are well positioned to support elders in these roles and draw from their guidance to develop programs that serve the needs of Indigenous communities. Human service professionals can collaborate with elders as co-researchers to expand the knowledge base on many of the issues that impact Indigenous families and communities. Elders can work in partnership with helping professionals and be catalysts for positive social change:

> Gone are the days where social workers speak with the sons and daughters to learn of Grandma's ailments; Elders have found their voice and they not only speak for themselves but for their families and communities to ensure a healthy future for their grandchildren.
>
> *(Lewis, 2016, p. 279)*

Services for veterans

Realizing that no studies of the needs of Native Vietnam veterans existed, two Native veterans took the initiative, developed their own survey, and launched the Vietnam Era Veterans Intertribal Association. Their working group under the auspices of the VA's Readjustment Counseling Services authored a 1992 report and they held a four-day retreat on the Yakama Reservation for veterans and VA caregivers. The latter provided a therapeutic experience for veterans and a space where caregivers and VA counselors could learn about Native traditions and ways of healing. This initiative has continued ever since (Holm, 2017).

As per the traditional relationships between warriors and their communities noted earlier, returning Native American veterans have often sought culturally grounded mechanisms for healing. Many of them have found honoring or healing ceremonies to be effective in working through PTSD symptoms. Through reciprocal relationships, veterans heal and sustain their communities and cultures, and vice versa (Holm, 2017).

The VA has developed a Tribal Veterans Representative (TVR) program to address barriers to obtaining VA services. TVRs are volunteers appointed by their tribal councils, veterans, and members of the communities they serve. They undergo extensive training then reach out to Native veterans who are not currently connected with VA services. The TVRs have credibility as community members and veterans themselves, which enables them to build trust and rapport in ways that other government officials cannot. After beginning in Montana, the program has now trained over 800 TVRs and has expanded to other parts of the country, including Alaska. Providing these services to veterans has a wider effect as it also improves the wellbeing of their families and communities (Kaufmann et al., 2014).

Recall that Native Americans have higher rates of service-connected disabilities (Kaufmann et al., 2014). In response, additional services have grown from some TVR programs, such as a veteran transportation system from the Blackfeet Reservation to a hospital in Helena, Montana, and a veteran resource center on the Flathead Reservation. The VA has also established American Indian telemental health clinics that offer counseling with off-site clinicians for veterans in remote areas where no regular VA services are available (Kaufmann et al., 2014).

The societal and policy context for elder wellbeing

Indigenous communities traditionally had their own mechanisms for supporting families in meeting the long-term needs of elders, such as the Longhouse societies in western Washington. Now tribal governments are responsible for developing socioeconomic institutions to support elders' needs. Some tribal governments have established elders' programs and provide support for caregivers, but these efforts comprise a far from comprehensive response to the needs of the growing elderly population (Ryser et al., 2014). Traditional values about caring for elders and tribal government responses are now accompanied by policies instituted through federal and state governments. To serve elders appropriately, the Older Americans Act and other external policies must be implemented in ways that recognize Indigenous cultural contexts. This is necessary in order to promote quality of life, good health, and stable socioeconomic conditions for tribal elders (Ryser et al., 2014).

Multiple entities—including tribal and state governments, federal programs, and individual family and community members—have responsibility for providing care for Native American elders and people with disabilities. State, country, and tribal informants spoke to researchers from the Center for World Indigenous Studies about the challenges they face implementing policies and providing services to this population. In particular, they noted issues with duplication of services, confusion about policies, cultural insensitivity, lack of culturally appropriate needs assessments, insufficient information about the population in need of services, ineffective cross-cultural communication, mismatched services, and inflexible, complicated state regulations as barriers to the provision of effective services (Ryser et al., 2014).

The Administration on Aging and the Administration for Community Living fund three resource centers for American Indian, Alaska Native, and Native

Hawaiian elders that develop and share information and expertise for Indigenous organizations and communities, educational institutions, and helping professionals (Browne, Carter & Gray, 2015). The National Resource Center on Native American Aging in the School of Medicine and Health Sciences at the University of North Dakota focuses on health disparities and conducted a needs assessment with more than 17,000 Indigenous elders. Its aim is to address mistreatment of Indigenous elders. The National Resource Center for American Indian, Alaska Native, and Native Hawaiian Elders at the University of Alaska, Anchorage, assesses elders' needs and promotes understanding of the cultural values that guide service and care expectations. It advocates for improving wellbeing and understanding historical trauma. The Ha Kupuna Resource Center for Native Hawaiian Elders, University of Hawaii, Manoa, focuses on building the knowledge base to inform effective policies and practices (Browne et al., 2015).

Health disparities experienced by Native American elders mean more care is required. The demand for caregivers will increase as this sector of the population grows. Caregiving intersects with cultural norms. Family and community members often feel that caring for elders is an expected, important, and valued role. It does, however, present a variety of challenges. Caregivers themselves are likely to experience health and economic disparities, and the intersection of disparities and caregiver burden requires policy attention.

In the aforementioned western Washington study (Ryser et al., 2014), 90 percent of the people who cared for elders had been exposed to physical and emotional trauma, both interpersonal and accidental. These caregivers were therefore at high risk and in need of support. The researchers recommended an eldercare conference with training as well as more coordination of policies and practices to support the caregivers. They saw a need to revise tribally organized area agencies on aging to increase the cultural suitability of support services and mechanisms for coordination between tribal and state agencies.

Intergovernmental cooperation agreements can help clarify responsibilities. This is particularly important given the various entities with responsibility for serving American Indian elders. There is a need for policies on compensation and to provide integrated personal health support for family caregivers. This can also enhance bidirectional cultural competency as agencies learn more about culture from tribal caregivers, and caregivers learn more about agencies' policies and services. Turnover in tribal government inhibits quality services, so these administrations should work toward stabilizing program staffing. Meanwhile, the state can also work toward improving services by simplifying regulations and allowing for more flexibility in their implementation (Ryser et al., 2014).

Colonial histories contribute to ongoing social and health disparities for Native people and elders (Balestrery, 2016). Conventional health and social organizations (i.e., community-based health and social services that deal with medical, substance misuse, behavioral, dental, food, and shelter needs) seek to address these disparities, yet these organizations are not culturally neutral and are often guided by long-standing cultural assumptions. Differences between Indigenous and mainstream assumptions can create misunderstandings, and points of tension can have a detrimental impact on services for elders (Balestrery, 2016).

Lewis emphasized that community programming and social policies must be grounded in strengths-based approaches to health and wellbeing. Elders wish to be engaged at all levels of planning, service delivery, and policy development for themselves, their families, and their communities. As traditional knowledge holders, their perspectives are not only relevant but may be more valuable than those of highly educated external scholars. It is important to engage elders and gather their input. They are particularly well suited to serve in advisory capacities, such as on elders' councils and in residence initiatives for social work programs.

Veterans' programming and policies

The VA is taking steps to minimize disparities in how Native American veterans are served. These include telemental health outreach for rural and reservation-based populations, TVR training, and developing an Office of Tribal Governments Relations. There is a Memorandum of Understanding between the IHS and the VA that articulates this commitment to improve care. Despite these initiatives, however, effective coordination of care delivered by federal entities remains an elusive goal (Kaufman et al., 2016).

The VA has policy and funding initiatives to improve access to healthcare for reservation-based veterans. These initiatives seek to provide interdisciplinary, non-institutional care to veterans with complex, chronic, disabling conditions. They work to optimize veterans' ability to access needed care in their communities and prevent decline that would necessitate hospitalization or admission to a skilled nursing facility (Kramer et al., 2018). Many of these veterans qualify for services through Medicare, the VA, and IHS.

Kramer et al. (2018) documented the demographic and health characteristics of veterans accessing these community-based services and evaluated service effectiveness. In particular, they sought to determine whether outcomes were equitable for Native and non-Native service recipients. They found that IHS recipients were significantly younger (mean age 67.5, compared with 77.7 for non-Natives), and less likely to live alone (13.6 percent, compared with 33.7 percent). Among Native American veterans, 40.9 percent lived with their spouse, compared with 47.9 percent of non-Natives; 39.8 percent lived with relatives, compared with 11.8 percent of non-Natives; and 5.7 percent lived with non-relatives, compared with 4.9 percent of non-Natives. None of the Native Americans lived in group residences, compared with 1.7 percent of the general veteran population. The Native American veterans had more unduplicated diagnoses and more emergency room visits prior to enrollment in the community-based program (50 percent, compared with 34 percent of non-Natives). Similar to their non-Native counterparts, 30 percent had impairments in two or more ADLs. Participation in the community-based program reduced both hospitalizations and emergency room visits. Consistent with previous studies, these Native veterans reported fewer hospitalizations than their non-Native peers. The introduction of the program led to more IHS beneficiaries enrolling in VA medical benefits.

Filing a claim for veterans' benefits can be daunting. Only authorized individuals and organizations are able to provide assistance with claims, but accessing this help can be difficult for veterans on reservations. For example, reservations in Montana are an average of almost 100 miles away from the nearest Veterans Service Officer. In response to this problem, the VA, in consultation with tribes, amended regulations to allow tribal organizations to assist with applications. This change addresses concerns about travel distance and the cultural competence of available assistance (Wandler, 2017).

The consultative process between the VA and tribes included grappling with how regulations might affect tribal sovereignty and the federal Indian trust responsibility, under which the federal government accepted responsibility for the wellbeing of tribes. Any regulation that required tribal governments to spend non-federal assets was viewed by the tribes as a violation of sovereignty and their right to self-governance. Certifying tribal entities such as TCUs to determine eligibility and process applications alleviated this concern (Wandler, 2017).

The VA and IHS are working to align their organizations more closely, draw on their respective expertise, develop policies, and coordinate services. For example, the VA has developed a model of home-based primary care to provide interdisciplinary services for veterans who are unable to leave their homes. This has been implemented with various models, with tribes sometimes retaining primary care responsibilities. In addition, the VA has funded efforts to develop home-based care in partnership with tribes, IHS, and tribal health facilities. This is done through co-management agreements between federal agencies and tribes (Kramer et al., 2015).

Model programs and trauma-informed care

Both Cross and Lewis noted that few models of best practices with elders have become widely known, although there may be individual tribal services that provide quality services for elders. In particular, they reflected that trauma-informed care has yet to be systematically integrated as a guiding principle in services for Indigenous elders. There are, however, some local examples of innovative services.

In one notable example, the public library and tribal college on the Winnebago Reservation created a position of *tribal aide to elders*. This program connects with elders and home-bound individuals to mitigate their isolation (Ford & Hughes, 2017). The aide delivers library books, provides transportation, teaches basic computer skills, facilitates a book club, provides accessibility devices, and offers other activities to keep elders connected. This initiative was originally funded by the Institute of Museum and Library Services Enhancement through a grant designed to enhance existing services among Native American tribes and Alaskan Native villages. It is now funded by the Little Priest Tribal College. The library aide is engaged in the community, makes home visits, and attends funerals. He or she stocks the library cart at the senior center but also goes above and beyond typical library services by helping patrons to research wheelchairs, accessible vehicles, and internet providers. In the first two years of the program, library circulation to older adults increased from almost zero to 27 percent (Ford & Hughes, 2017).

Cross noted that her tribe has an elders' residence—Andahwod—on the reservation. It has only 37 places but provides a wide range of services and is well integrated into the community. For instance, it offers clinics, health education, and a monthly breakfast for the whole community. It also organizes behavioral health visits to those who may need services and provides transportation to the reservation-based health clinic. Young children from the local school attend interactive events and the tribe holds its high school graduation at Andahwod. The home organizes dances and breakfasts with elders as well as many other activities and services. Cross and her brother joke about making advance reservations for places, given the large cohort of aging baby boomers. This seems to be an appealing place for all members of the community. Indeed, the Chippewa word Andahwod translates as "where we live."

Cross noted key elements of quality services for elders. She emphasized the importance of a comprehensive assessment as the foundation for all services and pointed out that there must be a process for checking health on a regular basis. Services must include traditional care, transportation, and physical and mental health appraisals. They should help elders to be more mobile and care for themselves, with support. Furthermore, they must give elders a sense of purpose, inspiring them to remain passionate and engaged with life.

Lewis noted that the National Congress on American Indians has been attentive to the needs of elders and that the Alzheimer's Institute in Phoenix is developing some programs for Native Americans with dementia. While there may be some innovative grassroots programs, as yet these have not been highlighted in newsletters or other publications, so they do not currently inform best practices and trauma-informed care with elders.

Conclusion

This chapter has reviewed demographic information on Native American elders and contrasted the status of elders and veterans in Indigenous and non-Indigenous communities. Subject-matter experts Lewis and Cross have shared their perspectives on elders' challenges and resilience as well as best practices for serving this cohort. It is both notable and troubling that both of these experts were unfamiliar with services for elders that implemented the principles of trauma-informed care, particularly as members of this population have likely been exposed to significant trauma, including periods in boarding schools. This is clearly an area that requires more attention, both in highlighting innovative local programming and developing well-articulated best practices.

As Lewis noted, Native communities have always prioritized their elders. Now that mainstream society is beginning to look at community aging, it could learn a lot from Indigenous perspectives. Indeed, elders are not just service recipients but can offer significant guidance in developing programming and policies for the wellbeing of all community members. They have plenty to offer youth, families, and communities, so helping professionals would do well to seek their assistance.

As the number of elders increases, helping professionals and policy makers must be responsive to their needs. Indeed, demographic trends clearly demonstrate a need to be proactive. Lewis drew attention to some small communities in Alaska where all of the residents are over the age of 55 and raised the question, "How will they age well?" The answer, should it be found, may well inform other communities.

Elders are perceived differently in Indigenous and non-Indigenous contexts. These differing worldviews have a variety of implications. Indeed, it is important to reflect on how mainstream perspectives on elders and the aging process have deeply permeated our thinking. Forgetfulness and the things that tend to be forgotten provide a poignant example. The World Health Organization has identified dementia as a public health priority, mirroring Western narratives that classify aging as a stage of deterioration. It is telling that they seem to be "casting elders with memory loss as a greater socio-political risk than the historical amnesia of the settler state; a striking statement in this particular political moment, as the settler state implodes from the relentless animus of its own denial" (Grande, 2018, p. 174).

6

EDUCATION FOR A CONTEMPORARY WORLD

Learning and knowing from Indigenous and non-Indigenous perspectives

This chapter approaches education as knowledge transmission in its many forms and settings. A wide range of topics is covered, including traditional and institutionalized approaches to teaching and learning, both historically and today. This is balanced by a review of efforts to integrate Indigenous knowledge and methods in mainstream education to facilitate better outcomes for Native American students. The chapter also examines examples of Indigenous-controlled education and the social climate and socialization aspects of educational settings.

Input from subject-matter experts Dr. Katie Johnston-Goodstar and Dr. Lori Quigley informs a discussion of what educational professionals and policy makers need to know about Native students. Based on their extensive experience, they offer their perspectives on major issues in Native education. In addition to challenges, they share stories of resilience and integration of trauma-informed principles. Both Quigley and Johnston-Goodstar were shaped by their own experiences in educational systems, then sought careers where they could make a difference for future Native students. Their different but complementary pathways bring insight to various elements of education and the experiences of Native American students.

Johnston-Goodstar is an associate professor in the School of Social Work at the University of Minnesota. She studies the social, political, and historical contexts of Indigenous youth development. Drawing on Indigenous and social justice youth development frameworks, she collaborates with youth in participatory action research (PAR) to explore social justice issues, decolonization, and community building. She is currently studying Native youth perspectives on school climate and its influence on traditional indicators of academic achievement, such as truancy, grades, and progress toward graduation.

Johnston-Goodstar strongly identifies as a youth worker. Much of her early career involved street-based outreach to Native youth. This included informal, participatory education where she helped youth connect to services. This blossomed into working with an Indigenous charter school in northern Minnea-polis, a place where many youth gravitated after being poorly served in mainstream schools. As she pursued her professional degrees, she found her fit in macro social work facilitating community education and public awareness. Her lived experi-ences as a Native American in the educational system have consistently influenced her career path.

Quigley is Vice President for Academic Affairs and Chief Academic Officer at Medaille College. She grew up on the Allegany Territory of the Seneca Nation of Indians and is a member of the Wolf Clan. She has been the principal grant writer for several Native education initiatives, totaling nearly $4 million. In 2004, she received a presidential appointment to the National Advisory Council on Indian Education, which she chaired until June 2010. She researched the history and sociological impact of the former Thomas Indian School and was an advisor on the documentary *Unseen Tears: The Impact of Native American Residential Boarding Schools*.

Quigley's mother, a representative on the White House Initiative on Indian Education, was a powerful role model who brought her daughter to Indigenous education conferences from the age of 14 onwards. Quigley soon picked up where her mother left off, participating in the first statewide Native education conference in New York. She saw the importance of convening people from across the state and used her credentials and background to support the state organization, even when no budget was available.

Indigenous knowledge and traditional approaches to teaching and learning

Traditional knowledge transcends what can be written. Writing and categorizing are inherently limiting and inadequate representations of traditional knowledge (Wiebe, 2016). Indigenous knowledge is characterized by holistic thinking, subjectivity, and a focus on community wellbeing rather than the linear, hierarchical, individualistic, objective stance that undergirds Western thought (Roberts, Butler & Green, 2016).

> Indigenous knowledge is dynamic, derived from original instructions given to particular Peoples and reflected in Creation stories. It results from a continuous scientific process—observation, experimentation, documentation, evaluation, education, and adaptation. It has the capacity to blend with western scientific knowledge and should be considered complementary to current scientific and technological efforts to solve problems in today's world.
>
> *(Nebelkopf et al., 2011, p. 267)*

Language, words, and names are crucial components for understanding Indi-genous knowledge and how it is organized and recorded. These reflect the shared understandings of Native Peoples that are documented in songs, stories, and speeches. Words and names are chosen with great care and deliberation to reflect the multifaceted aspects of the world and relationships between all beings and surroundings (Littletree & Metoyer, 2015). Indigenous Peoples have ways of recording knowledge that include stories, medicine wheels, winter counts, wampum belts, and totem poles. Viewed within cultural contexts, these are interconnected aspects of knowledge that inform and guide contemporary societies (Littletree & Metoyer, 2015). Indigenous knowledge is sacred and purposeful (Brayboy & Maughan, 2009).

Indigenous thought is grounded in circles, cycles, and a relational worldview that affirms that we are all related. Relationships grounded in lived experiences are central to Indigenous epistemology and are the basis for gathering information about the world (Brayboy & Maughan, 2009; Littletree & Metoyer, 2015). This epistemology is the foundation of education. An Indigenous worldview frames how things are categorized, such as what is perceived to be living, medicinal, or economic. There are rarely dualistic distinctions like those that are found in Western thinking between male and female, physical and metaphysical, sacred and secular, body and mind, or human and non-human (Littletree & Metoyer, 2015). Rather than these differences and distinctions, there are connections and relationships. Ancestral knowledge guides contemporary actions and future possibilities. Connections are central to how we view our place in the larger cosmos and the responsible use of knowledge (Brayboy & Maughan, 2009).

Learning is grounded in a state of consciousness. All aspects of the world (e.g., plants, landscape, and animals) are in the active role of teacher (Brayboy & Maughan, 2009). Relationships are pervasive, profound, and require attention and reciprocity. Knowledge is powerful. It is important to use it as a guide so that all actions are taken in a thoughtful way (Brayboy & Maughan, 2009).

Knowledge about and for Native Peoples

Outsiders have typically not recognized Indigenous knowledge and ways of knowing. Likewise, Native people have rarely had access to information that others have recorded about them, even though they have a right to know what others have documented about their ancestors, histories, and stories (Littletree & Metoyer, 2015).

The subject headings that are used to categorize data about Native Peoples and other means of accessing this information are inadequate. For example, they often reflect bias, and there is inconsistency in how Native American names are categorized. Cosmology is frequently categorized as "Myth" and an author named "White Horse" may be listed under either "W" or "H." Information about Native people is often grounded in the perspectives of the colonizers and may use inaccurate or offensive language.

Language reflects values. For instance, depending on the author's perspective, an event could be referred to as a massacre, a battle, or an incident. This raises the question: who has the power to label and name? Conversely, who is marginalized? For many years, the site where the US 7th Calvary shot approximately 300 mostly unarmed Lakota encamped at Wounded Knee Creek was called a battlefield. Only recently was the historic marker changed to use the term massacre rather than battle. In an earlier encounter involving the 7th Calvary, a site in Montana known to many Native people as Greasy Grass or Little Big Horn, was known by most Americans as Custer Battlefield. This is perhaps the only example of a site being named for a *losing* general.

Native people are often not considered authorities on their own experiences. Rather, the presumption of credence and validity is given to outsiders. The way information is recorded and catalogued often silences Indigenous voices, relegating them to stereotypes and historical artifacts rather than reflecting their contemporary realities as living Peoples and cultures (Littletree & Metoyer, 2015). Quigley emphasized that Native people are experts in their own experiences, so there is no need for external validation. Yet, the struggle to have Indigenous research and knowledge accepted continues. When the National Museum of the American Indian, part of the Smithsonian Institution, opened in Washington, DC, Quigley attended the opening ceremony and found Dr. Jolene Rickard's exhibit portraying the diverse faces of contemporary Native Americans empowering and affirming. However, this wonderful day was diminished when a *Washington Post* article criticized the Smithsonian for supposed insufficient consultation with "esteemed historians." In other words, the knowledge and competence of Native people—even well-known experts with doctoral degrees—were considered inadequate.

Indigenous Peoples around the world continue to assert their own stories, ways of knowing, and ways of categorizing information. For instance, librarians have developed alternative methods for organizing information that reflect Indigenous understandings. There are now multiple Indigenous approaches to library classification, including those developed by the Maori of New Zealand and the Aboriginal and Torres Strait Islanders of Australia (Littletree & Metoyer, 2015).

The Mashantucket Pequot Thesaurus of American Indian Terminology Project integrates Indigenous epistemologies in subject headings for Native American topics. The four domains in this thesaurus reflect the four directions and spiritual, physical, social, and mental aspects of Native American philosophies. By integrating Indigenous and non-Indigenous ways of thinking, the project makes Indigenous content more accessible to both Native and non-Native researchers (Littletree & Metoyer, 2015).

The value of knowledge

Western knowledge continues to be granted more credence and esteem than Indigenous knowledge. This perpetuates imperialism, colonialism, and power differentials. Even when Native perspectives are sought, Western knowledge is deemed superior and Western assumptions about good and bad, right and wrong, or standards of progress predominate (Roberts et al., 2016).

In some limited contexts, scholars and practitioners have recognized that Western knowledge is insufficient and have developed collaborative approaches with

Indigenous partners (Von der Porten, De Loe & McGregor, 2016). For example, the US National Climate Assessment recently collaborated with Indigenous Peoples to gather comprehensive information on climate change. The team that was assembled included tribal members, agencies, academics, and non-governmental organizations who partnered to solicit, collect, and synthesize traditional knowledge and data from Native people across the United States. They recognized both synergy and discord between traditional knowledge and Western science and sought to integrate Indigenous perspectives in sustained ways through respectful partnerships and engagement around climate change and Indigenous vulnerabilities (Maldonado et al., 2016). However, while Indigenous expertise about environmental issues is increasingly recognized and valued, the social sciences and education lag far behind in this regard.

In another example, traditional knowledge about the cultural landscape was crucial in designation of Bears Ears as a National Monument in 2016. The Bears Ears Tribal Coalition is a multi-tribal entity contributing to a new model of federal land management. These tribes remain ready to share information about the meaning of sacred and culturally significant sites as well as Indigenous knowledge about sustainable living within this arid landscape. Having lived in this area for millennia, they have a wealth of information to share (Utah Dine Bikeyah, 2018).

The perspectives of elders and traditional knowledge holders are often discounted while people educated in Western systems are perceived to be experts. Quigley recounted a painful instance when well-intentioned educators relied on external sources rather than Indigenous knowledge holders. In an attempt to include Native American content on a standardized test for fifth-grade students, the drafters of the test inadvertently included questions about ceremonial practices that, according to traditional teachings, must not be depicted or described in non-ceremonial contexts. The Native students who took the test had mixed responses: some were able to answer the questions easily due to their familiarity with the subject matter, but others experienced shock and were unable to complete the exam on account of its highly inappropriate content. This example speaks to the challenges of trying to include diverse content in education.

Valuing input from non-Native scholars and devaluing Indigenous knowledge, wisdom, and perspectives can have serious, unintended consequences. Whether recognized and valued by outsiders or not, Native people continue to expand their knowledge base. Indigenous models of evaluation have been developed incorporating Native perspectives on worth and importance. Culturally responsive evaluation methods are grounded in Indigenous knowledge and offer an alternative to research imposed on Native people. Evaluation is important in measuring the impact of programs for Native people (Roberts et al., 2016).

The need for a cyclical evaluation model grounded in relationship building and knowledge and skill building prompted the development of the Roadmap for Collaborative and Effective Evaluation in Tribal Communities for use within tribal child welfare programs. Likewise, the Indigenous Evaluation Framework was developed by the American Indian Higher Education Consortium, informed by the knowledge of elders and cultural experts as well as educators and scientists. This framework is anchored in four core premises: Indigenous Peoples are grounded in particular places; it is important to acknowledge gifts; family and community must be honored; and sovereignty is central (Roberts et al., 2016). Consequently, Western knowledge is not privileged over Indigenous knowledge in these decolonized evaluation models.

Differing worldviews and education

Different conceptualizations of knowledge and methods of knowledge acquisition are more than arbitrary distinctions. They have significance for what is taught, how it is taught, and how learning is facilitated or impeded. Educational settings must grapple with how different ways of learning and knowing manifest in the classroom and wider academic environment. Educators are faced with the power of multiple possibilities. Education can be administered with the heavy hand of colonialism or facilitated through a synergistic partnership. Conceptualizing Western and Indigenous ways of knowing as opposites obscures their complexities, is ineffective, and closes the door to possibilities. Both can be worthy, useful, and integrated in ways that are complementary rather than contradictory (Brayboy & Maughan, 2009).

One of the challenges noted by Quigley was the need for more Indigenous people in the field of education. Native people can bring diverse perspectives and help transform the curriculum. It is important to note, however, that Indigenous people seeking to become educators often face many challenges and barriers. The implications of conflicting knowledge systems become obvious in the context of teacher training, which can be rigid, narrow, and unaccommodating of different ways of engaging the world (Brayboy & Maughan, 2009). However, it need not be this way. For example, a science lesson anchored in Indigenous knowledge could explore how local plants grow using observation and experiential methods. The importance of place, space, and context can be integrated to engage students in learning values as well as content. Culturally based teaching can have fluidity between classroom and home. A science lesson about growing plants can include classes at night, looking at the stars to determine the right time for planting, and learning tribal cosmology (Brayboy & Maughan, 2009). In this example of culturally grounded pedagogy, a Native American student teacher noted that she goes beyond a simple science experiment to contextualize the act of growing plants. In this way, Native students are exposed to a culturally grounded way of thinking about and connecting with the world in which they live. The study of science can be personal and engaging rather than sterile and presumably objective (Brayboy & Maughan, 2009).

Native American students tend to have a learning style grounded in cooperation and sharing based on a naturalistic, holistic worldview. Visual learning opportunities and group work can be helpful, facilitated by hands-on active participation after observation. Native students often take some time to think, reflect, and gather evidence before performing tasks or answering questions, demonstrating a concern for accuracy over speed, and they tend to be more humble than their non-Native peers in public displays of knowledge (Gentry et al., 2014; Morgan, 2010). They may be quiet, with slow, soft speech, use indirect and nonverbal communication, and are usually introspective rather than inquisitive. Culturally responsive teaching can affirm the background of these students and consider their cultures as strengths. Quigley noted that there are diverse learning styles among Native Americans, and felt that many students—Native and non-Native alike—would benefit from hands-on learning.

The Indigenous value of silence is often misinterpreted in mainstream educational institutions. While many Native people focus on listening and observing rather than speaking, dominant society norms often interpret this as a lack of involvement or participation. There may be an assumption that a silent student is not listening or engaged when the opposite may be true (Singson et al., 2016). Indeed, students who do not actively participate verbally may be penalized and receive lower grades. Rather than making assumptions about the meaning of silence and other forms of nonverbal communication, educators must employ critical thinking about what it means to be engaged in learning and how to recognize it in diverse students.

Many Native students are not afforded the same educational opportunities as their non-Native contemporaries. Native youth with high potential typically go unrecognized, leading to underdevelopment of their talents and potential. Poverty decreases the chances that gifted students will be recognized as such. Many reservation-based youth face multiple obstacles to academic achievement, including poverty, marginalization of their cultures, and living in remote areas where schools and communities have limited basic resources and little access to the technology that is taken for granted in other settings (Gentry et al., 2014).

While scholarship documents how differences in worldview affect learning for Native students, educators must recognize that significant diversity exists in the lived experiences of contemporary Native Americans. As Johnston-Goodstar pointed out, intergenerational experiences of colonization have, in some cases, led to a shift in worldview. The impact of trauma must be recognized and considered in determining effective pedagogy. One study (Gentry et al., 2014) used focus groups of educators and administrators from three tribes to examine how the literature on learning styles of Native Americans compares with contemporary experiences on Dine', Lakota, and Anishinaabe reservations. The researchers found both similarities and contrasts between published material and contemporary observations. They also noted differences in experiences both between and within tribes. The Dine' focus group identified a need for positive male role models to support gifted and talented youth. They noted that a dearth of academically successful role models contributes to a high drop-out rate. Professional development that enhances the cultural knowledge of educators, especially non-Natives, was considered crucial for bridging the cultural disconnect and helping Native students reach their academic potential. Focus group participants also noted that traditional values and learning styles are now inconsistent in many Native communities. While still meaningful within some families and communities, they have been replaced by materialism and pop culture in others. There may also be a middle ground. Youth may reject formal religion but turn to gang affiliation in their search for spirituality and belonging. They exhibit a lack of patience and self-control, as well as increased materialism. On the other hand, the Dine' matriarchal clan system is apparent in group projects where students often self-select to work with others from their clan.

While language is consistently mentioned as a core element of culture and its continuity, the Gentry et al. (2014) study revealed nuanced perspectives. Under the Navajo Sovereignty in Education Act of 2005, the core curriculum is supplemented with content on Navajo language, culture, history, government, and character. In contrast, the educators in the focus group viewed the Dine' language as an oral language that was never intended to have written form and therefore an impediment to learning. They noted that students often lack fluency in both Dine' and English. Indeed, very few students are fluent in their Native language, according to Ojibwe, Lakota, and Dine' educator focus group participants.

School districts' disregard of students' culture and learning styles is often reflected in high drop-out rates (Morgan, 2010). That being said, it is important not to base assumptions about learning styles of Native youth on stereotypes or information that does not fit current generations. When non-Natives think of Native youth only as artistic, quiet, naturalistic, musical, and spiritual, they often miss their strengths in verbal and mathematical areas (Gentry et al., 2014).

Quigley strongly emphasized the importance of understanding the diversity among Native people. While there are commonalities, it is important to eliminate stereotypes and avoid assumptions. There are differences between urban and reservation populations and even within tribes. As Quigley noted, "We have many faces." It is important that teacher training programs include some basic courses on Native Americans. This is a requirement in some states but not others, including New York. Yet, all teachers must have an understanding of where their students are coming from in order to build good relationships with them.

Institutionalized learning and assimilation

The United States' trust relationship with Native Americans includes provision of education under more than 150 treaties (Meza, 2015; Raffle, 2007). The government's education strategy was grounded in paternalistic oversight and delegation of operations to churches where Native children were dehumanized in an attempt to transform them into US citizens (Harrington & Chixapkaid, 2013).

The earlier discussion of boarding schools need not be repeated in full here, but it is helpful to review the major characteristics of residential education as it was implemented among Native Americans. The Indian Removal Act of 1830 led to the appointment of a Commissioner of Indian Affairs in the US Department of War. The primary duties of this Commissioner involved overseeing the vocationally focused education system for Native people and addressing issues for Eastern tribes that had been removed from their land. The perception that day schools were ineffective at disconnecting Native children from their cultures and Americanizing them led to the promotion of boarding schools (Harrington & Chixapkaid, 2013). These institutions sought to eradicate Native cultures, languages, value systems, and spirituality while requiring students to practice Christianity and speak English, essentially changing the way Native youth thought and emphasizing the superiority of US ways (Marker, 2009).

US education for Native people explicitly undermined Indigenous cultures and knowledge systems, yet some Native people viewed education as an important tool for survival. In general, the boarding schools were harsh, demeaning places, but there was variation among them, and some students had better experiences than others. The schools could provide an escape from hunger and devastated communities as they at least offered basic food, shelter, and clothing.

Johnston-Goodstar noted that few people are aware of the BIA's parallel policy of reservation-based family education, which was undergirded by the same assimilationist philosophy as the boarding school system. In these programs, teachers would visit Native American families in their homes and cause untold harm in their efforts to impart "civilized" values and education.

From its inception, education for Native children has devalued Indigenous people and their ways of being by forcing them to abandon their cultures and learn to live as non-Natives (Harrington & Chixapkaid, 2013). Contemporary education is still rooted in this legacy. While forced education in boarding schools is a thing of the past, Native Americans continue to be educated in mainstream schools with no attention to different learning styles or how cultural values may be expressed and respected in the classroom. Therefore, for many Native Americans, the social climate in schools continues to be stigmatizing. Native people experience disproportionate negative educational outcomes, ranging from overrepresentation in special education programs and suspensions to low graduation rates.

The federal trust responsibility for education continues to be acknowledged through legislation such as the Indian Self-Determination and Education Act, the Native American Education Improvement Act, and Native-specific provisions in the No Child Left Behind Act (Meza, 2015). Under the 1934 Johnson O'Malley Act, the federal government began to contract with states for provision of education to Native Americans. The Indian Education Act of 1972 created an advisory council and funding for schools and districts serving Native children. Most Native youth now live in cities and attend public schools, so state education policies have more impact than federal policies. The implementation of federal policy is dependent on how states and local school boards interpret the mandate to use federal funds to benefit Native students. This leads to significant inconsistencies from state to state (Meza, 2015).

The self-determination era saw Native Nations asserting their interest in shaping education for their youth. This interest was eventually codified in the Elementary and Secondary Education Act (Raffle, 2007), and Indigenous traditions, cultures, and languages were subsequently integrated in the terms of the No Child Left Behind Act (Brayboy et al., 2012). Even after these advances, however, Native education is still largely shaped by external priorities, and Native schools remain chronically underfunded. Moreover, they tend to suffer the earliest and deepest cuts during federal financial crises (Mitchell, 2013). Reservations have no taxable land for a funding base, so up to 60 percent of the funding for their schools comes directly from the federal government (Layton, 2013).

Tribal sovereignty is affected by education of future leaders, including language and cultural content. Native children are integral to the preservation of tribal sovereignty but as education systems continue to fail Native students and omit or undermine the foundational knowledge of their culture and language, the next generation of tribal leaders will be ill prepared (Meza, 2015). It is therefore imperative to support culture and language preservation as key elements of education.

School policies continue to be grounded in Western knowledge systems, learning practices, and values that legitimize socialization and assimilation. These policies create distance between Native students and non-Native teachers and administrators. Education has been based on a hierarchy of knowledge in which Indigenous ways continue to be perceived as deficient (Brayboy & Maughan, 2009) and school rules are intertwined with microaggressions (Cerecer, 2013).

Curriculum content

Continued devaluation of Indigenous knowledge is apparent in curricula and instructional resources. Information on Native Americans is often unrepresented, stereotypical, or misrepresented in textbooks, including in areas with large Native populations (Morgan, 2010). As an example, some texts in Nebraska refer to Native Americans as lazy and drunks. Native Americans are rarely represented as contemporary Peoples. Indeed, 87 percent of the references to Native Americans in state academic standards reference events prior to 1900, and only four states include information on the boarding schools (Clarren, 2017).

Of course, classroom literature shapes students' beliefs and attitudes about the world. Children understand that the topics they read about matter. Scholastic Reading Clubs are a way for teachers to expand classroom libraries and for parents to purchase books. However, a study of these clubs (Chaudhri & Schau, 2016) revealed few multicultural books and almost none on Native Americans. Stereotypical representations persisted among the texts, while literature by Native authors and illustrators was completely absent. There was not a single Native American book on the Scholastic order form in 2012–2013. The inability to read about people like themselves has a lasting legacy among Native youth. Likewise, non-Native youth are affected by this void, which reinforces the perception that Indigenous Peoples neither matter nor even exist in contemporary times.

Books for and about Native people are among the least published annually. This also affects non-Native Americans, leaving them undereducated and allowing stereotypes to flourish. Native American content is most likely to be offered around Thanksgiving, with books from the *Little House on the Prairie* series being the most frequently available items. These books are steeped in derogatory language, including comparisons between Native Americans and wild animals (Chaudhri & Schau, 2016).

Some educators who claim to value multiculturalism have internalized Western paradigms that devalue cultural knowledge systems and privilege dominant archetypes (Cerecer, 2013). This conflict can manifest in how Native history is taught and subsequently impacts student engagement. When the curriculum is modified to incorporate Native content, this is typically done around Columbus Day and Thanksgiving. Indeed, Columbus is still celebrated and legitimized. Such visible celebrations reinforce inaccurate historical narratives and stereotypical depictions of Native Americans. Contemporary Native people remain absent from the curriculum, as Native Americans are depicted as historical artifacts or noble savages. Schools still use curricular models where the contributions of people of color are covered in supplements rather than the core curriculum. They also support dominant narratives with ethnic history months (Cerecer, 2013). Leadership practices shape the identity of Native students, discount their agency and what they know, and undermine their engagement in academia.

Eurocentric ideologies serve as a framework for public education of all students. For Native Americans, conformity to this ideology was seen as necessary for them to be civilized. Education was a tool of cultural genocide that was designed to strip them of their cultural identity, and public educational programs and services continue to neglect the perspectives of Indigenous cultures and other people of color (Harrington & Chixapkaid, 2013). Research-based recommendations for curricular change are often ignored and public school settings continue to marginalize Native students.

The dominant academic knowledge system impacts school culture as students become conscious of whose knowledge is valued and whose is not legitimized. This has an impact on academic and social engagement and the likelihood of completing school (Cerecer, 2013). There are many forms of racism, including the imposition of someone else's priorities. As one Native educator asked,

> Why are the collective lies of Columbus still taught as history? Why do we continue to have to deal with the absence of teaching in our tribal languages, history, literature, or stories even in schools on or near our reservation communities? Why are we forced to adopt No Child Left Behind when maybe the saving of our languages should be our first priority?
>
> *(Peacock, 2011, p. 16)*

Yet, change is possible. Educators can support Native students by recognizing the legitimacy of various knowledge systems, refusing to frame knowledge hierarchically, and recognizing connections between Western educational practices and Indigenous ways of knowing (Brayboy & Maughan, 2009). Native youth are more likely to thrive, avoid trouble, and remain in school when their culture and language are incorporated in the classroom. Some states, including Washington, now incorporate Indigenous concepts for all students at all levels. A useful tool for these endeavors is the National Museum of the American Indian's Native Knowledge 360, which provides free online interactive lessons and educational resources for teachers of all grades and subject areas (Clarren, 2017).

Active participation of family members is integral to culture-based education (Harrington & Chixapkaid, 2013). Community can be a setting for student learning. Place-based and service learning projects are mechanisms to promote community wellbeing. Students can undergo rigorous assessment for a range of competencies and skills as well as career planning and preparation for global citizenship. Indigenous educational research can also be informative. Indigenous perspectives must be incorporated in policies, curriculum, pedagogy, and all aspects of education, with tribes taking an active role in shaping educational reform (Harrington & Chixapkaid, 2013).

School climate

Johnston-Goodstar emphasized the importance of school climate as she feels the impact of context on educational outcomes is vastly underestimated. Social and historical context are at the heart of contemporary educational issues. The way that the learning environment is experienced is crucial to student success, yet schools are often a source of trauma rather than a safe haven for Native students (Johnston-Goodstar & VeLure Roholt, 2017). Indeed, school is more dangerous for Native students than other youth (VeLure Roholt, Johnston-Goodstar & Eubanks, 2016).

Educators must find ways to create inclusive learning environments. Quigley noted that even some schools with significant Indigenous student populations have nothing that represents these students' culture in their buildings. She gave an example of a building with a prominently displayed picture of General Washington crossing the Delaware. This can perpetuate an alienating environment for Native students, particularly as Washington ordered a scorched-earth campaign that was designed to eradicate every Native American within the state of New York. In schools with significant numbers of Native students, there is no excuse for a lack of Native representation throughout the institution. Positive Indigenous images in the school environment foster a welcoming climate and academic success for Native people.

Teachers and administrators often know little of their Native students' culture, even when serving a reservation-based population. As Quigley noted, while Christian and sometimes Jewish holidays are acknowledged in the school calendar, there is no such accommodation of Indigenous religious observances. In another example, some school districts have expelled students who have missed school to attend tribal funerals. Additionally, in a 2013 Office for Civil Rights complaint, the Wiyot Tribe of California took legal action against their local school district for a range of inappropriate behavior, including teachers regularly touching their students' hair (Clarren, 2017).

Administrators internalize dominant epistemology and pass this on through their leadership (Cerecer, 2013). One student described how a school with little history of violence hired a police officer. Analyzed through the lens of microagressions, the student interpreted this as a need to secure *others* from *us*. Allocating scarce educational resources in this way is divisive and undermines students' trust of administrators. Instead of enhancing campus security, this appointment was perceived as branding Native students as problems requiring police attention. Such insensitivity inhibits opportunities for school staff to build trusting relationships with Native students, families, and communities (Cerecer, 2013).

Native students regularly experience microaggressions that reinforce a deficit perspective of their academic abilities. They internalize these negative beliefs about themselves and their place in school and society, undermining their confidence and abilities (Cerecer, 2013). Johnston-Goodstar echoed the need to understand and address microaggressions. Native youth experience microaggressions as well as blatant racism from their peers, teachers, and school administrators. Recently, Cerecer (2013) reported that many of them had experienced direct racism from their teachers over the previous year. This broader social context impacts their commitment to school and their ability to achieve academic success. One Native American educator recounted a painful story from his own childhood that ultimately inspired him to become a teacher:

> I was a little kid, and the playground at my school was a big, scary place. And it seemed that at every recess, a group of town boys would tease a Native girl who rode the reservation bus with the rest of us "injuns," as they called us, into school each day. Their words were sharp as knives, incessant. "Hey, squaw! You gonna scalp us?" She would plead with them to stop, but they would continue their taunting until she cried uncontrollably and chased them all over the playground. Ultimately she would tire and then cower in a corner like a wounded fawn, and her tormenters would encircle her like jackals and kill her spirit with the sharp spears of their tongues. Only once do I remember she caught one of them and beat holy bejesus out of him. When I saw this, the inside me, the part that never showed, rose and gave her a standing ovation. Most of the time, however, she would suffer the poison of their words. I remember as I watched and listened to the daily, awful scene, my stomach muscles would tighten and sometimes I would almost bend over in pain. I wanted to say something to them, to yell at them, beg of them, "Leave her alone. Please leave her alone, she has done nothing to you." But I never said a word. I was stopped cold by fear. Fear that they would turn on me, that I would become their target. So the years passed, and the unrelenting torment continued. And then one day, in the 6th or 7th grade, the girl just quit coming to school. Myself, I grew in stature and confidence and became good with my fists. I was not teased. Some years ago I was reading the hometown newspaper and noticed her name in the obituary column. She died young. I don't know the circumstances. Her former tormentors are now the city fathers—city councilmen, business owners, bankers, and teachers all.

(Peacock, 2011, p. 15)

In some cases, the incessant racism and psychological trauma in public schools became so bad that placement in boarding schools seemed a preferable alternative. A case in point is the situation of the Lummi, a Coast Salish tribe in Washington State. In the 1960s and 1970s, the Native students in the Puget Sound region of the state faced open hostility from both classmates and teachers following public outcry and resentment over legal victories in fishing rights cases. This produced a climate of institutionalized racism in the public schools. Escalating antagonism led to boats being rammed, gunshots fired over the heads of Native fishermen, and school interactions saturated with racism (Marker, 2009). Under these circumstances, Native communities pushed for their own schools that were physically and culturally safe, and tribal leaders advocated for increased access to Chemawa Indian Boarding School in Salem, Oregon. Chemawa had opened in 1880 as an authoritarian force for assimilation but moderated under the Collier reforms of the 1930s. By the 1970s, Coast Salish families viewed it as a potential safe haven where youth could have educational opportunities and celebrate their culture (Marker, 2009).

Dismantling policies and leadership practices that allow microaggressions and bullying of Native students is crucial to preventing their marginalization in academia. New policies and practices can be developed that reflect both Indigenous and Western academic knowledge systems, thereby supporting academic success for Native youth (Cerecer, 2013). Classrooms should be safe spaces for raising questions, sharing insights, and engaging in conversations. For Native students, it is critical to have positive relationships with adults in the classroom and throughout the school as these can mediate microaggressions. Culturally responsive school policies foster strong Indigenous academic identities and school retention (Cerecer, 2013).

Educational outcomes

Poor educational outcomes are often the result of a combination of student factors and school factors. Native American students frequently feel unwelcome at school due to poor connections with teachers, problems with peers, and perceptions that academic environments are culturally irrelevant (Sprague et al., 2013). Institutional discrimination, school climate, high-stakes standardized testing, and academic tracking present additional barriers (Cerecer, 2013). Students also internalize racial microaggressions and bullying, as illustrated in Peacock's (2011) story, above.

The irrelevant curricula and teaching methods that permeate much of Western education undermine Native students' academic achievement, ultimately leading to high drop-out rates. Rather than being a reflection on Native students, this is a failure of educational institutions to engage and educate Native youth (Harrington & Chixapkaid, 2013). Native students have the lowest graduation rates in the United States (Brayboy et al., 2012; Cerecer, 2013). Almost half of all Native American students leave high school without a degree, compared to less than one-third of non-Native students. The drop-out rate for Native youth in Canada is even higher at 66 percent, compared to 37 percent for non-Native students (Kanu, 2006). Most Native students typically do not take college preparatory classes, leading to some of the lowest college entrance and retention rates (Brayboy et al., 2012). Combined with demographic patterns of Native Americans as a young population, these trends converge alarmingly, resulting in a cohort of young adults with limited formal education who are unlikely to be competitive in the workforce. Therefore, it is imperative to launch a critical examination of educational pathways for Native students, remove barriers, and cultivate a hospitable and supportive climate to enhance educational success and graduation rates.

While in the United States Native students comprise approximately 1 percent of the total student population, they are disciplined roughly twice as often as White students, and represent 2 percent of school arrests as well as 3 percent of school incidents referred to law enforcement (Clarren, 2017). Johnston-Goodstar noted that Native youth are well aware of these disciplinary disparities. Her participatory action research with Native youth co-researchers revealed that they feel they are subjected to more surveillance than others. They were also able to name specific practices and people who perpetuate injustices.

Native American youth are disproportionately represented in disciplinary exclusions from classrooms. As a result, they lose more than four times as many school days as White students and are placed in alternative education programs for relatively minor offenses, such as attendance policy violations (Sprague et al., 2013). Lakota students are often placed in special education classes because of misunderstandings related to their communication norms, including quiet, slow speech and delayed response time (Gentry et al., 2014). They are also disproportionately sent to virtual schools with less math or reading content than traditional public schools.

Johnston-Goodstar's youth co-researchers explored the tensions that Native youth experience in educational settings. They examined how the academic achievement gap is framed and primary contributing factors. Their research documented that Native youth and families are typically depicted as the root cause of the problem: if they only had more resources; if families could get more involved; if student attendance could be improved. These were identified as explanatory factors and therefore targets for change. On the other hand, the youth researchers understood the achievement gap as rooted in everyday institutional practices that exclude Native students and make them invisible. They identified how Native American issues are not included as standard aspects of the curriculum or included only in archaic ways, such as dioramas of ancient practices. Meaningful contemporary issues, such as treaty rights, are ignored. This oblivious stance leaves Native students feeling unwelcome and lacking any sense of belonging in mainstream schools.

The Jefferson County School District in central Oregon serves the residents of the Warm Springs Reservation. In this district, more than one-third of all Native students in grades six–twelve were suspended at least once during the 2015–2016 school year, meaning they were more than twice as likely to be suspended as their White peers. In addition, while Native students comprise one-third of the school district's population, they represent almost two-thirds of the expulsions (Clarren, 2017).

Missing out on learning opportunities makes it hard to grasp concepts and may lead to youth dropping out of school. Fewer than two-thirds of Native seniors at Warm Springs graduate (Clarren, 2017). A tribal councilwoman who graduated from the district in 2005 believes Native students do not receive an equal education to their non-Native peers. The former superintendent of the district that includes Warm Springs linked high student disciplinary rates to teachers' lack of cultural understanding and affirmed the councilwoman's perception that the district is failing Native youth:

> The administrators "don't see us as people deserving the same sort of education and opportunities," she said. Miller [the tribal councilwoman] was suspended several times herself, once for swearing; a white student once called her a "prairie nigger." As a student, she added, "I felt worthless—like I wasn't worth the effort or patience to understand who I am and my history. This school district has failed us my entire lifetime, and it continues to do this today."
>
> *(Clarren, 2017, p. 13)*

Warm Springs is not atypical. Alienation, disproportionate disciplining, and high drop-out rates are all common outcomes for Indigenous students. In excess of 90 percent of Native students attend public schools, with most of the rest attending Bureau of Indian Education schools, institutions that have some of the lowest test scores and graduation rates in the country (Clarren, 2017). Indeed, Native Americans are the only population group that have not improved their standardized test scores for reading or math in grades four and eight (National Congress of American Indians, 2018).

Poverty creates barriers to educational success, but Native students do not fare well even when this is controlled (Clarren, 2017). They are more likely to be harshly disciplined, suspended, and expelled. Frequent suspensions and expulsions lead to gaps in learning, resulting in poor test scores. In 2015, only 10 percent of Native students were proficient in math by senior year. They are less likely than other groups to graduate in four years. Low graduation rates translate into fewer economic and social opportunities. For people of color, drop-out rates are also associated with higher risk of incarceration. Furthermore, negative school experiences, including expulsion or suspension, likely contribute to the suicide epidemic (Clarren, 2017).

Per-pupil spending on Native education is declining and there is little oversight of how federal money is distributed. The Johnson–O'Malley Program allocates money based on the number of enrolled tribal members in public schools, but Congress has not completed a population survey since 1994. During this time, the number of Native students has grown by approximately 4 percent per year, but without a population survey the old funding level must cover these extra students. In 1995, $125 was allocated per student, but that has now dropped to $63.80. Moreover, the Trump administration has recently proposed an additional 30 percent cut (Clarren, 2017). Title IV, the other major federal funding source earmarked for Native students, is rarely audited and there is no assurance that districts spend the funds on Native youth rather than the general student population. This funding amounts to more than $100 million annually and there is significant concern about mismanagement. Lack of transparency and oversight inhibit efforts to determine how the money is spent.

Schools receiving public funds must follow federal antidiscrimination laws including the Civil Rights Act of 1964. In 2017, a complaint filed by the ACLU of Montana with the US Department of Education and the US Department of Justice alleged a school district in Montana discriminates against Assiniboine and Lakota students. The complaint alleges systematic disadvantage including racial bias in how school disciplinary policies are enforced, verbal abuse by teachers and staff, inequitable access to school activities, and mismanagement of Native-specific federal funding (Clarren, 2017).

There are, however, glimmers of hope. Eileen Quintana, an educational administrator in Utah, introduced Ute dance classes at her school. Her dedication to supporting Native students is credited with raising graduation rates from 37 to 100 percent over the course of just 20 years (Clarren, 2017).

Johnston-Goodstar emphasized the importance of relationships—a key factor in supporting resilience. Teachers who demonstrate that they care about their students' lives outside of school can make an important difference. For example, a teacher who engages with a student may learn that their home is overcrowded and this makes it difficult to complete homework assignments. A student may share that their foster placement has changed, thereby disrupting their routine. An unstable living situation may result in multiple moves during the academic year. A teacher who demonstrates an interest in the student's home context can help them feel more comfortable and this can open the door to strategizing how to manage various challenges.

In 2016, President Obama signed a law that requires school districts to engage in meaningful and timely consultation with tribes on issues related to Native students or risk losing federal funding (Clarren, 2017). As a result, the Chickasaw Nation of Oklahoma is now notified by the school district when their students are absent. After notification, they implement a tribally led process with families and wraparound services to keep students in school (Clarren, 2017). At the time of writing, there was concern about how such initiatives will fare under the Trump administration, given its emphasis on vouchers and virtual schools where students learn primarily from computers.

Fostering a sense of belonging enhances academic achievement (Gilliard & Moore, 2007). Native students with Indigenous content in the classroom performed significantly better on exams than other Native students while demonstrating broader understanding, higher-level thinking, and greater self-confidence (Kanu, 2006). Offering a culturally relevant curriculum and engaging with families fosters a sense of belonging and respect and may also reduce school failure rates (Gilliard & Moore, 2007; Rivera & Tharp, 2006).

Native leadership and college participation are hindered by the lack of an adequate pipeline of well-prepared Native youth. Integrating Indigenous cultural learning objectives, resources, and instructional methods within the high school curriculum would help prepare Native youth for higher education (Kanu, 2006). Afterschool programs at Native American community centers would also be useful for supporting youth and creating a pathway to higher education (Maduram, 2011).

Higher education

Before the United States was founded, the colonies set aside land to build a college for "children of the infidels" (Brayboy et al., 2012, p. 7). Harvard, Dartmouth, and William and Mary, three of the nine original colonial colleges, included educating Native Americans in their mission statements. By the American Revolution, 47 Native Americans had matriculated and four had graduated from college. However, only 385 Native students had enrolled and 52 had graduated from US colleges by 1932 (Fox et al., 2005). College enrollment for Native Americans doubled between 1976 and 2002, but currently only 26 percent of 18–24-year-old Native Americans are enrolled in college, compared to 37 percent of their peers, and only 4 percent have completed undergraduate degrees (Brayboy et al., 2012).

Native American college students face many of the same challenges experienced by youth in primary and secondary schools. Indeed, problems are often compounded as those seeking college degrees may find they are ill prepared by their earlier education, particularly if they were tracked into vocational streams (Brayboy et al., 2012). They are typically an invisible cohort, representing just 0.8 to 1.1 percent of the total college population since 1976 (Singson et al., 2016). In addition, they often struggle to adjust to Eurocentric educational institutions and find them to be hostile environments (Singson et al., 2016). Constant exposure to racial microaggressions produces a form of battle fatigue (Brayboy et al., 2012). Native students are often forced to describe and defend their worldviews and their relevance in non-Native college settings. Attending college frequently raises their awareness of their own rootedness in Indigenous knowledge systems and how these contrast with the type of knowledge that is valued in Western academia. Understanding how Indigenous worldviews and knowledge systems are marginalized allows Native students to contextualize classes and faculty feedback on their work so they can make strategic accommodations to facilitate academic success while maintaining a sense of themselves as Indigenous people (Brayboy & Maughan, 2009).

Indigenous faculty also experience hostility and microaggressions in educational settings. Native faculty are often treated as tokens, their expertise goes unrecognized or is undermined, and they are consulted on topics that are unrelated to their field, simply because the subject is perceived to be a "Native issue." Quigley described how she was contacted multiple times about an administrative position on a reservation, even though it was not her area. She also spoke of an alienating and offensive memorandum from the Governor's Office and the state university system that any state employee could not speak to a Native American and those doing any work with Native Americans, currently or in the future, must declare this in writing. This memo was unprecedented and did not apply to state employees having contact with anyone other than Native Americans.

Educational content and teaching methods

Indigenous students often face challenges when pursuing their education in mainstream universities, even when these institutions specifically seek to serve Native students. For example, students in an Indigenous teacher training program identified significant differences in the ways their faculty approached knowledge and teaching and their own understandings (Brayboy & Maughan, 2009). The students felt their teachers spoke rapidly and tried to impress them with big words. They expressed the belief that

> teaching itself is a political act by pointing to the importance of word choice, pacing, and the implications of passing or failing a class for the Indigenous pre-service teachers who want to serve Indigenous elementary and secondary students. Teaching's political nature implicates the epistemic clashes inherent in how knowledge is used and how hierarchies of knowledge are produced and reproduced in educational institutions. These clashes raise critical connections between power and the (re)production and transmission of knowledge.
>
> *(Brayboy & Maughan, 2009, p. 2)*

For Native students to succeed, educators must transform these knowledge clashes. Universities must recognize a variety of forms and demonstrations of knowledge. Indigenous students are well aware of differences in how knowledge is created, produced, reproduced, and valued in mainstream institutions compared to tribal communities (Brayboy & Maughan, 2009). University teaching is perceived as linear in ways that make no sense to many Indigenous students. Non-Native faculty and students are seen as self-absorbed. Native students may prefer teaching styles that make circular connections, are holistic, and produce knowledge to serve others.

A disconnect between Indigenous and academic cultures presents challenges, but culture can be a crucial strength. Once Indigenous culture is valued, synergy can be developed to enhance learning. Rather than being a deficit, Huffman (2010) found that some of the most culturally traditional Native American students were the most academically successful. Ultimately, in the teacher training program noted above, Native students were able to transform how faculty understood both teaching and learning (Brayboy & Maughan, 2009).

The context of learning

Western education prioritizes classroom instruction, but the learning context can be equally important (Singson et al., 2016). Incorporating Indigenous values in residential settings can increase academic success. Some universities have taken steps to make campus settings responsive to the needs of Native American students. To provide hospitable environments for Native students, colleges must be attentive to respect, relevance, reciprocity, and responsibility (Singson et al., 2016).

Campus living spaces can play a significant role in helping Native students feel comfortable and remain in college (Singson et al., 2016). Recognizing the history of the land where a college is located can help engage students and facilitate learning within a spatial context. Universities can also develop policies that recognize Indigenous spiritual expressions and ceremonial release time, provide Indigenized halls of residence, develop Indigenous curricular offerings, and have a visible presence that acknowledges Native Americans (Singson et al., 2016).

University personnel and students must strive to recognize and counteract forces that continue to erase the history of the Indigenous Peoples whose land the institution occupies (Singson et al., 2016). Furthermore, it is possible to incorporate Indigenous sensibilities in architectural designs to make them more welcoming. The design of Wassaja Hall at the University of Illinois, Urbana–Champaign, is one such example. In naming this hall after a Yavapi alumnus, the university followed traditional naming protocols and also sought guidance from the Peoria—the traditional holders of the land. Making connections between the university and the Peoria helped educators understand Native history, which in turn equipped them to enhance the education of future residents of Wassaja Hall. Relationship building has led to initiatives like an alternative spring break visiting the Peoria in Oklahoma, where they have lived since their removal from Illinois. This has helped residential life paraprofessionals facilitate peer education on diversity and social justice. Students benefit from building reciprocity with both the Yavapi and Peoria through learning about the hall's namesake and increasing their understanding of and respect for the original people of the land where the college is located (Singson et al., 2016).

Another example is a culturally grounded dormitory wing for Native students at Arizona State University (ASU)—O'odham Ki ("People's House"). The goal was to create a communal living space to increase retention among first-year and transfer students. Previously, ASU Native students had a 52 percent retention rate, but this rose to 70 percent after completion of the new wing. This space promotes Native-centered programming, activities, and values (Singson et al., 2016). It is important to be familiar with and incorporate local protocols. At ASU, a prayer is conducted for students, families, and campus colleagues before students take up residence. Sacred practices like burning sage or cedar are accommodated by working with the local fire and police departments: fire alarms are temporarily disconnected and residents are given advance warning of ceremonies. O'odham Ki provides opportunities to learn about the experiences of other Native students and families, as well as resources and support. Non-Native students also learn from the tribal community, as both teaching and learning are two-way processes. The Native Student Association sponsors Native food on campus. This is a concrete and meaningful way to incorporate Native students into the college environment (Singson et al., 2016). O'odham Ki has become a home away from home, fostering a sense of belonging, mitigating loneliness, and minimizing feelings of invisibility.

In another example, South Dakota State University (SDSU) developed a smudging policy. Smudging is a form of ritual cleansing and prayer that can facilitate reflection, eradicate negativity, and help students cope with adversity. At SDSU, student services and residential life units collaborated to develop the policy, implement training, and develop accountability mechanisms that respected Native values while complying with campus rules and regulations. Similarly, making a campus community a welcoming environment can involve developing a policy for the use of traditional medicine. Crafting such policies demonstrates some universities' commitment to environments that respect and accommodate Native values and traditions (Singson et al., 2016). However, universities that are committed to serving Native students must also develop responsive policies and practices to recognize that Indigenous students may need to return home for ceremonies, funerals, or cultural sustenance.

Role models, support groups, and a broader Native presence in universities can all help facilitate Native students' success (Fox, 2005; Weaver, 2000) It is important to note, however, that Native faculty and staff also experience hostility in academic environments (Walters, 2013) and their low numbers inhibit this potential source of support (Cross et al., 2009). Only 0.5 percent of faculty in four-year degree-granting institutions and 0.7 percent in two-year colleges are Native American (Brayboy et al., 2012). Cohort models for Native American students such as those at the George Warren Brown School of Social Work at Washington University, St. Louis, and the Rural Human Services Program at the University of Alaska, Fairbanks, infuse support and Indigenous knowledge and ways of knowing into higher education.

Transforming academia

Some educators, both Indigenous and Non-Indigenous, have attempted to move beyond deficit perspectives and make education culturally responsive to Native people. There have been various efforts to infuse Native content, integrate Indigenous values into educational institutions, and foster culturally engaged and responsive teaching and school policies. All of these projects have potential, but they also face major barriers to success.

The 1928 Meriam Report called for the incorporation of tribal culture in American Indian education, but this and subsequent recommendations have not resulted in modified policies or practices. Education for Native youth is still largely controlled and defined by non-Native people, leaving the Native population to justify the importance of their knowledge and their priorities for what and how they want their children to learn (Harrington & Chixapkaid, 2013).

Making the school environment culturally relevant for Native American youth includes enhancing the cultural knowledge and awareness of teachers and administrators, using relevant language and social skills lessons, making decisions with valid data, modifying curricula, and enhancing home–school connections to facilitate education in the least restrictive environments (Sprague et al., 2013). Culturally responsive teaching engages Native students in learning, but many teachers find this hard to implement in a climate of high-stakes testing (Cerecer, 2013). Often, teachers are faced with priorities that undermine their abilities to focus on student need. In some contexts, teachers and administrators may be dismissed if students achieve low scores on mandated standardized tests.

It is important to promote parental participation in schools and check for mutual understandings (Sprague et al., 2013). An emphasis on culture, tribal traditions, and language can help positive development and cultivate a sense of belonging. The latter, in turn, fosters more appropriate student behaviors and outcomes. Acknowledging the validity of Indigenous knowledge can engage Native students. While these factors are important, Quigley noted that Native parents may feel unwelcome in schools, particularly if they had negative experiences during their own education. Schools must recognize and address such barriers to family engagement. This can be an important role for human service providers.

Indigenous students may bring different but equally valid ideas about knowledge and how it is constructed (Brayboy & Maughan, 2009). Native people are inventors, analytical thinkers, and members of fully functioning societies. The knowledge these societies have amassed can be shared in ways that transform how non-Native teachers understand teaching and learning. Indigenous educators must draw on multiple strengths to dismantle the ongoing deficit thinking that permeates colonized educational systems (Brayboy & Maughan, 2009).

Johnston-Goodstar noted the impressive resilience and hopefulness of her Native youth co-researchers. Their efforts in the face of considerable institutional and historic issues never fail to surprise her. She has never encountered someone who did not dream of a better future. Native youth are not inherently passive in the face of dismissive or hostile learning environments. Rather, many are resilient and engaged in attending to institutional issues and creating a better learning environment.

Native organizations also have a role to play in shaping education. They can provide a venue for Native peer education as well as youth leadership programs. Youth can be both inspired and inspiring, learning skills that can help them achieve their aspirations. For example, Johnston-Goodstar shared an example of a youth learning skills in documentary filmmaking as well as other youth seizing opportunities to make positive change in the world. Native people can be active participants in shaping education to meet their needs. As described in detail earlier, the Coast Salish people worked to reclaim the Chemawa Boarding School and make it responsive to their needs:

> Indigenous communities were not simply resisting racist schooling; they were also reaffirming and renewing their own traditional understandings of the uses of knowledge. Decolonisation, from the Coast Salish perspective, meant distinguishing local cultural knowledge from the imported knowledge of the empires. Resistance to the hegemony of school based knowledge often took the form of participation in those aspects of Coast Salish life that had been kept as private ceremony and away from state surveillance.
>
> (Marker, 2009, p. 7)

One way in which Indigenous Peoples have asserted control in mainstream higher education is the movement to *indigenize the academy*. This movement has led to academic content with direct relevance to tribal people, including priorities such as language preservation, health and wellbeing, traditional agricultural techniques, and environmental sustainability. Using Indigenous priorities to guide scholarship can inform legal and policy developments in areas such as land, water, and fishing rights. Disciplines such as literary criticism can examine traditional stories that inspire strategies for decolonization. Indigenizing the academy is a tangible form of empowerment that can lead to significant positive changes in the everyday lives of contemporary Native Peoples (Mihesuah, 2006).

Focusing on Indigenous priorities has inspired research into traditional foods, their cultivation, uses, and nutritional benefits. It has also spurred activism to protect sacred sites and medicines. Academia can benefit from understanding traditional methods of treating physical and mental health issues and recovering knowledge. The influx of Indigenous priorities in higher education has led to museum studies courses in which Native people learn to run their own museums. Particularly notable is the emphasis on language and policy to sustain nationhood. Indigenizing the academy fosters the reclamation of history and recognition of the impact of colonization on contemporary disparities.

Indigenous scholars and their allies are challenging racist and sexist academic institutions (Mihesuah, 2006). This involves reclaiming stories and confronting the ivory tower. In Indigenous value systems, knowledge must be practical and serve communities. Knowledge that is cloistered in the ivory tower is therefore unjustifiable. Indigenous theories and theorists can guide work in the academy. It is important to address the realities of tribal life, not just history, in the classroom. Students are stimulated by the prospect of making real change in their tribal communities, inspired by the importance of being useful (Mihesuah, 2006)

Universities have moral responsibilities to serve students and share knowledge with the neighboring community. Tribes can drive this process. One example is a tribally developed and funded service learning project that linked community needs and academia (Sykes, Pendley & Deacon, 2017). Through this project, students participated in community-based participatory research (CBPR). In addition to developing their research skills, this enhanced their tribal connections and identity, and they later became peer mentors for tribal youth. Therefore, this initiative not only helped engage and retain Native college students but also created role models to cultivate and support the next generation of students. Through such partnerships, tribes gain programming and enhance their research capacity. This model has been empirically evaluated and can be replicated.

Quigley described a collaborative venture between the Awkesasne Mohawk community, Sarah Lawrence College, and Salmon River that she termed a "200 percent" education model. Half of this grant project was devoted to helping Mohawk youth achieve 100 percent on state educational benchmarks. The other half of the grant focused on ensuring Mohawk youth were well versed in their culture, customs, and traditions. She compared this to the Two Row Wampum, in which each way is valued, and Mohawk youth became skilled in both types of knowledge. They were proud to be Mohawk and just as skilled, smart, competent, and ready to succeed in the mainstream world as anyone else.

Universities can create learning communities to help tribal freshmen feel welcomed, valued, and integrated in academia (Sykes et al., 2017). These can include on- and off-campus activities, such as language classes, dance demonstrations, service events, and field trips to tribal events. However, if these are presented as extracurricular activities or add-ons, this may inadvertently communicate that they are of less value than coursework. Therefore, under this model, culturally based activities may be squeezed out as academic demands increase. To counter this risk, cultural content can be institutionalized as an integrated component of credit-bearing coursework through methods such as service learning projects and CBPR.

Johnston-Goodstar spoke of the importance of ethnic studies and their potential to engage youth at the high school level. These programs can have a positive impact on attendance, grades, retention, and graduation. She specifically cited Mexican American studies programs with a strong Indigenous focus as helpful for Native youth. The impact of ethnic studies programs is currently being studied and has the potential to inform curricula, pedagogy, and teacher development.

Humboldt State, part of the University of California system, has a long tradition of supporting Native students, beginning with the creation of the Indian Teacher Education partnership between tribal members and faculty in 1969 (Smith, 2017/ 2018). By 1979, it had broadened its programming to include Native students in counseling and social work. These initiatives provide opportunities to Native people who had never considered college, including older students with families. The university president has a Native American advisory council that includes tribal leaders, staff, and graduates.

Tribally-controlled education

There are several examples of Native American Nations and communities developing their own educational institutions, including tribally run primary and secondary schools. For example, the Zuni took control of their school district in 1980. However, establishing tribal control does not automatically resolve every issue. Even after taking control, the Zuni continued to face a range of problems, including resistance from the school bureaucracy and educators, ongoing disrespect for Native students, and a disempowered Indigenous leadership and community (Rivera & Tharp, 2006).

The most visible form of tribally controlled education is the network of Tribal Colleges and Universities (TCUs). There are currently 32 fully accredited TCUs in the United States and an additional formal candidate for accreditation. These schools serve approximately 30,000 full- and part-time students, 78 percent of whom are Native American. Thus far, 86 percent of TCU students have completed their program of study. Meanwhile, fewer than 10 percent of Native students who go directly from reservation schools to mainstream universities attain undergraduate degrees (White House Initiative on American Indian and Alaska Native Education, US Department of Education, 2018).

TCUs can link traditional knowledge and contemporary life. They comprise a hybrid form of education that is well positioned to integrate Indigenous philosophies and knowledge in academia. By functioning under the sovereign authority of Native Nations, TCUs assert the inherent right of Native Peoples to control their own educational destiny (Crazy Bull, 2012). In spite of their vast potential, though, TCUs struggle with inadequate facilities and funding. By the mid-1990s, they were receiving less than half of their promised federal funds (Fox et al., 2005).

Navajo Community College (later known as Dine' College) opened in 1968 as the first college on a reservation and the first tribally run college (Kostelecky et al., 2017). It was founded during a period of self-determination and embodied a core philosophy of tribal control. College President Ned Hatathli noted that many non-Natives found it difficult to function in only an advisory capacity, rather than from a position of control.

Following the legacy of disrupted knowledge transmission and compulsory attendance at federal schools, Dine' College sought to teach Indigenous knowledge through Western educational models. All instructors must take courses in Dine' educational philosophy and how to incorporate Indigenous epistemology across the curriculum. Likewise, students take courses in Dine' language and history as general education requirements, regardless of major (Kostelecky et al., 2017).

There are various TCU models. While Dine' College was created by a single tribe, the Institute of American Indian Arts (IAIA) was launched as part of the federal Indian education program, and Southwest Indian Polytechnic University (SIPI) was developed by multiple tribal entities, beginning as a federal initiative under the BIA's Office of Indian Education Programs (Kostelecky et al., 2017). SIPI, one of just two federally operated colleges in the United States, admits only enrolled members of federally recognized tribes and is tuition free under the federal trust responsibility.

Tribal colleges are well situated to provide platforms for the difficult, emotionally draining topic of racism. This requires courage to move beyond angry emotions among those who continue to suffer racism on a daily basis and those who experience a sense of White guilt or feel they are unfairly blamed for their ancestors' actions. Tribal colleges have a crucial role to play in preparing the next generation of Native leaders and unshackling them from the bonds of racism, particularly internalized racism (Peacock, 2011).

It is important to note that Indigenous controlled does not necessarily mean Indigenous centered. College is a Western rather than an Indigenous model, so TCUs are inherently hybrid institutions. Even tribally based education faces challenges to ensure education centers Indigenous knowledge. Indeed, many of the materials found in TCU libraries are written by and for non-Native people (Kostelecky et al., 2017).

TCUs must grapple with issues such as which texts should be included in library collections and how services should be offered. For example, how do you deal with stereotypical, offensive, and inaccurate material? Does it matter that texts are often written for non-Native audiences? Historically, the type of knowledge production housed in libraries has been largely closed to Indigenous people and perspectives. Now, libraries must determine how to serve those people whose histories, ceremonies, and other forms of knowledge were written by and for outsiders and are currently held in library collections (Kostelecky et al., 2017).

Libraries have multiple missions and audiences. Relevant content for one audience may be damaging for another. For example, children's books that portray stereotypical or offensive views of Native Americans can be critically analyzed by Native studies, sociology, and education students. On the other hand, the same books may be read by families and inadvertently reinforce inaccuracies and stereotypes (Kostelecky et al., 2017).

The centrality of oral traditions for Indigenous Peoples also presents challenges for libraries. Transcribing important cultural information from oral traditions is a viable option only if the tribe has a written form of their language. Additional barriers exist if students are not literate in the tribal language. While recordings can preserve knowledge from oral traditions, access for students who are not fluent is obviously limited. Moreover, the recorded material may become the definitive version even if it is quite different from traditional stories that vary and contain unique flavors depending on individual storytellers and contexts (Kostelecky et al., 2017).

TCU libraries must find creative ways to be responsive to patrons and community members while maximizing usually sparse financial and human resources. For example, as a way to incorporate educational materials in the absence of published works, Dine' College library was designed with a storytelling room modeled on a traditional hogan that can be used for stories, prayers, and songs. In addition, the collection is supplemented with lectures and other events (Kostelecky et al., 2017).

In general, all libraries hope that their collections reflect the populations they serve, but this can create specific challenges for libraries in Indigenous institutions. For instance, many Native Americans may be confronted with stark and often hostile depictions of how they and their culture were and are viewed by non-Native academics and other outsiders. This can be a shocking and revelatory experience, regardless of whether the materials are accurate or inaccurate (Kostelecky et al., 2017). Of course, there must be increased access to accurate cultural knowledge for Native Peoples.

Non-Native scholars often consider key resources, such as those developed by the Smithsonian Institution, to be authoritative sources on Native people, history, and culture. These sources may have value for Native people, but they demand critical reflection about who created them, under what circumstances, and for whom. Documents created about Native people by non-Native people for non-Native audiences frequently contain distortions and misinformation (Kostelecky et al., 2017). Indeed, it is not unusual for Native people to find inaccurate information about their own tribes even in some of the most well-respected mainstream resources. Students may recognize places and family members, and engage with materials in ways that would likely not happen outside tribal institutions. Native students can bring their own perspectives and knowledge to critique the biases and assumptions inherent in written materials and other aspects of Western education (Kostelecky et al., 2017).

Dine' College chose to collect Navajo materials comprehensively, which resulted in a collection that includes many inaccurate, offensive, and culturally inappropriate resources, such as sand paintings and ceremonial information that should not be recorded, according to traditional protocols. (The recording of certain sacred matters may be perceived as actively harmful to both people and culture.) This raises the question of whether including inaccurate materials in a library collection, such as a fabricated Navajo memoir written by a non-Native author, inadvertently grants them legitimacy. While doing so certainly does not increase understanding of Dine' culture, it may at least contextualize and facilitate discussions of cultural appropriation.

Another quandary involved debates about whether to use mainstream cataloging, such as the Dewey Decimal Classification system. As one solution, the IAIA modified this system so that Native American topics are not primarily placed in history or anthropology sub-fields (Kostelecky et al., 2017). It was also decided to list tribal creation stories under religion, not folklore. Librarians must think critically about which aspects of their work need to be indigenized. Ultimately, the IAIA chose to classify tribal oral histories under history and Indigenous cosmology under religion, rather than categorizing either of them under mythology, as often happens in other libraries (Kostelecky et al., 2017). There is not one correct path to indigenizing libraries; rather, there are multiple models that can inform thoughtful decision making.

Reconciliation in education

Canadian universities are now striving to be more responsive to Native students in the wake of the Truth and Reconciliation Commission that sought to recognize the impact of the residential schools and move beyond their painful legacy (Lewington, 2017). These efforts are balanced by concerns about recruiting academically prepared Native students, eliminating academic disparities between Native and non-Native students, implementing culturally relevant curricula, and transforming academic cultures to make them more hospitable. Universities are working to make campuses more welcoming by integrating Indigenous knowledge, perspectives, and worldviews. Initiatives include feasts, peer mentoring, elders in residence, and on-campus Aboriginal centers. In Canada, Indigenous-focused programs increased by 33 percent between 2013 and 2015, with 86 percent targeting support for Native students, including transition programs and pre-university academic bootcamps (Lewington, 2017). Although there are some notable examples of Native-friendly programs in the United States, overall Canadian universities have done much more to modify academia to make it more accessible to Native students.

The Truth and Reconciliation Commission issued a call for more relevant curricula by indigenizing both content and pedagogy (Lewington, 2017). As an example, 35 percent of Thompson Rivers University's C\$1.2 million strategic initiatives budget was earmarked for indigenizing the curriculum, which led to hiring Native advisors and offering language support. Its Native retention rate subsequently increased from 54 percent in 2006 to 65 percent in 2016, which means it is now comparable with the rate for non-Native students. Other Canadian universities are developing new courses as part of their commitment to the Truth and Reconciliation Commission. Three of them now mandate Indigenous content. These have become safe spaces to acknowledge Indigenous knowledge, content, and pedagogy. Universities and Indigenous communities have negotiated formal agreements on shared issues to ensure this momentum continues (Lewington, 2017). However, although these commitments are encouraging, Native advisors remain cautious about recruiting additional Native students until there is hard evidence that they will be entering hospitable, supportive environments.

Efforts at reconciliation are not without their challenges, as illustrated in a statement issued by the University of Saskatchewan's Indigenous Student Council in February 2018. The members of the council noted that ongoing calls for reconciliation had yielded few practical results. Despite months of effort, the students continued to feel unempowered as decision makers. As a result, they demanded student activism, non-participation, and Indigenous student withdrawal from administrative committees and councils. They noted:

> We are told to maintain hope and toe the line of Reconciliation and Indigenization. However, we have not seen any real systemic change occur on campus. We are controlled, regulated, and limited in our ability to govern and develop the solutions our Indigenous students need. We are looked upon as impoverished threats unable to govern ourselves, we see security cameras directed at us as we attempt to study in one of our safe havens, the Gordon Oakes Red Bear Student Centre. We are tired of the colonial dynamic unfolding on our campus, the systemic racism, and the blatant racism we face everyday.
>
> *(Migchels, 2018)*

Innovative models and trauma-informed education

The principles of trauma-informed care apply in educational and other settings. The fact that education has historically been weaponized against Indigenous Peoples, leading to significant intergenerational trauma, makes applying trauma-informed principles in educational settings imperative. Johnston-Goodstar noted that most grassroots Native education programs are trauma-informed, although mainstream organizations are less so. Native-led organizations have developed strong efforts to revitalize languages and utilize Indigenous pedagogy in their programming. While Quigley was unaware of specific models of trauma-informed education, she noted the importance of these principles. All educators and administrators must recognize trauma and its implications for education. She noted that long before the ACE study, Native Americans were well aware of the lingering effects of trauma.

Generations of Native Americans have been unsafe in educational settings. Issues range from the persistent physical, emotional, and sexual abuse in many boarding schools to contemporary disparate treatment and microaggressions. Native Americans should be able to exercise choice in their education, and Indigenous knowledge and traditional learning styles must be considered on a par—and potentially synergistic—with Western knowledge and knowledge-transmission methods. Collaboration is a prime way to incorporate multiple learning strategies and enhance opportunities for Native students.

Small acts of informed kindness can make a big difference. Quigley described a Native college student who came to see her after the death of his partner. He could have walked away from higher education and not returned, but Quigley took the time to sit with him, listen, and share her understanding of traditional teachings of condolence. Recognizing the student's distress and offering support during this time were crucial. Quigley's concern helped him feel safe, understood, welcome, and valued. He later graduated.

Historically, and often today, education has been heavy-handed and has imposed values and expectations that are foreign to many Indigenous Peoples. Enhancing trustworthiness means recognizing this legacy and actively dismantling policies and practices that inhibit trust and disengage Native people from educational processes. Indigenous knowledge and cultures must be valued, and Indigenous educators and students empowered to teach and learn in multiple ways that respect traditions and prepare the students for the challenges faced by contemporary Indigenous people and communities.

Educators and administrators must grapple with what it means to have trauma-informed education. First, they must recognize how past educational practices and policies have traumatized Native American people and how colonial practices continue in contemporary educational settings. Many schools and districts have reached out to Quigley for guidance. As she put it, certain issues trigger an "ouch." Teachers and administrators need to understand that a Native student's presence in school is sometimes a success in and of itself, regardless of academic achievement, and that success must be recognized. Quigley also recounted a painful story of a Native woman who lost her college housing when her grades declined. Having lost the stability of her apartment she fell into a downward spiral and died shortly after her eviction, leaving five children motherless.

Trauma has been acknowledged within the apologies that some governments and religious institutions have issued regarding their implementation of education as a tool of cultural destruction. However, the impact of Truth and Reconciliation Commissions and subsequent apologies remains unclear. Canadian First Nations may feel the apologies fall short of their expectations and view them as incongruous with their cultural practices. In this sense, the dominant culture may feel some relief after issuing the apology while First Nations people remain frustrated:

> The politics of apology and recognition are thorny—the "political economy of trauma" may do more to benefit the dominant cultures who are apologizing, maintaining their dominance and power, or may help usher in a new period of greater equality … Studying narratives of historical trauma can help disentangle the ways in which contemporary actions perpetrate or repair historical wounds.
>
> *(Mohatt et al., 2014, p. 133)*

Decolonizing education must be a shared process rather than guided from the top down. Cerecer (2013) made the following recommendations for roles for teachers, administrators, and governments in moving toward societal change:

- fund professional development opportunities for educators to enhance cultural responsiveness;
- assess institutional policies to determine how they may hinder student academic success; and
- create an advisory board of students, parents, and community members to provide feedback and guidance to principals and teachers.

Institutions must take responsibility for the achievement gap, rather than continue to marginalize Native students.

Resources are available to transform education to meet the needs of Native people. For example, Education Northwest in Portland, Oregon, incorporates research to develop solutions to help teachers and administrators address the educational needs of Native youth. Its resources include an Indian reading series. It also has a supplemental reading and language development program with books for grades one to six, lesson plans, and teacher manuals. All of these resources are available free of charge. It also offers a self-assessment tool for schools to determine if they are meeting the needs of Native students (Harrington & Chixapkaid, 2013).

Indigenous education scholars have offered critiques of current models and developed alternatives. Most American educational research benchmarks all student performance to White, middle-class peers. By definition, this model marks all others as "different." Instead of a deficit model, Indigenous educational researchers call for recovering power to articulate a vision of quality education for Indigenous youth. Indeed, this is one of the most significant issues for Native Peoples (Harrington & Chixapkaid, 2013). Educators must recognize how local communities understand Indigenous identity, oral traditions, and the natural world in order to contextualize and be guided by their educational priorities. Only through understanding Indigenous epistemology can education move beyond its colonial history as a failed assimilation project (Marker, 2009).

Quigley's tenure as Chair of the National Indian Education Association (NIEA) gave her an opportunity to travel across the country and see many innovative educational programs. She witnessed true commitment among many educators, both Native and non-Native. The NIEA became an advocate at the federal level to share and increase these gains. Interagency collaborations through organizations such as the Administration for Native Americans and Native American Rights

Fund should be welcomed. Native educators are often challenged within their own communities as well as by the dominant society, but opportunities to network and share innovative practices with students and communities hold much promise.

Conclusion

This chapter has reviewed a wide range of topics, including sources of knowledge, how they are valued, and methods of teaching and learning. It is important to recognize that past colonial models of education were oppressive and traumatizing for Native people, but we must also acknowledge that many colonial assumptions persist in contemporary education. By moving toward empowered learning using decolonized, trauma-informed educational models, it is possible to affirm and cultivate the potential of Indigenous learners.

"A decolonizing approach ... requires that Indigenous scholars reclaim the mental universe from pre-contact times and cause it to brush up against the official story from the centre of the empire" (Marker, 2009, p. 759). A way forward may be found with guidance from the *Ganonyok*—also known as the Haudenosaunee Thanksgiving Address. This address is used to open and close many ceremonies and gatherings. Among the many aspects of the natural world, this recitation acknowledges the importance of and gives thanks to enlightened teachers. These may be major figures who have delivered messages of peace, such as Jesus, Mohammed, and the Buddha, but also contemporary people, both well known and local, who provide the guidance and instruction that are necessary to live in the modern world. Traditional teachings have always recognized the importance of teachers.

Teaching and learning are central to Indigenous ways of being. Today, it is imperative that we recognize and shed the colonial aspects of education. We must cultivate enlightened teachers, administrators, and policy makers and move forward with curricula and school climates that value all learners as well as various bodies of knowledge and forms of learning. Coalitions and allies can play a central role in creating this new reality. It cannot happen solely for Native people or in Native contexts. One Native educator eloquently articulated a shared change process with other marginalized populations:

> The struggle for equality will continue with ... [our grandchildren's] generation ... they will need to actively fight racism and all its forms of intolerance. I know that they will need to take Dr. Martin Luther King, Jr.'s dream, our collective dream to be free at last, and make it real, that we hold these truths to be self evident that all people are created equal. That is what we need to do as educators. We need to prepare young people for a world they cannot even imagine, a world that does not even exist, for a day when freedom will ring from every tribal center in every one of our villages, and throughout our tribal nations.
>
> *(Peacock, 2011, p. 17)*

7

TO BE WELL

Explorations of health and balance

This chapter explores manifestations of health and wellbeing, beginning with how these are defined and framed within a policy context. Various aspects of wellbeing are explored, including physical health, violence, mental health, and substance misuse. There is synergy among these areas and all must be in balance to achieve wellness. Concerns with one aspect of health, such as substance misuse, are often intertwined with others, such as mental health issues and violence, as well as broader issues, such as family and community wellbeing. Programs and services are explored to highlight innovative and promising initiatives to reduce health disparities and implement trauma-informed care.

The chapter is informed by the perspectives of Dr. Margaret Moss and Dr. Maria Yellow Horse Brave Heart. These subject-matter experts have spent decades conducting research and providing physical and mental health services for Native people. Both bring the multifaceted perspectives of service providers, researchers, and members of Indigenous communities. They are therefore well positioned to highlight key issues and practices for promoting wellness among Indigenous Peoples.

Moss, a member of the Three Affiliated Tribes, is a nurse with a background in law whose work focuses on American Indian health, health policy, and health disparities, particularly social and structural determinants of health. She is Assistant Dean for Diversity and Inclusion in the School of Nursing, University at Buffalo, State University of New York. She has been a Health Policy Fellow through the Robert Wood Johnson Institute of Medicine and a National Congress of American Indians delegate to the White House Conference on Aging. Her book *American Indian Health and Nursing* (2016) was the *American Journal of Nursing's* Book of the Year.

Moss's nursing career began with the Veterans Administration (VA). While working at a VA hospital in Santa Fe, New Mexico, she became immersed in serving Native Americans from local pueblos. This cultural context was quite different from her own background in the Great Plains and her experience with Native Americans in urban areas. While working in the medical/surgical unit at Santa Fe, she encountered common health issues, such as diabetes and alcohol misuse, as well as a wide range of issues that nursing school had not covered, such as plague, suicide, pregnant teens, and serving elders. One woman clutched an ear of corn, a powerful spiritual symbol, as she was being wheeled into surgery. These experiences led Moss to write her first book in order to help newly qualified nurses address the gamut of medical issues experienced by Native Americans. Her growing understanding of the importance of culture and observations that elders preferred returning home without services to entering a nursing facility led her to conduct an ethnography with Zuni elders. She recognized the need to integrate cultural practices in nursing facilities but was frustrated when the societal emphasis on community-based care hindered the development of culturally responsive units. Seeing the need to influence policy, she completed a law degree to complement her advanced nursing degrees.

Brave Heart, whose scholarship on historical trauma was introduced in Chapter 1, is Hunkpapa/Oglala Lakota and a clinical social worker whose work centers on Indigenous collective trauma, grief and loss, and cross-cultural mental health. She is widely credited with bringing historical trauma and related healing interventions to the attention of helping professionals and Indigenous communities. She founded the Takini Network, a Native American non-profit organization focused on healing intergenerational trauma, and is a research associate professor and Director of the Native American and Disparities Research Program at the Center for Rural and Community Behavioral Health in the Department of Psychiatry at the University of New Mexico.

Brave Heart's early experience in clinical social work led her to question assumptions that poor people and people of color could not benefit from insight-oriented, psychodynamic work, which engendered her long-standing commitment to culturally responsive behavioral healthcare. Her clinical work has always been informed by and integrated with a deep commitment to serving Native American communities. In 1978, shortly after completing her master's degree in social work, she became aware of the concept of historical trauma. As she looked at historical and family photographs, she became overwhelmed and conscious of carrying collective grief. Around this time, she connected with a Jewish Holocaust survivor and the children of survivors and recognized their commonalities. She found her professional direction through a synergistic combination of interest in psychoanalytic work, community commitment, personal connections with collective grief, and affirmation that this professional path was meaningful. She learned to pay attention to signs that give spiritual and emotional guidance. Even when these fail to fit a traditional academic mold, she feels they guide her in fulfilling a higher purpose in historical trauma healing work.

Perspectives on wellness

Culture can shape how wellbeing is experienced. Indigenous people who remain culturally grounded may conceptualize health differently than non-Indigenous people, providers, and health delivery systems. A review of health and wellbeing for Native people must begin with a common understanding of these terms.

Indigenous cultures typically view health and wellbeing in holistic ways. A study of Anishinaabe women (Brown, 2016) identified health as comprised of various facets of life, including environment, space, and wellness of the earth. Therefore, wellbeing was intimately connected with the environment and participants in the study equated land with life. In other words, the survival of humanity was tied to the survival of land. Wellness was understood as a balance between people, land, and spirit.

Indigenous conceptualizations of health are intertwined with a strong sense of identity. For Native Americans, cultural identity is not necessarily anchored in external or legal definitions. Rather, it can be linked to traditional understandings of Indigeneity and community membership. For example, living in an urban environment and enrollment status did not influence whether Native Americans accessed traditional healing to maintain or enhance wellness (Moghaddam, Momper & Fong, 2013). Western knowledge systems may inform Native American health but should not supplant Indigenous knowledge and ways of helping as the starting point for thinking about health (Cavalieri, 2013).

An overview of Native American wellbeing

In some states, the life expectancy for Native Americans is 20 years below the national average (Whitney, 2017). These contemporary health and mortality disparities are rooted in historical trauma (Brown, 2016; Warne & Lajimodiere, 2015). Historical trauma is linked to chronic diseases and poor mental health, and it may help explain undiagnosed chronic pain (Struthers & Lowe, 2003). It has also been identified as part of the explanatory framework for disproportionate rates of substance misuse, violence, and suicide in Native American communities (Morgan & Freeman, 2009). Additional research is needed to understand how historical grief and loss as well as collective and individual lifespan trauma undermine intergenerational health and wellbeing for diverse groups of Native people (Brave Heart et al., 2011).

Contemporary trauma, including high adverse childhood events (ACE) scores, has also been linked to health disparities (Warne & Lajimodiere, 2015). For example, Indigenous youth are exposed to many losses, which means they have more experience of grief than their non-Indigenous peers (Nicolai & Saus, 2013). Native youth also have high rates of exposure to violence as well as significant behavioral health disparities, such as parental alcohol misuse (Goodkind et al., 2012). Frequent exposure to racism, discrimination, and heteronormativity are correlated with a range of negative health outcomes, such as cardiovascular disease, respiratory problems, smoking, chronic pain, HIV risk behavior, depression, and poor self-perceptions of physical and mental health (Moghaddam et al., 2013). Psychological reactions to stress are connected to chronic diseases like diabetes that are prevalent in Native American populations (Tiedt & Brown, 2014).

Clearly, both historical and contemporary trauma influence wellbeing. In North America, Indigenous Peoples experience greater health and social problems than their non-Native peers, perhaps because of their disproportionate exposure to both historical and contemporary stressors (McQuaid et al., 2015). Generations of Native Americans are exposed to stressors such as physical and sexual abuse, racism and discrimination, and fear of child removal (Myhra & Wieling, 2014). The Trauma History Questionnaire (American Indian Version) was administered at the Denver Indian Family Resource Center. Of those screened, 93 percent reported trauma histories (Lucero & Bussey, 2015).

Native Americans experience high rates of both intentional and unintentional physical injury (Tsosie et al., 2011). When asked what she viewed as longstanding issues in Native American health, Moss emphasized the disproportionate impact of unintentional injuries, such as motor vehicle accidents. Beyond this, she noted that suicide and homicide are especially high on some reservations, but their magnitude is obscured in nationwide statistics. A study of 30 Native Americans at a trauma center (Tsosie et al., 2011) found high levels of lifetime trauma as well as moderate levels of PTSD, depressive symptoms, and alcohol use. Within this group, 33 percent sought assistance from a Native healer or spiritual advisor, and 60 percent participated in traditional activities, ranging from following a subsistence lifestyle to traditional dancing and crafts, to facilitate healing.

Interviews with more than 3000 Native Americans living on or near a reservation documented that many live in adverse environments with a high risk of trauma exposure and resulting health sequelae (Manson et al., 2005). In this study, both women and men had comparable rates of trauma. This finding contrasts with other studies that consistently document gender difference in trauma exposure in other populations. The researchers suggested that widespread use of alcohol in these communities may account for the difference, but further empirical investigation is needed to support or contradict this theory.

The Manson et al. (2005) study further found that American Indian men and women witnessed traumatic events, experienced trauma to loved ones, and were victims of physical attacks more often than the general US population. Respondents who had more education also had more trauma exposure. This was especially true for Native people in the Southwest. The researchers posited that education may expose American Indians to life beyond the reservation, exposing them to more adverse events or educational status that contrasts with that of reservation peers. In turn, this may lead to interpersonal conflict. Poverty was associated with less trauma exposure, while employment status bore little relation to trauma exposure. Widowed, divorced, or separated respondents had more trauma exposure than those who were married or had never married. The researchers noted that being widowed can be a form of traumatic loss, while separation or divorce can indicate discord and associated trauma, whereas never marrying may indicate a smaller interpersonal network and consequently less exposure to trauma. This community-based sample may provide a clearer picture of Native American trauma exposure than research using clinical samples. It is noteworthy, however, that the associations documented in the study need further investigation to enable an understanding of connections between variables such as education and trauma.

The extraordinary diversity among Native American Peoples makes generalizations based on research prone to significant error (Whitesell et al., 2012). Moss noted the importance of looking at regional and tribal data in order to understand health issues. In particular, the fact that most research focuses on reservation-based populations is problematic because these groups no longer comprise the majority of Native Americans. Even though the Manson et al. (2005) study took an important step by questioning a large non-clinical sample, it does not inform an understanding of Native Americans living away from tribal territories. Validated treatment options are also lacking. Evidence-based treatment protocols for many mental health issues, such as bipolar disorder, schizophrenia, ADHD, and depression, have been developed with efficacy studies that did not include Native Americans (Goodkind et al., 2012).

Moss and Brave Heart both highlighted a number of issues that helping professionals must consider. In particular, they emphasized the importance of understanding that Native American people are diverse and distinct from mainstream society. Brave Heart mentioned that treaties reflect Native Americans' distinct legal status, whereas Moss stressed the importance of understanding the differences *among* Native Americans. Native people do not share one generic, common culture. There are substantial differences across regions, distinctions between urban and reservation-based Native people, and contrasts between and among tribes and bands.

Discrimination and the structural determinants of health

The dismal statistics on Indigenous health must be viewed within context. There are many aspects of the physical and social environment that impact health. These include substandard housing, persistent boil-water advisories, widespread environmental contamination, and discrimination within educational systems. Understanding health disparities requires understanding these ongoing social determinants of health (Wiebe, 2016).

Moss estimated that structural determinants account for 85 percent of wellbeing and provide a crucial framework for understanding health issues. Limited educational opportunities, poverty, substandard housing, food insecurity, and a lack of transportation are urgent concerns in many Native American communities. Until we address these social determinants of health, medical interventions are likely to have little or no positive impact on communities. Moss gave an example of health professionals assisting diabetics by counseling them about taking exercise and medication yet failing to recognize that some patients live in areas where it is unsafe to walk, while others may not have a refrigerator to store the medication. In such instances, the patients are unable to comply with instructions issued by providers who fail to recognize that life circumstances affect health.

Health is closely linked to structural disadvantage. For example, high rates of motor vehicle fatalities are related to the quality and maintenance of roads and vehicles. Roads on reservations are often poorly maintained, and economic factors force some Native people to drive poorly maintained vehicles. Limited emergency response services also contribute to poor health outcomes and road fatalities (Sarche et al., 2017).

Health delivery systems rarely consider the experiences of Indigenous Peoples, including the impact of colonization and trauma. The evidence linking trauma and violence to various health problems has not translated into changes in how healthcare is designed or delivered to Native Americans. A decolonizing lens can be applied to examine the root causes of people's health and social issues and to make adjustments accordingly (Browne et al., 2016).

About one-quarter of Native Americans report facing discrimination at health clinics or doctors' offices (Whitney, 2017). Ongoing discrimination in healthcare is fed by stereotypes and stigma, such as racialized assumptions about Native Americans and alcohol (Browne et al., 2016). These stereotypes interact with media messages and assumptions in everyday conversations to undermine Indigenous rights and influence thinking about which patients are credible and deserving of healthcare (Browne et al., 2016).

Discrimination against Native Americans in healthcare settings exists everywhere, but is particularly prominent in regions with large Indigenous populations. For example, it may take years and extensive advocacy before post-surgical follow-up care is obtained (Whitney, 2017). Differential treatment in healthcare settings is common for Indigenous people around the world. Orr (2018) described a well-publicized example of an internationally renowned Australian Aboriginal musician who died from internal bleeding after being left unexamined and unattended on a hospital gurney for hours, based on a presumption of drunkenness.

One study of urban Native Americans (Moghaddam et al., 2013) found that discrimination in healthcare settings is significantly associated with the use of traditional healing. In this study, a quarter of respondents reported discrimination in a healthcare setting, and half used traditional healing. Women aged 35–44 were most likely to use the latter. It is unclear to what extent these women access traditional healing due to personal preference or experiences with discrimination in other healthcare settings. While traditional healing is an important resource for many Native people, they should also have access to other forms of medical treatment without bias, stigma, or discrimination.

Because of discriminatory treatment in healthcare settings and elsewhere, Indigenous people may be reluctant to seek services in Western medical settings. Historical discrimination, along with forced sterilizations that continued into the 1970s, has contributed to continuing physical and mental health disparities (Tiedt & Brown, 2014). In Australia, some hospitals implemented specific procedures and appointed social workers dedicated to taking Aboriginal children into foster care and adoptive placements, often without any justifiable cause. Additionally, in the past, some hospitals assigned Aboriginal patients to beds in morgue wings rather than the main wards.

This history continues to affect Aboriginal people's willingness to be admitted to a hospital as well as their tendency to leave a hospital against medical advice (Orr, 2018).

In addition to longstanding health disparities, such as heart disease and stroke, Moss noted that suicide, use of opiates and other drugs, and violence against women are becoming increasing concerns for Native people. Brave Heart made connections between longstanding and emerging issues. For example, diseases like tuberculosis, which were unknown in tribal communities prior to European contact, had devastating impacts at the start of colonization and rates remain elevated today. She noted that heart disease, breast cancer, and asthma are all significant concerns in Native communities and are often linked to or exacerbated by environmental factors, such as pollution, mining, pipelines, and weapons development.

During the first 16 sessions of the United Nations Permanent Forum on Indigenous Issues, 22 recommendations were issued specific to women's health and reproductive rights, but relevant data and progress have been limited (United Nations Population Fund, 2018). Recommendations related to a life free from violence are often general and geared toward raising awareness of human rights violations. Some emphasize the impact of armed conflicts on Indigenous women and children, including their vulnerability to trafficking. While such recommendations are a welcome starting point, meaningful change requires action.

Moss identified the large number of missing and murdered Indigenous women (MMIW) as a major emerging health issue. Many advocacy organizations and families continue to demand that the Canadian government be held accountable for MMIW. There have also been calls for action at the United Nations. A national inquiry began in Canada in early 2016 and a final report was imminent at the time of writing in late 2018 (United Nations Population Fund, 2018). Indigenous women experience comparable vulnerabilities in the United States and other parts of the world, yet these have drawn significantly less attention.

Policy parameters

Federal policies, both general and health specific, are ever present in the lives of Native Americans. Policies and programs that stem from treaty obligations and the federal trust responsibility continue to have a powerful influence. Indeed, many treaties contain provisions for the delivery of health services. The federal Indian Health Service (IHS) is a legacy of these ongoing obligations in the United States. In Canada, the federal government maintains a fiduciary responsibility for First Nations' health, articulated in paternalistic language as a moral—as opposed to a legal—obligation (Wiebe, 2016). This has led to a discretionary, piecemeal patchwork of responsibility for Indigenous health services.

The early policy of confinement to reservations had severe health consequences for Native Americans. High rates of infectious diseases are linked to poor sanitation, poor food quality and handling, and inadequate medical care (Tiedt & Brown, 2014). Additionally, the Bureau of Indian Affairs (BIA) withheld food and supplies to force compliance with its rules, leading to significant psychological, physical, and spiritual distress (Tiedt & Brown, 2014).

Notwithstanding the establishment of the IHS, healthcare remains fragmented, funding is severely inadequate, and health disparities persist (Tiedt & Brown, 2014; Whitney, 2017). Indeed, the IHS is sometimes perceived as more of a bureaucratic barrier than a meaningful service (Whitney, 2017). There is always doubt over whether the Indian Health Care Improvement Act, an amendment to the Social Security Act that provides the legal foundation for provision of health services for American Indians, will be adequately funded (Lane & Simmons, 2011). Funding for tribal healthcare does not keep pace with either inflation or population growth, so allocated funds are often exhausted midway through the year. In 2016, the IHS budget was just $4.8 billion—equivalent to $1297 per person—while an average of $6973 was spent per inmate in the federal prison system (Whitney, 2017).

There is a complex, inconsistent set of tribal, state, community, federal, and local mental health services for Native people (BigFoot & Schmidt, 2010). Little treatment is available for sufferers of PTSD and there is a growing demand for trauma-informed care. The IHS, urban, and tribal organizations are poorly equipped to screen for trauma and trauma-related problems among service users (Bassett, Buchwald & Manson, 2014).

Health policies need to be reframed and must become more attentive to areas such as the wellbeing of young children and women. The foundation for lifelong emotional and physical wellbeing develops in early childhood, yet most of the research on children's development and health has focused on adolescence (Sarche et al., 2017). Young children's health therefore requires more attention from policy makers, funders, and researchers. Assessing and addressing the health needs of young children is a crucial element of enhancing wellbeing for Native people. Likewise, policies and programs to prevent violence are scarce (United Nations Population Fund, 2018), in part because of the institutionally entrenched structure of cultural subordination.

Physical wellbeing

Prior to colonization, Native Americans suffered from some infectious diseases, malnutrition, and traumatic injuries, but contact with Europeans brought a host of new diseases to which they had no immunity, including influenza, typhoid, mumps, chickenpox, smallpox, measles, and diphtheria (Tiedt & Brown, 2014). Within 400 years, these diseases from Europe had spread across the entire continent, killing up to 90 percent of the Indigenous population. This decimation weakened Indigenous communities physically, spiritually, emotionally, and psychologically, leaving them with a deep and lasting legacy of unresolved grief (Warne & Lajimodiere, 2015). This grief has been transmitted across the generations and contemporary health is often rooted in historical conditions. Therefore, understanding history facilitates an understanding of contemporary circumstances. More than half the population died in tribes where smallpox infections were deliberately spread (Warne & Lajimodiere, 2015). Distrust based on such historical experiences subsequently influenced perceptions of more recent health crises, including HIV, with some people believing the virus may have been intentionally introduced.

Health concerns disproportionately affect socially disadvantaged groups. There may be a gene–environment interaction or factors related to allostatic load—the wear and tear on the body associated with chronic stress—that perpetuate this inequity and enhance the chronic disease burden of disadvantaged groups (Tiedt & Brown, 2014). For Native Americans, multiple traumatic events across generations have led to hypervigilance and increased sympathetic nervous system activation that compound the effects of daily stressors. Widespread, collective, intergenerational experiences lead to a biologically based stress response. In turn, the stress response of parents affects how they interact with their children, creating a loop of reinforcing social behaviors across generations (Tiedt & Brown, 2014).

Native Americans are more likely than Whites to experience traumatic brain injuries (TBIs), regardless of age and gender. For Native men, the rate of violent TBI is 46.6 percent, compared to 21 percent of White men. For Native women, the rate is 32.2 percent, compared to 8.5 percent for White women. Violence-related injuries are the leading cause of TBI death for Native Americans, although most TBIs in older adults are the result of falls or other accidents, rather than violence. When older adults experience TBIs as a result of violence, the perpetrators are usually family members (Linton & Kim, 2014).

Heart disease is the leading cause of death for Native and non-Native Americans alike (Wilson, 2018). However, the Strong Heart Study (Jernigan et al., 2010) found that the incidence of heart disease among Native Americans is double that of the general population. Moreover, the risk factors for cardiovascular disease, such as obesity, hypertension, and diabetes, are all increasing among Native people. In 2005–2006, 79 percent of Native Americans had at least one risk factor, and 46 percent had two or more. Therefore, it is unsurprising that Native people have the highest incidence of cardiovascular disease in United States. The mortality rate is also increasing for Native people even as it decreases for all other groups. The prevalence of obesity is particularly worrying, and low levels of physical activity are an additional concern. Native Americans engage in less physical activity during their leisure time than any other group. Obesity rates for Native children exceed those of their non-Native peers and increase as youth age (Sarche et al., 2017). Over 80 percent of Native American adults aged 20–74 are overweight or obese (Indian Health Service, 2018a). This has significant implications for a variety of health issues, including diabetes, high blood pressure, respiratory problems, and some types of cancer. Psychological distress and lack of familial support have both been linked to excess weight. On the other hand, culturally based spirituality was associated with lower weight in a weight-loss program for pre-diabetics (Dill et al., 2015).

Native American men and women both experience diabetes at least twice as frequently as White men and women or the general population (Cho et al., 2014; Simonds, Omidpanah & Buchwald, 2017). Moreover, they tend to develop diabetes at a younger age, which obviously increases their vulnerability to diabetes-related complications (Cho et al., 2014). Diabetes was the fourth-leading cause of death for Native people in 2009, and the seventh-leading cause of death for Whites

(Cho et al., 2014). Diabetes-related mortality is decreasing for all groups, yet, depending on age, Native people remain 2.5 to 3.5 times more likely than Whites to die due to the condition (Cho et al., 2014).

Overall, Native Americans have the highest rate of smoking of all ethnic groups in the United States (Jernigan et al., 2010), although there are wide variations in cigarette use depending on gender, tribe, and region (Odani et al., 2017). Prevalence is higher among males, young adults aged 18–25, low-income people, and those without a high school degree. A 2014 study found that 5.3 percent of Native American middle school youth and 45 percent of high school students had used electronic cigarettes. Nearly one-third of these youth had never smoked traditional cigarettes (Rhoades et al., 2017).

The average time Native Americans—adults as well as youth—spend looking at screens (e.g., televisions, computers, smartphones) exceeds 3.5 hours a day. This is a health concern as screen time is associated with obesity and other health risks. Native youth report more screen time than White youth. One meta-analysis (Foulds et al., 2016) revealed that screen time was highest among young, male Native Americans and overweight or obese individuals. Canadian Indigenous youth reported less screen time than their US Native American counterparts. Television watching was the most reported type of screen time. Native and non-Native youth reported similar time playing video games, but the former spent less time on computers or the internet.

Disparities also exist in oral health (Cladoosby, 2017). People of color are less likely to see a dentist and more likely to suffer from untreated tooth decay. Indeed, the rate of tooth decay among two- to four-year-old Native youth is five times the national average (Sarche et al., 2017). More than 70 percent of Native youth aged 2–5 have a history of tooth decay, compared to just 23 percent of White children. Adult Native Americans suffer from untreated caries at more than twice the rate of the general population. They are also more likely to have severe periodontal disease, missing teeth, and generally poor oral health (Cladoosby, 2017).

Food insecurity

Adequate nutrition is important for the maintenance of good health. Forced relocation and government food programs impeded access to healthy foods. When Native Americans were forced onto reservations, they often lost access to their traditional food sources. Instead, they received highly refined government-subsidized food that has been linked to diabetes—a previously unknown malady in Native American populations (Tiedt & Brown, 2014). Food options that are available through commodity programs may contribute to chronic disease and mortality disparities (Warne & Lajimodiere, 2015). Food insecurity is an ongoing issue with underlying causes that include limited availability of healthy food and poverty (Jernigan et al., 2017).

Food insecurity is defined as uncertain or inadequate access to nutritious and safe food. Roughly 30 percent of all Native families—and 40 percent of those with young children—experience food insecurity, compared with approximately 16 percent of the general US population (Jernigan et al., 2017; Sarche et al., 2017). Native Americans in California, Montana, Alaska, and South Dakota suffer particularly high rates. The Tribal Health and Resilience in Vulnerable Environments (THRIVE) study found that 56 percent of tribal members in rural Oklahoma suffered inadequate food quantity and 62 percent inadequate food quality (Jernigan et al., 2017). Those with inadequate quantity and quality were more likely to develop diabetes, obesity, and hypertension.

Food assistance programs, such as the Supplemental Nutrition Assistance Program (SNAP) and Women, Infants and Children (WIC), do not eradicate food insecurity. Furthermore, commodity distribution to tribal communities creates unhealthy food preferences and fosters diet-related diseases (Jernigan et al., 2017). Discriminatory practices lead to food inequity. Native community members have reported that some non-Native store owners raise prices, do not verify SNAP- and WIC-eligible products, and even refuse to serve Native customers. These discriminatory practices obviously exacerbate food insecurity for Indigenous people (Jernigan et al., 2017).

In 1996, the United Nations Human Development Index ranked Canada first in the world on indicators of wellbeing, yet its First Nations communities were rated only 63rd. This inequity continues as many Indigenous households lack running water, sewerage systems, and nutritious food (Thompson & Lozecznik, 2011). As an example, food insecurity in northern Manitoba is roughly eight times the national rate, which has prompted community members to highlight this inequity in a video project. Making the video also served an empowering function. The project highlighted the importance of traditional foods, the extent of food insecurity, factors that undermine the right to healthy and culturally appropriate food (a.k.a. food sovereignty), and food-centered community development strategies (Thompson & Lozecznik, 2011). Traditionally, fishing, hunting, gathering, and gardening provided an abundance of diverse food sources. Treaty rights protect sustainable livelihoods and food security, but these are often undermined and/or not respected. For example, Native communities suffer from water regulation as dams deplete fish populations (Thompson & Lozecznik, 2011).

Regulations create additional barriers to food security. While school cooks prefer to serve locally available, culturally appropriate food, all meat and fish must be inspected at a federal food facility before it can be served at schools, hospitals, or other public institutions. However, no such federal food processing facility is available in northern Manitoba (Thompson & Lozecznik, 2011). Other heavy-handed applications of federal policy also contribute to food insecurity. When community health representatives at Garden Hill First Nation set out a fishing net as part of a health program to feed community members, the net was confiscated later that day by Manitoba Conservation (Thompson & Lozecznik, 2011). A survey found that 13 of 14 northern Manitoba First Nations communities had only one food store with limited and expensive options. In addition, food is often damaged during shipping to remote and isolated areas. Some communities have no store at all and a lack of all-weather roads limits access to stores in other communities. Therefore, simply purchasing food can involve overnight travel with hotel, taxi, and train expenses, all of which can add hundreds of dollars to the price of the food (Thompson & Lozecznik, 2011).

Environmental health risks

Environmental contamination poses significant health risks. Wild foods continue to be important for some Native people, but Indigenous communities in northern Canada experience significant mercury exposure through their consumption of these foodstuffs. Children that are prenatally exposed to mercury are known to suffer adverse neurodevelopmental outcomes, and long-term postnatal exposure is probably similarly damaging, although this requires further study (Pirkle, Murkle & Lemire, 2016).

As noted earlier, northern Indigenous communities experience significant food insecurity as a result of a rapid transition toward store-bought foodstuffs combined with decreasing access to local resources (Pirkle et al., 2016). Programs to reduce mercury exposure are at odds with this growing food insecurity. Pirkle et al. (2016) point out that many Indigenous people continue to draw cultural and economic sustenance as well as food and medicine from the ocean, rivers, and lakes, yet food from these sources is frequently contaminated with mercury. Sources of mercury exposure and the availability of wild foods vary across regions, so location-specific, nuanced, interdisciplinary approaches are needed to guide health promotion programs. It is important to note that not all wild food is equally contaminated. Mercury exposure is a global health concern, but Native people in the far north may be particularly at risk. That said, much remains unknown about the health risks; for example, it is difficult to judge safe levels of toxins in fish (Pirkle et al., 2016).

A legacy of radioactive and toxic chemical exposure disproportionately affects Indigenous communities. Toxic chemicals, such as mercury, bioaccumulate and biomagnify as they pass through the food chain, ultimately ending up in Indigenous communities' traditional and subsistence foods (Goldtooth, 2010). Policies do not adequately protect the Indigenous Peoples of the world, particularly children.

Environmental risks go far beyond food supply. Uranium mining, power generation, and fossil fuel extraction have resulted in contamination that will persist for generations, even if operations were to cease today. These enterprises have significant detrimental impacts on Indigenous health and cultural practices. For example, people from the Laguna Pueblo and the Navajo Nation in New Mexico have developed cancer from exposure to radioactive uranium waste. Members of the Three Affiliated Tribes on the Fort Berthold Reservation in North Dakota and Navajo people from the Shiprock area of their reservation have developed respiratory illnesses caused by coal-fired power plants and oil refinery emissions. Likewise, members of the Ponca Nation in north-central Oklahoma have contracted acute respiratory illnesses due to exposure to toxins (Goldtooth, 2010). Many environmental risks are generated by neglecting the wellbeing of poor, politically isolated Indigenous communities while prioritizing unsustainable resource extraction. Native people are considered expendable and their lands are viewed as sacrifice zones (Goldtooth, 2010; Wiebe, 2016).

In Canada, entire Native communities have no access to safe drinking water. Many people around the world view Canada as a desirable place to live with a pristine natural landscape, yet that myth is challenged and disparities are highlighted by repeated drinking-water advisories on the country's reserves. Health issues tied to environmental concerns must receive attention as part of the federal obligation to provide comprehensive healthcare to Indigenous peoples in Canada (Wiebe, 2016).

Violence

While violence is a prominent factor in the lives of many Native Americans, this must be understood within a societal context rather than as an individual pathology. A legal system that does not protect tribal citizens should be regarded as an institutionalized failure (Sarche et al., 2017). The social environment both facilitates and perpetuates violence, so large-scale societal change is required to eliminate violence:

> The ideologies, attitudes, behaviors, and practices of oppression at multiple levels provide unwavering structural support for disempowering acts of violence and abuse against women, and many other groups. Too often analysis of pressing social problems fail to critique the interlocking dynamics of subjugation or the intersectionality of social structures and power relations in creating, reinforcing, and perpetuating oppressive practices such as violence against women.
>
> *(Chenault, 2011, p. 1)*

Structural violence and human rights

Structural violence plays a major role in fostering and sustaining inequities. It is systemic and may be defined as "disadvantage and suffering that stems from the creation and perpetuation of structures, policies, and institutional practices that are innately unjust" (Browne et al., 2016, p. 2). Structural violence fosters conditions that perpetuate health and social disparities.

The lives and health status of Indigenous Peoples and communities around the world are steeped in it, both historically and today. Structural deficits created through measures such as placement on reservation lands with inadequate means for sustenance and state-sponsored child removal have profound effects over multiple generations. Poverty, substandard housing, systemic racism and discrimination, lack of employment opportunities, and limited access to education are some of the legacies of colonization. Structural violence also contributes to the individual and institutional racism experienced by Indigenous people around the world, while individualized health services fail to address resulting disparities and inequities (Browne et al., 2016).

Interpersonal violence within Indigenous communities can be understood as anger turned inward as a result of historical trauma. The violence often plays out within the context of families and interpersonal relationships. Although visible on a micro level, it has structural roots in society:

> Violence against women, and certainly violence against Indigenous women, is rarely understood as a human rights issue. To the extent that governments, media and the general public do consider concerns about violence against women, it is more frequent for it to be described as a criminal concern or a social issue. It is both of those things of course. But it is also very much a human rights issue. Women have the right to be safe and free from violence. Indigenous women have the right to be safe and free from violence. When a woman is targeted for violence because of her gender or because of her Indigenous identity, her fundamental rights have been abused. And when she is not offered an adequate level of protection by state authorities because of her gender or because of her Indigenous identity, those rights have been violated.
>
> *(Amnesty International, 2004, p. 3)*

Colonialism, subjugation, oppression, and subsequent trauma create a legacy of disproportionate rates of domestic violence among Native Peoples. This violence is further fueled by poverty, racism, substance misuse, and isolation, particularly in rural areas (Jones, 2008). History led to clustering Native Americans in economically marginal, rural areas. Subsequent alcohol and drug use can be at least partially explained as responses to trauma. Co-morbidity and the complexity of the violence issue mean that multimodal responses and interprofessional collaboration are essential (Jones, 2008).

Interpersonal violence

As noted in Chapter 4, violence is a significant concern for many Indigenous people. The violent crime rate for Native Americans aged 12 and older is 2.5 times the national average (American Indian Law and Order Commission, 2015). The anarchic violence that is a common feature of contemporary Native communities is a direct legacy of colonization. Violence is rooted in self-hatred, often turned upon family and community members, and exacerbated by alcohol and drugs that were unknown in traditional cultures. Internalized oppression manifests in community divisions and devaluing tribal members who understand and express their culture in different ways (Kipp, 2004).

Native American women and men experience the highest rates of intimate partner violence—including rape, stalking, and physical abuse—of any groups in the United States. The rates are 46 percent for Native women and 45.3 percent for Native men (Burnette & Figley, 2017). In Canada, Indigenous women aged 25–44 are five times more likely to die from violence than other Canadian women (Amnesty International, 2004), while Native American women are ten times more likely to be murdered than others in the United States (American Indian Law and Order Commission, 2015). Economic stability or lack thereof can interact with risk of interpersonal violence. For example, revenue from casino payments can change the power dynamics within a family and may lead someone to remain in a violent domestic relationship if their partner receives money. Likewise, a batterer may not let their victim go if they are the recipient of casino payments (Jones, 2008).

One in three Native American women is sexually assaulted in her lifetime (Edwards, 2017)—four times the national average. For Native Alaskan women, the rate of sexual assault is 12 times the national average (American Indian Law and Order Commission, 2015). Some Native men internalize violence as a norm and direct it at their partners as a result of oppression they experience from wider society (Jones, 2008). The impact of interpersonal violence transcends individual partnerships and affects whole families and communities (Burnette, 2016).

Violence often occurs across the lifespan. One study of Native women in New York City (Evans-Campbell et al., 2006) found that 65 percent had experienced some form of interpersonal violence. Of these, 28 percent experienced child abuse, 48 percent rape, 40 percent domestic violence, and 40 percent multiple victimizations. High levels of emotional trauma are associated with all of these experiences. A history of interpersonal violence is correlated with depression, dysphoria, help seeking, and high-risk sexual behavior. Of the women in this study who experienced violence, 75 percent had accessed traditional healing and 70 percent had accessed conventional mental health services. Those who experienced sexual assault were most likely to access both types of assistance.

Indigenous youth in the United States are up to ten times as likely to experience violent crimes than the national average (American Indian Law and Order Commission, 2015). Native youth also experience more violence within schools than their peers (Johnston-Goodstar et al., 2016). Exposure to violence creates additional vulnerabilities. For example, in Canada, a disproportionate number of Indigenous children enter the sex trade in order to survive (Amnesty International, 2004).

Distrust of law enforcement officers often makes Native Americans reluctant to report violence. Police may be personally implicated in violence against Indigenous Peoples or at least demonstrate a lack of concern for their safety and wellbeing (Amnesty International, 2004). Violence is likely underestimated due to inconsistencies in police record keeping, and rape often goes unprosecuted. Many of the Native people who experience the latter believe that "it is more painful and dangerous to testify than it is to silently grieve" (Alexie, 2017, p. 178).

Aboriginal and Torres Strait Islander women in Australia are ten times more likely to die of violent assault and 32 times more likely to be hospitalized due to violence than their non-Indigenous peers (United Nations Population Fund, 2018). As in the United States, violence frequently goes unreported, often due to distrust of the system. Suicide rates are also escalating rapidly. Aboriginal Australian women described their powerlessness, a deep sense of cultural loss, and a lack of control over their own lives. They called for a holistic approach that recognizes cultural connection as a central element of social and emotional wellbeing. In turn, this holistic approach could foster sustainable improvement in health indicators (United Nations Population Fund, 2018). Access to justice for Indigenous women experiencing violence is elusive, regardless of national context.

Various Indigenous women's organizations around the world have drawn attention to violence and its impacts. The Companion Report to the UN Secretary-General's Study on Violence against Women, authored by the International Indigenous Women's Forum in 2006, was a milestone in documenting violence against Indigenous women (United Nations Population Fund, 2018). Gender-based violence, including gang rape, is a common threat for Indigenous women and girls. For example, during armed conflicts in Guatemala, the military, acting under state orders, participated in the mass rape of Indigenous women as well as other widespread human rights violations. Indigenous Peoples continue to face multiple challenges in obtaining justice in the wake of such atrocities (United Nations Population Fund, 2018).

Mental health

Active trauma symptoms can be overwhelming, draining both emotional and physical energy. Individuals with high trauma loads may be unable to manage day-to-day responsibilities as well as additional requirements imposed by institutions such as the child welfare system (Lucero & Bussey, 2015). Social contexts and families affect children. Native infants are more likely to be rated "of concern" on the Infant and Toddler Social Emotional Assessment Scale (Sarche et al., 2017). Mothers with stronger Indigenous identities rate their children as more socially and emotionally competent, although girls are rated significantly higher than boys (Sarche et al., 2017).

As noted in Chapter 1, Native Americans have high rates of PTSD and related symptoms. The leading causes of PTSD are combat and interpersonal violence, and symptoms include physical pain, lung problems, general health issues, substance misuse, and problematic gambling. The risk factors and co-morbidities for Native Americans are similar to those of other populations, but they experience much higher rates (Bassett et al., 2014). The rate of PTSD among Native youth is officially 22 percent, which is equivalent to the rate of US military personnel who served in Iraq and Afghanistan (American Indian Law and Order Commission, 2015; Attorney General's Advisory Committee on American Indian/Alaska Native Children Exposed to Violence, 2014). However, it should be noted that most of the studies into Indigenous PTSD have been conducted with Native Americans of the Plains or Southwest, and it is unclear if these results are generalizable.

To reiterate, about 40 percent of people who are exposed to a traumatic event develop PTSD. This equates to 6.6 percent of the US population, but prevalence varies by both type of trauma and gender. PTSD and related nightmares are particularly notable among veterans: 97 percent of Northern Plains veterans with combat-related PTSD report nightmares (Shore, Orton & Manson, 2009). This is a much higher rate than for non-Native combat veterans. Clinicians working with

Native American veterans experiencing PTSD and nightmares need to understand the cultural context of their dreams. There are tribal differences in the meaning, role, and context of dreams, but generally they serve important emotional and spiritual functions. Some are believed to contain messages for the dreamer, spirits may communicate through dreams, and dreams may reveal the future (Shore et al., 2009).

The prevailing social climate that devalues Native American Peoples and cultures can lead Native people to internalize negative self-images. Media representations of Native Americans depicted in stereotypical and historical ways influence how young Native people think about what is possible for themselves (Leavitt et al., 2015). It is important to counteract demoralizing influences with empowerment and restore lost roles. Traditional roles have been undermined by government policies, leaving Native men marginalized and with no visible representation in society. Moreover, while they were stripped of these traditional roles, patriarchal systems of government were introduced that privileged men's leadership in tribal governance and fostered male dominance in Indigenous communities. Boys and young men may be socialized into domineering forms of masculinity portrayed in mainstream media and based on observations of their non-Native peers (Ball, 2010).

Just as internalized oppression can lead Native Americans to denigrate aspects of Indigenous cultures and Peoples, it can also lead them to turn this oppression upon themselves. This can result in depression, high-risk behavior, and self-harm. Intergenerational trauma contributes to high rates of suicide among Native American people (Indian Health Service, 2018b). Native Americans have the second-highest suicide rate in the country at 13.5 per 100,000 individuals, just behind Whites (15.2 per 100,000). This rate is more than double those for other populations of color (American Foundation for Suicide Prevention, 2018). It should be noted that many suicides go unrecognized or unreported, and that Native American suicide rates vary significantly depending on age, gender, tribe, and region. Therefore, in addition to the gaps in what is known about suicide among Indigenous people, it would be inappropriate to generalize about all Native Americans on the basis of information that is collected on one sub-population.

Substance misuse

Traumatic experiences are often directly linked to substance misuse (Myhra & Wieling, 2014). Historically, colonizers used alcohol to debilitate Native people. Susceptibility to misuse was exacerbated by traumatic exposure and access was facilitated by settlers who deliberately encouraged intoxication as a way to cloud judgement and enable unscrupulous dealings (Carlson, 2010). Indeed, Benjamin Franklin made explicit references to rum as likely to clear the land of Indigenous Peoples (Szlemko, Wood & Thurman, 2006).

Substance misuse is intertwined with disproportionate rates of violence, suicide, accidental injuries, and death (Sarche et al., 2017). Native Americans tend to have higher rates of alcohol use because they are exposed to more risk factors, such as poverty, family history of alcohol use, and peer behavior (Szlemko et al., 2006). People exposed to trauma, especially at a young age, often seek to escape traumatic memories through the numbing effects of drugs and alcohol (Lucero & Bussey, 2015). For combat veterans with PTSD, alcohol may be used in the hope of encouraging sleep and blocking out nightmares (Shore et al., 2009).

Contemporary trauma and substance misuse are exacerbated by intergenerational historical trauma, which is heightened by the cumulative effects of detrimental and racist policies directed against Indigenous Peoples. This combination of contemporary and historical stressors affects the wellness of Native Americans and their ability to meet life challenges successfully (Lucero & Bussey, 2015).

While many researchers and practitioners believe historical trauma makes a substantial contribution to Native American substance misuse, others believe that contemporary trauma may play a larger role (Lane & Simmons, 2011). Native youth may lack alternative coping skills and turn to drugs to manage stress. A lack of culturally relevant mental health and substance misuse resources in urban areas contributes to youth drug use and consequently increases the risk of contracting HIV (Pearce et al., 2015).

Identity is often shaped through experiences of racism. This has an impact on an individual's sense of self and belonging. In Myhra's (2011) study of Native American sobriety programs, all but one participant had experienced foster care or adoptive placements with White families. Many had heard only negative things about Native people and reacted with shame and disappointment when learning they themselves were Native. One poured baby powder on herself, proclaiming that she was not Native American, while another expressed fear. For the latter woman, realizing she was a member of the group she had been groomed to fear was both confusing and traumatizing. Most said they wanted to numb themselves against racism, discrimination, and the cumulative stress related to historical trauma through alcohol and drugs. In foster care and adoptive placements, most experienced significant abuse and were exposed to derogatory comments about their biological families. Many ultimately returned home seeking answers and reconnection.

There is a complex picture of substance use in Native communities. In general, the research documents higher rates of use and earlier onset in adolescents, but disparities vary across the studies. Some show adult substance use is lower in Native communities than the general population, but those who do drink often have a pattern of heavy, episodic drinking (Whitesell et al., 2012). As noted earlier, Native Americans also tend to have high tobacco use. There is diversity in rates and patterns across Native American groups for all substances, with some tribal communities displaying higher rates, while others have lower rates than the general population (Whitesell et al., 2012). Discharge from IHS hospitals with an alcohol-related diagnosis is higher for Northern reservations than those in the Southwest and occur twice as often for men as women, illustrating that level of use can vary according to both gender and region (Szlemko et al., 2006). Native adults suffer a higher rate of alcohol-related death than the general population, although once again this varies across tribes. Native adolescents have a higher lifetime prevalence of alcohol use than their non-Native peers, as well as earlier onset of use. They also tend to drink alcohol in greater quantities and experience more negative consequences (Szlemko et al., 2006).

The link between substance misuse and historical trauma is not fully understood (Myhra, 2011; Szlemko et al., 2006). No single theory of alcohol use adequately captures all of the risk and protective factors. It is important to examine both risk and resilience, including how these may be transmitted intergenerationally, and how alcohol use varies across tribes. In spite of the grim statistics, it is worth reemphasizing that not all Native Americans misuse alcohol. Indeed, they have an unusually high rate of abstinence from alcohol use.

Interventions

Moss emphasized that helping professionals cannot claim to provide culturally competent care without understanding their clients' cultures. She pointed out that many Native American people are misidentified in federal, state, and regional records, although it is impossible to know the magnitude of these errors. Moss recalled receiving care at a reservation-based hospital then noting that the discharge paperwork identified her as White. She pointed out the irony that "many people live their whole lives as Native, then die as White" because miscoding identity at death happens much more frequently for Native Americans than any other ethnic group. As a nurse educator, she tells her students, "Ask everyone in front of you how they want to identify. You *must* ask."

Brave Heart noted that ignorance persists among service providers, even in areas with large Native populations. Native Americans encounter many daily stressors that may trigger past trauma, including microaggressions and offensive content in the media, such as the common assertion that "we are a nation of immigrants." Brave Heart also emphasized that Native American people have experienced and continue to experience extensive trauma. In very traumatized communities, problems like interpersonal violence can be common occurrences. Service providers must be prepared to handle difficult or even overwhelming life circumstances in ways that do not stigmatize Native people. They should be equipped to provide a range of referrals and must approach Native clients with cultural humility and a willingness to learn from them. It is important to recognize the strengths of tribal cultures in spite of impositions and losses. There is wisdom grounded in culture. In the past, traditional practices were prohibited and prevalent racism brainwashed some Native people to believe that their practices were wrong, yet they persist and remain sources of strength and resilience.

An increasing number of helping professionals and scholars attribute the disproportionate psychological distress experienced by Native Americans to the trauma that is always inherent in colonization (Duran, 2006; Brave Heart & DeBruyn, 1998). Intense traumatic events may lead Native people to dwell on historical losses (Tucker, Wingate & O'Keefe, 2016). Understanding intertribal differences can help clinicians identify which Native Americans are most likely to experience historical loss thinking and depressive symptoms.

Ineffective helping professionals and service gaps

Mental health disparities persist and interventions have been largely ineffective for Native Americans. Providers must recognize historical trauma and its multifaceted effects in order to understand and address these concerns (Struthers & Lowe, 2003). Healing from historical trauma must include culturally appropriate strategies.

Children's mental health needs often go unmet. Native American children do not receive the same treatment options as their non-Native peers. For example, Native youth are more likely to receive mental health treatment through the juvenile justice system and inpatient facilities, be treated in a facility with few specialized children's mental health professionals, and enter systems with inconsistent attention to established standards of care (BigFoot & Schmidt, 2010).

The mental health needs of Indigenous adults are also inadequately addressed. Treatment options for Native Americans with mental health concerns are often limited and may be distant from tribal communities. Privacy may be a concern in small tribal communities, the quality of care may be substandard, and services may be hindered by a lack of communication and trust in providers (Tsosie et al., 2011).

Lack of attention to the unique history and social conditions of individual tribes has been cited as a reason for the failure of substance misuse interventions (Lane & Simmons, 2011). Indeed, treatment for alcohol misuse that does not consider the historical context can actually aggravate the effects of historical trauma. Evaluation and treatment approaches continue to be rooted in European American cultural values, mirroring attempts at assimilation that have caused and exacerbated significant trauma (Szlemko et al., 2006).

In a study on sobriety (Myhra, 2011), many Native Americans thought of themselves as outsiders in society, attributing their substance use to feelings of alienation. Some began learning Indigenous cultural and spiritual practices for the first time or made efforts to reconnect with family members as part of their healing and recovery. These actions helped them find a place in their communities, but they also have the potential to exacerbate a sense of disconnection if they lead people to question their legitimacy as Indigenous community members.

Disproportionate rates of violence and health disparities often obscure tremendous resilience and transcendence of oppression (Burnette & Figley, 2017). The White Buffalo Calf Woman's Society opened the first reservation-based domestic violence shelter in the United States on the Rosebud Reservation in 1977 (Jones, 2008). Unfortunately, such services have not been replicated everywhere. For instance, women from Alaska's 229 federally recognized Nations are served by just one adult shelter; this in a state where domestic violence rates are ten times higher than those in the lower forty-eight (American Indian Law and Order Commission, 2015). Moreover, there are no juvenile shelters in Alaska.

Services for domestic violence survivors are crucial, but preventive services and societal change that minimizes the risk of violence are equally important. A study of domestic violence among Native Americans in southern California found that better employment opportunities could help prevent family violence in isolated rural areas (Jones, 2008). More preventive mechanisms must be identified, followed by services and societal initiatives that are specifically designed to reduce violence.

Mitigating injustice and closing the public safety gap

There are glimmers of hope with respect to policy change. Complicated jurisdictional issues were among a number of factors that led US federal courts to decline to prosecute 67 percent of the sexual assault cases that occurred on reservations (Edwards, 2017). The Tribal Law and Order Act (TLOA) now provides for more transparency when cases are declined (American Indian Law and Order Commission, 2015). This Act received bipartisan support and was signed into law in 2010. It holds federal agencies more accountable for services in Indigenous territories and provides more flexibility for tribes to design and implement their own criminal justice systems, including more sentencing options and enforcement training (American Indian Law and Order Commission, 2015). However, the American Indian Law and Order Commission acknowledges that the greatest challenges to equal justice for Indigenous Peoples on tribal lands are due to structural, longstanding issues that cannot be addressed under the terms of the TLOA. Remaining obstacles include systemic underfunding, ongoing jurisdictional complexity, and inadequate numbers of federal judges and courts. In addition, federal officials still have limited accountability and there is a lack of respect for tribal sovereignty. The TLOA did at least create an independent commission to advise Congress and the President on structural changes to enhance safety (American Indian Law and Order Commission, 2015).

After a comprehensive assessment of public safety and criminal justice for Native Americans, the American Indian Law and Order Commission (2015) held the federal government largely responsible for the public safety gap in Native America, both directly and indirectly through the transfer of criminal jurisdiction under PL 280 (a law, described in more detail in Chapter 8, that allowed some states to assert legal jurisdiction on reservations). Responsibility for justice is remote rather than community-based, which also undermines safety. There are few resources and little local accountability. The Commission described its recommendations for jurisdictional reform as "bringing clarity out of chaos" (American Indian Law and Order Commission, 2015, p. 23) and insisted that all tribes, including those in PL 280 states, should be able to resume federal criminal jurisdiction, except for laws with general application. In addition, both Native and non-Native criminal defendants should have the right of direct appeal from tribal court to federal court for alleged constitutional rights violations. Further jurisdictional reforms could empower tribes to define their own laws, sentences, and remedies, liberating them from decades of reliance on courts and services that are geographically and culturally distant from tribal communities. Currently, the amended Indian Civil Rights Act gives criminal jurisdiction to tribal courts with regard to non-Native perpetrators of domestic violence, although Indigenous children enjoy no such protection. It is imperative that tribes are given full criminal jurisdiction over all perpetrators of physical and sexual abuse against children (Attorney General's Advisory Committee on American Indian/Alaska Native Children Exposed to Violence, 2014).

Understandings of violence must be rooted within the larger societal context rather than relegated to individual responsibility or seen as the norm for particular groups. Violence in communities of color is often an excuse for victim blaming and reinforcing deficit perspectives and stereotypes that paint entire communities, cultures, and Peoples as dysfunctional. This, in turn, is used to justify ignoring these communities' needs and rationalizing violence as a cultural norm rather than a phenomenon that is fed by ongoing societal factors, such as racism and oppression (Chenault, 2011).

The elements of successful interventions

Awareness of intergenerational trauma may influence how Native Americans understand and experience contemporary trauma. Those who experience trauma and substance misuse often know that their parents and ancestors did, too. They may develop a sense of pride in and grief on behalf of elders who survived adversity, even after experiencing trauma at their hands. With this frame of reference, abusive elders may be viewed as survivors rather than perpetrators. Rather than denying that elders have been abusive to others, this stance embodies forgiveness and recognition that descent from an ancestral line of survivors can be a source of strength and motivation for healing and renewal (Myhra, 2011).

As we have seen, Native Americans have high rates of recreational tobacco use, obesity, and inactivity. They also have low fruit and vegetable consumption, cancer screening, and seatbelt compliance, along with high-fat, low-fiber diets (Cobb, Espey & King, 2014). To improve Native health, the IHS must be fully funded and urban populations must be adequately included in services (Jernigan et al., 2010).

Beyond recognizing that a client is Native American, Moss stressed that there must be a mechanism to offer culturally appropriate services, such as smudging. She also noted the importance of cultural navigators to bridge services for Native Americans. Brave Heart mentioned the importance of understanding health beliefs and knowing history. Native Americans tend to be closely connected with their ancestors, so service providers must recognize and validate the wounding that is still experienced from historic events such as the 1890 massacre at Wounded Knee. Emotions affect physiological wellbeing. It is important to recognize that Native Americans remain *First Nations* with land and water rights because trauma may be triggered if this is not done.

Helping professionals should not help people adapt to their oppression. Empowerment is crucial. Native Peoples must have the resources and power to identify and implement their own priorities. Helping professionals must prioritize sovereignty and support the development of Indigenous theories, research programs, and psychotherapeutic interventions. It is insufficient for well-meaning helping professionals to work toward cultural competence. Unless sovereignty is actively supported, Western thinking will continue to be privileged and the legacy of colonization will persist (Cavalieri, 2013).

Context influences both risk and protective factors, so contextual issues, including historical and contemporary trauma, must be considered when addressing health concerns. The social work emphasis on understanding and influencing the social environment is a useful perspective to adopt when assisting individuals and reducing disparities. Interventions that strengthen families, communities, and health service systems are critical in reducing health risks (Whitesell et al., 2012).

Most research is *deficit* based and focuses on risk factors for health conditions. Shifting to a *strengths*-based approach acknowledges successful outcomes and the vast majority of Native people who do not have active substance use problems. It is also important to examine protective factors and develop interventions that build on individual, community, and cultural strengths (Whitesell et al., 2012). The social work profession's emphasis on strengths is compatible with this community mandate.

There is a need for integrative theories that span a range of academic disciplines (Whitesell et al., 2012). Valid screening and assessment tools for Native Americans must recognize that complex trauma is likely and that its origins may not be easily identified. An integrated lens that includes biological, psychodynamic, and socio-cultural theories can inform treatment and ideas about intergenerational trauma transmission (Myhra & Wieling, 2014). Regardless of whether the origin of the trauma is historical, contemporary, or a combination of the two, and whether its sequelae manifest in physical maladies, mental health issues, family dysfunction, or some other area, the impact must be considered in all settings and interventions. From a prevention perspective, however, distinctions between historical and con-temporary trauma are crucial. Recognizing and addressing sources of ongoing trauma are essential and likely to necessitate large-scale systemic change.

Recovering traditional roles and mechanisms for supporting wellbeing can be important in reclaiming and maintaining wellness. Disrupted traditional gender and parenting roles have inhibited men from becoming responsible community mem-bers and fathers. Many men whose families were affected by residential schools see themselves as lacking the necessary knowledge and skills to raise their own children (Ball, 2010). Some fathers have identified the historical disruptions caused by colonization as the source of the challenges they have experienced in developing positive, non-domineering masculine identities. Meanwhile, women have experi-enced different but equally challenging pressures. Both men and women can reclaim balance and wholeness through traditional paths to recovering Indigenous roles and values (Ball, 2010).

Individual resilience is influenced by community and context. Connection to culture can buffer the relationship between historical trauma and contemporary health disparities (Brown, 2016). Health providers have reintroduced traditional healing as effective, empowering, culturally grounded interventions (Moghaddam et al., 2013). Likewise, dream catchers form part of the tradition of many tribes. They can be used to filter out bad dreams for people struggling with nightmares (Shore et al., 2009).

Indigenous-focused programs do not necessarily reject Western knowledge and ways of helping. Critical thinking is important. Native cultures have always adapted and integrated new elements that are compatible with Indigenous values (Cavalieri, 2013). This is a form of conscious self-determination. There are many ways of pursuing and maintaining wellbeing. All options, Indigenous and Western, should be available for Native people. There are four general approaches for equity-based healthcare:

- develop partnerships with Indigenous Peoples;
- initiate action at all levels;
- pay attention to local and global histories; and
- remain vigilant of unintended consequences of strategies (Browne et al., 2016).

A sense of belonging is a protective factor that can reduce shame, sometimes resulting from boarding schools, reservations, or relocation transmitted through the generations and linked to substance misuse (Myhra, 2011; Szlemko et al., 2006). Traditional cultural practices and spirituality can support resilience and act as a protective buffer against substance misuse and mental health issues while promoting prosocial behaviors (Goodkind et al., 2012). This supports the inclusion of cultural elements in interventions and prevention efforts.

Moss advocated smudging, sweat-lodge ceremonies, and prayer as appropriate approaches for some Native patients. Spending time with elders can also be empowering as we begin to understand how they survived detrimental circumstances. Reclaiming traditions and spirituality are primary sources of hope that foster resilience. Talking circles, sweat lodges, and many tribally specific dances have therapeutic benefits for recovery from alcohol misuse (Szlemko et al., 2006). Some Native Americans have also found culturally adapted versions of Alcoholics Anonymous helpful, while protecting and respecting the Seventh Generation has been used as a powerful prevention message. Some tribes have revitalized traditions in ways that no longer tolerate alcohol misuse.

Culture promotes healing and wellness, and buffers against stress. This can be a preventive mechanism to counteract the boredom that is often cited as a reason for experimentation with drugs and alcohol (Myhra & Wieling, 2014). Holistic health approaches that include family preservation and traditional parenting are necessary. Historical loss thinking can be reframed to emphasize the importance of traditional culture. This can engender pride and empower clients to reflect on the strength and resilience associated with survival, which in turn counteracts depression (Tucker et al., 2016).

Brave Heart identified hope and resilience in recovering traditions and celebrating survival. However, she cautioned against an oversimplified glorification of resilience that dismisses the impact of trauma or sees it only as a thing of the past. Failing to acknowledge trauma can cause people to shut down. Individuals may feel stigmatized if they are perceived as insufficiently resilient. It is important to acknowledge that not everyone feels resilient and not to shut down people or diminish their voices.

Moss also emphasized that hope and resilience can be fostered by reclaiming traditions. This does not mean acting as if it is still 1800, but rather reclaiming core aspects of culture. Learning some language, even if not to the point of fluency, can be empowering. Many Native people have sought healing and wellness by reclaiming language as a central aspect of their culture. Language is power, so reclaiming it has been identified as a form of resistance and survival that counteracts cultural genocide (Lucero & Bussey, 2015).

While individuals and their needs differ, Moss noted that reclaiming any aspect of traditional culture, language, or spirituality can have health benefits. She observed that Indigenous Peoples in the Southwest are more likely to speak their languages than their counterparts in the Plains and less likely to take up smoking. Similarly, suicide is less prevalent in tribes that did not experience removals and managed to retain more of their culture. Moss has observed these connections between culture and wellness throughout her career and is currently exploring them in ongoing research.

Innovative and promising health initiatives

Both Moss and Brave Heart were asked to share their perspectives on resilience and stories of hope. The latter emphasized that the historical trauma framework has always been about hope. Acknowledging Native Americans' collective history and wounding normalizes experiences of ongoing grief and allows people to appreciate that many of their struggles are not their fault, leading to expressions of "No wonder!" Health and social disparities are not the result of individual pathology or because Indigenous people are backward; rather, they are the result of continuing oppression. Recognizing the causes of trauma and acknowledging that grief is a normal part of life allow Native people to feel better and celebrate that they are still here, recognize the wisdom that is held in traditional cultures, appreciate that all life is sacred, and let go of distorted stereotypes.

There have been multiple efforts to develop effective, culturally congruent models to support the mental health of Native Americans. The Center for Substance Abuse Prevention gathered Native educators and clinicians in the early 1990s to develop an evidence-based practice model for substance misuse prevention (Nebelkopf et al., 2011). SAMHSA has regularly offered funding to Native American programs to develop preventive mechanisms and services for physical and mental health. Likewise, Native American nursing summits have gathered data on culturally appropriate nursing services for Native Americans (Struthers & Lowe, 2003). Focus groups with Native nurses have identified several important dimensions in this framework, including caring, traditions, respect, connection, holism, trust, and spirituality.

Brave Heart noted that technology can be used to enhance wellness. Webinars, telemental health initiatives, and the behavioral health modules that are offered through the Indian Health Service can be effective vehicles for educating health professionals and delivering services. Brave Heart also highlighted the work of

Dolores Subia BigFoot, a child psychologist who directs the Indian Country Child Trauma Center, which develops culturally grounded trauma treatment protocols, outreach materials, and service delivery guidelines. Likewise, the Johns Hopkins School of Public Health has a Center for American Indian Health that has formulated initiatives to engage with Indigenous communities in the areas of adolescent health, alcohol and drug misuse prevention, early childhood development, entrepreneurship and workforce development, environmental health, injury prevention, maternal and child health, nutrition promotion and diabetes prevention, and sexual and reproductive health. In addition to its administrative locations in Baltimore and Albuquerque, it has established bases in the tribal areas of the White Mountain Apache, Navajo, and Santo Domingo Pueblo. From Brave Heart's perspective, these centers are prime examples of trauma-informed care and best practice for Native American health services.

Moss identified Wisdom Steps (www.wisdomsteps.org), a model program developed by eleven Minnesota tribes, three urban areas, and the Minnesota Board on Aging as an intervention to encourage elders to exercise and have regular check-ups. A conference attended by 500 elders featured informative presentations and distributed wellness information. In addition, participating elders were honored and each received a small gift.

In another example, Native community members and researchers collaborated to develop the Our Life intervention with the aim of promoting good mental health among youth and families by recognizing and encouraging healing from historical trauma, connecting with cultural traditions, parenting and social skill building, and working with horses to strengthen family relationships (Goodkind et al., 2012). The underlying philosophy of the program was that cultural grounding, self-esteem, coping skills, and parenting strategies can buffer daily stressors such as poverty and discrimination that lead to depression, PTSD, and substance misuse among Native youth. It encouraged parents and youth to collaborate in order to mitigate these stressors.

The "indigenist" stress-coping model, developed by Karina L. Walters, recognizes that historical trauma, cultural buffers, and health disparities are interrelated and seeks to enhance resilience by strengthening cultural identity, spirituality, and traditional healing. For example, traditional drumming can promote healing from depression. Recognizing and participating in sacred activities can also be revitalizing and healing (Brown, 2016).

A youth wellness intervention in the Pacific Northwest focused on cigarettes, marijuana, alcohol use, and other health issues. Through this intervention, youth learned to prepare traditional, nutritious food. Summer canoe journeys emerged from a grassroots tribal movement to renew culture and were implemented as a way to reach tribal youth. Participating tribes have a zero-tolerance policy toward substance misuse. Youth on the canoe journeys pledge not to use cigarettes, drugs, or alcohol. Anyone who violates this policy must face their tribal elders, who determine a punishment. If the participant does not accept this sanction, he or she must return home immediately and enroll in a substance-misuse program (Lane & Simmons, 2011).

Many scholars and activists point to decolonized diets and lifestyles as important aspects of Indigenous liberation (Brown, 2016; Lucero & Bussey, 2015). Food can be considered a type of medicine and growing it can be a form of prayer (Lucero & Bussey, 2015). The Iroquois White Corn Project was developed in the mid-1990s to reinstate white corn as a staple of the Haudenosaunee diet, rather than a food-stuff that was consumed only occasionally or ceremonially. The availability of white corn and other so-called slow foods (i.e., high-quality, locally sourced food grounded in local traditions) was conceptualized as a crucial piece of addressing Native nutrition and the diabetes epidemic. This was based on a vision of physical health, spiritual nutrition, and economic development. A wide-ranging market was developed that included world-class chefs. This enabled Indigenous farmers to support themselves and their families. The initiative garnered multi-year grants through the First Nations Development Institute. At its peak, individual consumers and over 100 restaurants and markets used white corn products. The project's founders died in 2005 and 2006, which led to temporary dormancy, but the Iroquois White Corn Project is now revitalized and operating from Ganondagan, the only historic site in New York State devoted to Native people (Iroquois White Corn, 2018).

In northern Manitoba, the Nelson House Country Food Program creates jobs, promotes community cohesion, and increases access to healthy food. Residents are employed to hunt and fish, and the resulting food is then distributed free of charge to community members, with priority given to elders, people on low incomes, those with disabilities, and single-parent families. The project serves approximately 1500 of the 2500 members of the community. In addition to providing sustenance, it promotes and maintains traditional culture. Community members are involved with regulating and protecting natural resources and work in harmony with Manitoba Conservation. Native community members and researchers created a participatory video on food sovereignty that both teaches and inspires and advocated for its distribution within schools (Thompson & Lozecznik, 2011).

Urban Native Americans in the San Francisco Bay Area are partnering with researchers to incorporate traditional healing in diabetes prevention after a Lakota corporate executive experienced a ceremony with a Navajo healer that helped his irritable bowel syndrome and left him with a general sense of revitalization (Zonana, 2016). They are testing whether incorporating Indigenous cultural elements may be more effective than standard treatments. In particular, culturally grounded interventions seek to address the cumulative historical trauma that drives unhealthy behavior among urban Native people (Zonana, 2016). This project resulted in community empowerment, a plan to construct a community center, and revitalization of and support for cultural identity.

In Alaska, Indigenous communities have been at the cutting edge of establishing village-based paraprofessional networks through a Community Health Aide Program (CHAP). In 2005, they expanded this initiative to include dental therapists, who provide routine services under off-site supervision by dentists (Cladoosby, 2017). This is an effective means to increase provider capacity in remote settings.

Moreover, Indigenous people now receive services from members of their own community who understand their language, culture, and history: 87 percent of the dental therapists in the program are Indigenous and 78 percent practice in their region of origin. In addition, in marked contrast to previously high turnover rates, the retention rate for dental therapists in Alaska over the first 11 years of the program was an impressive 81 percent (Cladoosby, 2017). There have also been efforts to incorporate dental therapists as part of a team approach to address the needs of underserved populations in Minnesota, but the American Dental Association has lobbied to slow their recruitment. The ensuing legal battles have raised issues of state jurisdiction over tribes as sovereign Nations. Blatant racism has also come to the fore. In spite of the positive initiative supporting dental health in Alaska, the President of the Alaska Dental Society recently asserted that Alaska Native oral health disparities were due to a lack of personal responsibility and suggested that "[a]ny culture that allows such disease will soon disappear and rightfully so" (quoted in Cladoosby, 2017, p. 83). This disturbing comment highlights the deep-seated racism that continues to influence policy discussions and inhibits access to good healthcare.

Access to dental care is a matter of equity. The battle for adequate care has affected tribal communities in multiple states. For example, the Alaska Dental Practice Act resulted in a legal limbo in which the dental therapists serving Native Peoples were subject to state authorization. In 2007, the Alaska Superior Court ruled that this protectionist law conflicted with federal law in that it disrupted the federal–tribal, government-to-government relationship and obstructed implementation of the federally sanctioned CHAP (Cladoosby, 2017). The Swinomish Indian Tribal Community Chair and President of the National Congress of American Indians took an unequivocal stand. He noted that tribal leaders have both a responsibility and the authority to act on behalf of tribal members, particularly children and elders with serious health needs who are denied adequate care due to the activities of professional lobbying groups (Cladoosby, 2017).

The Swinomish Tribal Council, with full community support, created its own dental health provider licensing board to adapt the federal CHAP code. This was a clear exercise of its inherent sovereignty, rooted in its responsibility to care for tribal members. The licensing board now requires providers to demonstrate cultural competence, and there is a growing momentum for similar initiatives in other regions (Cladoosby, 2017).

Promoting wellness through policy and structural change

Structural and policy change are necessary components of reducing health disparities and enhancing wellness. For example, juvenile justice systems must be reformed. Juveniles in federal detention should not only be allowed parole and secondary education; they should also have access to wellness and diversion programs as incentivized rehabilitation (American Indian Law and Order Commission, 2015).

Moss voiced the need for structural change in order to reduce health disparities. Specifically, she identified the importance of funding. The federal government must recognize and honor treaty-based promises. She noted that the IHS usually receives only 40–50 percent of the funding it requires to address health needs, yet it is well documented that Native Americans suffer more illness than the general population and are disproportionately affected by chronic diseases. Substantial policy change is a crucial component of ameliorating these health disparities. Indeed, even though the American Indian Law and Order Commission identified a severe public safety crisis among Native Americans, it emphasized that this is not an intractable problem. It highlighted "breathtaking possibilities for safer, strong Native communities achieved through home-grown, Tribally based systems that respect the civil rights of all US citizens and reject outmoded command-and-control policies in favor of increased local control, accountability and transparency" (American Indian Law and Order Commission, 2015, p. 46).

Both Moss and Brave Heart emphasized the need for leadership in various health arenas. The former pointed to multiple vacancies and interim appointments within the IHS, creating and perpetuating a void in leadership at a time when advocacy is crucial. Leadership is needed at all levels. Brave Heart spoke of the need to be courageous on behalf of our people and to take on the difficult work of healing. As whole Nations, we must be "brave enough to talk" about all the pain and suffering. This work begins internally, with Indigenous people identifying the needs and priorities in their own communities. Simultaneously, external allies, service providers, and policy makers must insure that the necessary infrastructure and funding are available for these priorities to be recognized, honored, and addressed.

Trauma-informed care

Brave Heart noted that we are living in an era that can be particularly triggering for Native Americans. She pointed out that recent confrontations, such as the militaristic response to "water protectors" near Standing Rock Reservation in 2016, may elicit memories of historical trauma, such as the Wounded Knee Massacre.

As noted above, violence, blatant racism, and microagressions are all common occurrences for many Native Americans and other Indigenous Peoples around the world. Service providers must work to create a climate of safety for Indigenous clients but perhaps more importantly must work toward societal change to promote their security. Violence reduction must happen within a context of renewed support for sovereignty. Reducing oppression will, in turn, reduce the triggers that exacerbate mental health concerns and substance misuse.

We must all work toward increasing trustworthiness within a context of collaboration. This chapter has presented examples of communities striving to increase healthy food options and access to dental care that were undermined or quashed by rigid regulations and powerful lobby groups. Such actions are antithetical to collaboration and perpetuate an environment where trust is impossible. Striving for trauma-informed healthcare necessitates confronting such barriers.

Empowerment includes supporting sovereignty and the ability of Indigenous Nations and communities to develop and implement health services that meet the needs of their members. Service providers must facilitate access to a variety of options for preventive and healthcare services. These principles apply not only in the United States but around the world.

Conclusion

This chapter has examined holistic perspectives of wellness within an Indigenous worldview as well as statistics on health disparities experienced by Native Americans. These are understood within the context of structural determinants of health and federal health policies anchored in the federal trust responsibility. The chapter also reviewed considerations for interventions, promising initiatives, and trauma-informed care.

It is worth noting that some health disparities are actually increasing. Progress toward reducing morbidity and mortality for Native Americans often lags behind advances for their non-Native peers. The state of wellbeing for Indigenous Peoples is alarming, but at the same time it is important not to lose sight of resilience and strength. These are important considerations for both clinicians and policy makers. It is crucial to be aware of how structural determinants of health and the policy context affect health, and both should be targets for change.

Meaningful large-scale change in Indigenous wellness will be impossible without political will. There are many small-scale, creative programs that bolster wellness, but these are largely unknown outside their immediate localities. Innovative, culturally relevant, trauma-informed interventions must be highlighted and brought to the fore as models. One way to do this is for academics, researchers, and other allies to reach out to communities and learn more about local programs. While honoring local priorities, they may be able to assist communities to obtain funding and technical support for their initiatives, ultimately highlighting and potentially replicating model programs. Making a genuine difference will require addressing structural determinants of health and eliminating the ongoing oppression and discrimination that continue to fuel trauma. Both structural change and trauma-informed interventions are essential in promoting wellness among Native Americans.

8

THE WELLBEING OF COMMUNITIES, PEOPLES, AND THE NATURAL WORLD

Indigenous Peoples often identify themselves according to their social relationships and community connections. Interdependence is valued and individual wellness inextricably intertwined with community wellbeing. A sense of group consciousness can underpin identity and is reflected in these connections to the social and natural environment. If the larger community and environment are unhealthy, this limits the wellbeing of all individuals. Accordingly, individualistic understandings of concepts like self-sufficiency must be reframed for relevance within Indigenous contexts.

The phrase "Native community" is frequently used to refer to people with a shared Indigenous identity grounded within this group consciousness, not necessarily defined by geographic boundaries. For example, members of an urban Native American community may or may not be clustered within a particular neighborhood. The same phrase may refer to a tribe, a reservation, or particular settlements on a reservation. It is also important to understand that "community" can carry a variety of meanings. It is not one thing. There are often multiple perspectives and interests within Indigenous communities (Wiebe, 2016).

This chapter explores wellbeing within the social environment. It includes an examination of expressions of contemporary sovereignty and Indigenous governance, and the impact of wider society on Indigenous wellbeing. Economic status and development opportunities are explored. The chapter also examines the importance of the physical environment for American Indian wellbeing, including a discussion of the meaning of the natural world and trauma associated with environmental damage.

Subject-matter experts Ada Deer and Dr. Eddie Brown shared their perspectives for this chapter. Both bring decades of experience working in tribal communities and as presidential appointees in the US federal government. They possess expertise in federal policy development and change as well as tribal governance. Their insights and examples of their ground-breaking work are shared below.

Brown, Professor Emeritus within the College of Liberal Arts and Sciences at Arizona State University (ASU), is Yaqui and O'odham and an enrolled member of the Pascua Yaqui Tribe. He has served as a political appointee and cabinet member at the highest administrative levels within federal, state, and tribal governments. For instance, he is the former Assistant Secretary of Indian Affairs, United States Department of Interior, Executive Director of the Tohono O'odham Department of Health and Human Services, and Director of the Arizona Department of Economic Security. He also served as Executive Director of the American Indian Policy Institute at ASU and Associate Dean/Director of the George Warren Brown School of Social Work, Kathryn M. Buder Center on American Indian Studies, Washington University, St. Louis. He has studied the impact of welfare reform on American Indian families and children, the mental health of American Indian youth, diabetes prevention in tribal communities, Title IV-E state–tribal agreements, and state ICWA compliance issues. He is nationally recognized for his knowledge and skills in working with tribal governments and community development programs. He served as Co-chair of the National Congress of American Indians' National Research Center's advisory board and currently sits on the board of directors of the Tohono O'odham Nation's gaming enterprise.

Brown was raised off-reservation and grew up with limited tribal connections and little sense of what it meant to be Native American. In college, he met American Indian students and alumni from across the United States and Canada, many of whom later held high-level positions. He became active in the student body and politics, soon questioning how best to make an impact on behalf of American Indian people. He considered business and law after feeling insulted when someone suggested social work as a career, but soon learned that classes in community organizing, social policy, planning, and administration could be pathways to change. The 1960s and 1970s saw significant policy developments, such as the Indian Child Welfare Act and the Indian Self-Determination Act. Brown was inspired by American Indian activists, and after earning his doctorate he was asked to craft a proposal that was subsequently funded to develop a mechanism to give tribes direct access to federal funding allocated for state block grants. For a tribe to seek money from a state would violate the government-to-government relationship between the tribes and federal government. Brown was soon asked to fill a new position created by Governor Bruce Babbit to define how Arizona would interact with tribes in various arenas.

Deer was the first member of the Menominee Tribe to earn an undergraduate degree at the University of Wisconsin and the first American Indian to earn a master's degree in social work at Columbia University. A lifelong activist, she has assumed leadership roles in the restoration of her tribe after their termination (see discussion of the termination policy in Chapter 2 and further details of the Menominee termination later in this chapter). She was the first woman to hold the post of Assistant Secretary of Indian Affairs, United States Department of Interior, and the first to be elected Chair of the Menominee Tribe. Among numerous honors, she received the Helen Marks Dicks Excellency in Advocacy Award from the Wisconsin Women's Network for her advocacy and commitment to advancing the status of women and girls. She recently retired from the positions of Distinguished Lecturer at the School of Social Work and Director of the American Indian Studies Program, University of Wisconsin.

Deer's life path was heavily shaped by her parents. Her father attended boarding school after the death of his mother in the flu pandemic following World War I. Thereafter, his life was dominated by two emotions: rage and shame. Deer's mother, a White Quaker nurse, was enthralled with American Indians, appreciated cultural differences, and took an interest in tribal affairs. By the time Deer was in grade school, her mother was taking her to meetings of the advisory council—the governing body composed of twelve Menominee men. Deer remembered these meetings as "people talking big stuff." In high school, Deer was intrigued by what she learned about governance. She received the Menominee Tribal Scholarship for college and was determined to repay her tribe for this honor. She was a sophomore at the University of Wisconsin when the Menominee Termination Act was passed. Her mother badgered her with letters about the termination, emphasizing that no one understood the implications of this piece of legislation. Deer's passion for helping people, her interest in government, and her concerns over tribal termination were the catalysts for a life and career grounded in activism.

Contemporary sovereignty and governance

Native Americans are unique among groups in the United States given their membership of distinct tribal Nations with histories and their continued ability to self-govern. While significant encroachment has hindered self-governance, many contemporary Indigenous communities strive for empowerment, restoration, and healing. They seek to strengthen their ability to act as sovereign entities with defined boundaries and powers.

Washburn (2017) argues that the federal understanding of the trust responsibility has moved from a foundation of paternalism to a sense of obligation to support and revitalize tribal governments. This includes advocating for and protecting sovereign powers. For example, he highlights the shift of criminal jurisdiction to tribes as a reversal of longstanding policy. He also points to federal contracting with tribes to fulfill trust functions—a change that has led to more relevant and effective programs. The current US role as the principal underwriter of tribal services can be viewed as a means of fulfilling the federal trust responsibility.

Rebuilding a Nation: an examination of Menominee termination and restoration

Deer recounted the process of termination and restoration of her tribe. The Menominee were the first American Indian tribe to be terminated by the US federal government. The termination Bill was passed by Congress in 1954 after the tribe won a $8.5 million judgement for violation of the federal trust responsibility over timber sales. When the money was added to the tribal budget, a US Senator enticed Menominee people with the lure of immediate cash. The money was distributed as $1500 per capita payments. Unbeknown to most people, however, these payments were linked to tribal termination. Deer noted that when tribal members understood the proposed legislation had implications beyond payment from the breach-of-trust lawsuit, 800 of them signed a petition to reverse their votes, but by then it was too late.

The subsequent termination was devastating. Deer reported that some people died when they could not get medical care and others left the area when they no longer had a reservation. Some former tribal members were unable to pay their taxes and their land was sold. Under the terms of the termination, Menominee people became certificate holders who were able to elect members to a voting trust, which, in turn, elected a board of directors. Menominee people were largely shut out of their own governance, and a land developer began selling vacation plots on the former reservation. Deer was aghast that land was being sold and the people had no say in the matter. She heard that Menominee people were organizing meetings and felt compelled to get involved.

Final implementation of Menominee termination took effect in 1961. Deer sought guidance from a legal services organization to explain the implications and decided that "something has got to be done—the question is what?" She reasoned that since termination was a law, another law could be passed to rescind it. She understood this would mean going through Congress and was advised that the timeframe for change was quickly waning.

Deer and other activists waged a proxy campaign seeking agreement from Menominee people to vote their certificate shares. They visited prisons and urban areas and ultimately secured enough proxies to elect two members to the voting trust, including Deer herself. Although many were involved in the effort, Deer became the spokesperson for the activist group Determination of Rights and Unity for Menominee Shareholders (DRUMS) as many other members had limited education.

Deer noted that the Menominee had to determine the type of government they wanted. In consultation with lawyers from the Native American Rights Fund, they developed a constitution and a body of law. Once they had drafted the terms of their restoration, they met with Senator Ted Kennedy, explained the termination, and sought his support. Deer dropped out of law school and volunteered to go to Washington, DC, where she lobbied many Senators to get the Act introduced in Congress. Due to the efforts of many Menominee people, the Act passed the House in 1973, received full Senate approval, and was signed into law by President Nixon on December 7, 1973. It is difficult to overestimate the significance of the Menominee Restoration Act. It was a landmark in federal Indian policy that paved the way to overturn other terminations.

Restoration of tribal status was momentous, but it was just the beginning of a long internal process. Deer chaired her tribe's restoration committee, which had to empower and engage people, elect officers, and form other committees. For example, there was a constitution committee (which Deer initially chaired), while eligibility for tribal membership and a mechanism to process applications were determined by an enrollment committee. Likewise, a health committee was formed and charged with developing a clinic and services.

Contemporary Nation building and partnerships

Nation building is a key component of sovereignty and governance. Large-scale restoration parallels individual empowerment. Asserting sovereignty is a crucial element in healing from trauma for Native communities. Rather than being passive, Native Americans are empowered agents, actively engaged in building a future for subsequent generations (Hartmann & Gone, 2014). In the past, tribal efforts have been hindered by a hostile context. During the early twenty-first century, a combination of federal commitment to self-determination and successful economic development for some tribes led to more external recognition of the authority and legitimacy of tribal governments. New interpretations of the federal trust responsibility have led to non-interference in tribal prerogatives, increased consultation, and strengthening of government-to-government relationships (Washburn, 2017). Notwithstanding these shifts, however, vestiges of federal paternalism remain, including mandates that tribal initiatives must be subject to federal approval.

For much of US history, the trust responsibility has translated into substantial federal control. Federal officials made many decisions on reservations, leaving little authority for tribal governments. This shifted with passage of the Indian Reorganization Act (IRA) and its recognition of the limits of federal power in addressing the needs of Native Peoples. This Act represented an updated perspective on the federal trust responsibility that incorporated a central role for tribal governments in identifying their needs and serving their people (Washburn, 2017). Although these advances dissipated in the era of termination, the War on Poverty and its emphasis on grassroots self-determination represented another pendulum swing back toward tribal empowerment.

More recently, federal control has continued to recede and there has been more recognition of tribal priorities and decision making. Under the Obama administration, the courts held the federal government less accountable for its actions and inaction, while Congress and the President increased funding for programs associated with the federal trust responsibility (Washburn, 2017). It is also noteworthy that the federal government has settled dozens of lawsuits brought by tribes alleging breach-of-trust actions rather than try to defend them in court. This could be considered a transfer in responsibility for federal trust obligations from the courts to the political branches (Washburn, 2017). Under these circumstances, presidential administrations are likely to have more sway over how the trust responsibility is implemented.

Brown spoke extensively about the importance of partnerships. As an American Indian with a doctorate at a time when many new programs were being developed, he was frequently asked to work with federal and state authorities on government projects related to Native Americans. He worked closely with Senator Inouye, Chairman of the Senate Indian Affairs Committee, and Senator McCain from his home state of Arizona. Brown became something of a jack of all trades, helping shape initiatives on aging, health, and tribal self-determination. His doctorate gave him credibility in non-Native contexts and he was frequently called to testify about the issues and needs of Native Peoples. He was particularly involved in developing programs and policies related to American Indians in Arizona. His early work with the state helped convince other states to work with American Indian liaison officers. States must provide mechanisms for tribes to participate in each and every area where they have a stake. In short, there must be a seat at the table for Indigenous Peoples. This is now much more common than in previous decades.

Brown particularly emphasized the need for tribally driven partnerships between universities and American Indian communities. Research priorities must be set by tribal Nations. As an American Indian academic, he was able to open the door for community-based partnerships in which tribes are fully involved in all aspects of data collection, review, and publications. In a similar model, five Indigenous Nations partnered with the Obama administration to develop protections and National Monument status for Bears Ears—a sacred area for multiple tribes in the Southwest (Utah Dine Bikeyah, 2018).

Barriers to self-governance

In spite of supportive policy shifts, there remain substantial barriers to recognition of sovereignty and implementation of self-governance for Indigenous Peoples. The ongoing legacy and impact of colonization must not be underestimated. On close examination, it is apparent that this continues to influence definitions of who is Indigenous, tribal membership, land boundaries, governance models, rights to traditional lifestyles (e.g., hunting and access to medicines), and external recognition. Even documents and treaties that Native Americans cite as protecting their rights are based on external laws and legal systems and rely on someone else's ratification (Carlson, 2010).

While most Native American tribes have retained some form of self-governance that is now being reinvigorated, other Indigenous populations have rather weaker foundations on which to build. For example, the Metis in Canada are currently recognized as rights-bearing people along with First Nations and Inuit. Their right to self-governance is recognized in federal policy, yet they have had difficulty realizing this right and their right to land without a constitution. Therefore, they are now in the process of drafting one in the hope of forging a government-to-government relationship and increasing recognition of their legitimacy. Many Metis view this constitution as a tool to define and strengthen their internal governance as well as a way to improve their position externally (Dubois & Saunders, 2017).

Another Canadian example is instructive. The Indian Act defined Native governance structures according to colonial models that included politically divisive elections (Carlson, 2010). Under the colonial system, tribal membership links people to certain tracts of land. The mandate that people belong in certain places leaves many feeling they can no longer connect with other land and/or family members elsewhere. This restricts freedom of movement, including relocating, visiting, and seasonal resource gathering. There is continuing community pain from the seemingly arbitrary locating of people. Dividing reserves undermines regional affiliations as well as family identities (Carlson, 2010). Various churches have also contributed to defining and fracturing communities. They not only rejected so-called paganism but specifically sought to remove communities from perceived social evils and vices of frontier society, such as alcohol, which first created then exacerbated isolation. Likewise, registration criteria under the Indian Act led to declining populations and further undermined political capacity and an ability to assert rights. This reinforced the colonial perception that Indigenous populations were a vanishing race and the belief that their concerns would vanish, too (Carlson, 2010).

Territorial control

True sovereignty would encompass control over citizens, laws, and programs as well as land, water, and other natural resources. Governance questions—such as who should manage, benefit from, or suffer the impact of resource extraction?— often arise in the context of environmental issues. Increasing recognition of Indigenous title and land claims raises the profile of these questions and obliges industry, various levels of government, and environmental groups to enter into dialogue with Native Nations. This brings foundational issues of governance and sovereignty to the fore (Low & Shaw, 2011).

Native people demand both rights and recognition. There is significant potential in transnational agreements that have been developed around environmental concerns, such as endangered species, water management, preserving biodiversity, and climate change. Various co-management practices have also been developed on regional levels that bridge cultures, values, and knowledge systems. These issues often arise in postcolonial situations and must be addressed by Indigenous Peoples and settler societies around the world (Low & Shaw, 2011).

Control over territory is a central aspect of sovereignty and self-governance but one that has been severely undermined by colonization. The complexity of Native American land ownership promotes a self-perpetuating, expanding, inefficient cycle of federal control. Native American land has been subjected to checkerboarding (see discussion of the Dawes Act in Chapter 2) and Indian law's idiosyncrasies, resulting in an extraordinary level of regulation that leads to both rigidity and uncertainty. This complexity has led to landowner withdrawal, bureaucratic growth, and democratic inertia. Fractionated heirship continues to be problematic, too (Shoemaker, 2017). Fractionation is a form of extreme co-ownership that is due to generations of distributions to multiple heirs and inflexible transfer options. Congress actively sought to eliminate this problem between 1992 and 2010, yet it roughly doubled in that period and continues to increase. For example, a 40-acre trust parcel with 439 co-owners in 1987 had 505 co-owners by 2004. The complexity of the reservation land tenure system contributes to economic and social disparities. More than half of jointly owned trust lands are either idle or generate no income, but it is often too expensive and too difficult to navigate the legal landscape:

> Everything we know about property and sovereignty applies differently in the unique legal spaces of American Indian reservations ... Different sovereigns define and regulate different properties within reservation territories. Property jurisdiction varies parcel by parcel depending on factors invisible to an outside observer, including the owner's identity and the land's legal tenure status. Within reservations, land is owned by both Indian and non-Indians and held in both "fee" and "trust" tenure statuses. Indian-owned fee lands are subject to tribal and some state law. Indian-owned trust lands are federally governed, with some tribal role. Non-Indians' fee lands are subject to varying degrees of state and tribal control, depending on a list of still other factors. The result is a strange and hard-to-predict mix of tribal, state, and federal property jurisdictions swirled together within reservation spaces.
>
> *(Shoemaker, 2017, p. 489)*

The current land tenure system on reservations is rooted in allotment and external values of individualism and property ownership. Under this complex system, a house can be in fee status owned by one person while the land on which it sits is in trust status owned by multiple people. Land with differential status becomes extraordinarily problematic when probate is necessary. Federal control and complicated jurisdictional issues undermine innovative, culturally grounded opportunities for environmental stewardship. Recent land tenure reforms promulgated by the federal government are presented as beneficial but are likely to have adverse consequences and increase the complexity. Support for true tribal sovereignty and self-governance would allow tribes to develop more effective solutions to meet their own needs (Shoemaker, 2017).

Like land rights, water usage and governance are often a murky mixture of tribal, state, and federal authority. Maine's authority to regulate water on tribal territories remains especially contentious, particularly in the context of Indigenous fishing rights (Marass, 2017). Many tribes do not have their own water quality standards. One way to close the regulatory gap would be for the Federal Environmental Protection Authority to promulgate standards (Lee, 2017). However, this option would fail to maximize the potential inherent in Indigenous sovereignty.

In other parts of the country, states cannot assert authority over water on tribal lands. For example, there are 19 pueblos along the Rio Grande in New Mexico. Legal cases have ruled that their water rights fall under federal rather than state law and are thus prior to other interests. Most cases that have been litigated have ended in negotiated settlements, which means no definitive ruling is rendered on the nature or extent of pueblo rights (Hughes, 2017).

First Nations communities in Canada view drinking water quality as a persistent problem, and one-quarter of all drinking water systems in these communities pose significant risks to human health (Baird et al., 2015). Unsurprisingly, boil-water advisories are common. Various funding initiatives have led to some progress, but the problem has yet to be resolved. Disparities in water quality are more than an ecological issue for Indigenous communities; they are a matter of justice. The relationship between these communities and water is substantial and complex, integral to all aspects of creation.

The challenges and promise of decolonizing governance structures

Decolonization is a prerequisite for healthy Native communities and nation building. Many current tribal systems replicate mainstream approaches to criminal justice, law enforcement, and prosecution systems in problematic ways (Chenault, 2011). Rather than imported, colonized models, Native people can draw on traditional values and approaches to develop their own models that are relevant for their contemporary circumstances.

Contemporary tribal governments are interconnected with federal, state, and local governments and will never return to the isolation that existed before colonial contact. On the other hand, some tribal governments are stronger now than they have been since the inception of the United States. A contemporary tribal renaissance has led to improvements in both federal and tribal governments. A secondary benefit of tribal governments running federally sponsored programs is an increase in their administrative capacity and skills (Washburn, 2017).

As Native Nations work to decolonize their governance structures, most are not starting from scratch, as Deer described with respect to the Menominee. All, however, have an opportunity for reform and revitalization. The experiences of Coast Salish communities in Canada provide an instructive example of the process of decolonizing tribal governance. These communities took steps to replace elected governance systems dictated by the Indian Act with a model based on their own traditional principles and system of extended family governance (Carlson, 2010). This was done with the recognition that Indigenous political authority remains compromised after 150 years of assimilationist policies. Under these circumstances, it was challenging to reassert self-governance. Understanding colonial influences provides a lens for Indigenous people to evaluate what works and what does not work when establishing traditional decolonized governance:

> What neither I nor the Shxw'ōwhámé community members fully appreciated, however, was the extent to which such improvements would be limited by the administrative, financial, and political isolation of each Stó:lō reserve community from the others. More than a century of colonial efforts at assimilating Stó:lō people had resulted in First Nations communities that were, in large part, products of colonial policies aimed at atomizing Indigenous societies and subverting Indigenous culture and governance. Reserve boundaries,

policies regarding the distribution of federal financial resources, missionary-sponsored inter-denominational feuds, and the reification of band membership lists, along with other facets of colonial history, had worked to constrain the revived siy:ám council. In particular, these colonial legacies undermined the council's ability to meaningfully involve those members of Stó:lõ extended families whose members were not recognized under the Indian Act as members of the Shxw'õwhámé band.

(Carlson, 2010, p. 3)

Indigenous sovereignty and governance in different contexts

Governance issues are distinct for Alaskan Natives in the wake of the Alaska Native Claims Settlement Act (ANSCA). Their inability to control their traditional lands hinders self-governance. As noted above, ability to control territory and membership is central to sovereign authority, but ANSCA separated these powers, leaving Alaskan tribes as "Sovereigns without territorial reach" (Kimmel, 2014, p. 180). Under these circumstances, tribal governments are unable to address issues related to community wellbeing. Alaskan Native tribes must be empowered and given the necessary resources to protect the safety and wellbeing of their members (Attorney General's Advisory Committee on American Indian/Alaska Native Children Exposed to Violence, 2014).

Unlike other US land settlements, ANSCA did not reserve governance rights on traditional lands. Its implications remained uncertain for decades until the 1998 Supreme Court decision in *Alaska v. Village of Venetie Tribal Government* deemed Alaskan Native communities to be state-chartered, state-regulated private business corporations. Under this ruling, their lands were not "Indian Country" subject to tribal governance. Therefore, ANSCA lands are beyond tribal control and subject to state regulation and taxation. Subsequent cases affirm that Alaskan Natives maintain authority over domestic relations, but even these continue to be contested by the state of Alaska (Kimmel, 2014).

This Supreme Court ruling has significant consequences. For instance, tribes are no longer permitted to manage the subsistence resources on which they depend. Unlike other tribes, Alaskan tribes have no authority to regulate environmental quality. Additionally, they do not have the authority to tax or regulate activities that may contribute to climate change. They do not even have the legal authority to improve public safety and protect their members (Kimmel, 2014).

Subsistence is at the heart of Indigenous Alaskan culture. Native people, like all rural Alaskans, are now considered stakeholders, not rights holders, in subsistence management of the 104 million acres set aside under the terms of ANSCA. On the other hand, Alaskan Natives (unlike other Alaskans) are recognized as rights holders in the taking of marine mammals, subject to federal management under the Marine Mammal Protection Act. This has led to co-management agreements between Indigenous groups and federal agencies (Kimmel, 2014).

Lack of territoriality has a deep impact on public safety. This is crucial, given that Alaska ranks first in the United States for suicide and intimate partner homicide. More than half of Alaskan women have been victims of sexual violence, yet only 30 of the state's 220 rural Native communities have courthouses and most lack public safety officers. In addition, 75 of these 220 Native villages have no law enforcement whatsoever. Access to law enforcement or shelter often means plane rides and other associated costs, leading to significant vulnerability. Lack of territorial control also has specific and dire legal consequences for tribes that are now unable to protect their communities. For example, the 2013 reauthorization of the Violence Against Women Act excludes the participation of Alaska Native tribes because there is no support for tribal jurisdiction. Therefore, the Indian Law and Order Commission Report articulated that reestablishing territorial sovereignty for Alaskan tribal governments is a crucial step in improving public safety. Alaskan Native tribes continue to fight for self-governance, including a proposed federal regulation to reestablish recognition of their lands as "Indian Country" (Kimmel, 2014). They are also asserting traditional knowledge as partners in resource management.

Indigenous people in Hawaii also have significantly less ability to assert their sovereignty and exercise self-governance than Native people in the continental United States. The federal government has exerted political and territorial control over Hawaii since 1898. Overthrow of the monarchy and annexation replaced Hawaiian control and citizenship, yet local voices have always asserted sovereignty (Siler, 2012). Hawaiians push back against being commercialized, exoticized, and having their homeland defined as a US vacation paradise. They insist on federal recognition as Indigenous people, recognition of injury, and reparations (Trask, 1993) within the context of universal human rights. Some of them are organizing politically for an independent land base, while others are pushing for completely self-governing structures or Nation-within-Nation status, as per Native Americans. In 2014, the Hawaiian Role Commission took a step toward exploring self-governance options by identifying the criteria for people to be declared Native Hawaiian and therefore able to participate in a process of organizing a governance structure. It held a convention that provided an opportunity to discuss these citizenship criteria, external recognition, and beneficiaries of the Hawaiian Homes Commission Act (Nu'uhiwa, 2013).

In Canada, Indigenous leadership has often been resistant to imposed federal policies. There are fundamental differences between the worldviews of Aboriginal and settler Canadians. Federal and provincial governments view Native communities through the lens of federalism, with each component of the Canadian government managing particular, discrete responsibilities toward Aboriginal people. They typically treat them as stakeholders rather than equal government partners. Indigenous people believe they operate on a Nation-to-Nation basis, yet policy making is grounded in federalism and the settler worldview. A new model of multilevel governance has the potential to restructure Crown–Aboriginal relationships (Alcantara & Spicer, 2016). The Kelowna Accord, a 2005 example of multilevel governance, promised $5.1

billion in support of Aboriginal issues. This ultimately went unimplemented when federal leadership changed, but it can still be a transformative model for policy making (Alcantara & Spicer, 2016).

The broader societal context

Sovereignty and the right to self-governance are crucial, but it must also be recognized that contemporary Indigenous people do not live in isolation. The broader societal context has a significant impact on Indigenous wellbeing. It is important to be conscious of the multiple dynamics of oppression that have historically supported colonization and continue to do so. The extensive systemic changes inherent in colonization affected and continue to affect Indigenous worldviews and social structures. Moving toward decolonization, social justice, and Indigenous empowerment demands close examination and understanding of the underlying ideological and structural dynamics of colonialism. Societal change at multiple levels grounded within a context of Indigenous resilience is imperative (Chenault, 2011). In spite of these challenges, it is both possible and necessary to work within this context.

The societal context shapes not only how Indigenous Peoples are perceived but how we perceive ourselves. This is evident in discussions of names and who has the right to name. Along with exerting claims to "discovered" lands, colonial explorers named the Peoples they encountered "Indians." While Indigenous Peoples have often retained names for themselves, they have also been given names by others. For example, the people of the Haudenosaunee Confederacy continue to use this label for themselves. They were also known as the Iroquois by the French and Six Nations by the British. All these names remain in use today by both Native and non-Native people. It is clear, however, that individuals often have strong preferences and may find some labels inappropriate or offensive.

Although many Indigenous people in the United States refer to themselves as "Native American," there are others who strongly believe it is appropriate to use the terms "Indian" or "American Indian," particularly as these are typically used in treaties, laws, and policies. Deer noted that "Indian" appears in the US Constitution and she believes it is important to continue to use it. She pointed out that "Indian" or "American Indian" is also used in many national organizations, including the oldest association of tribal governments—National Congress of American Indians (NCAI)—the National Indian Educational Association (NIEA), and the Association of American Indian Physicians (AAIP). While there are differing positions on preferred terminology, it is important to recognize the right to assert preferences in how we self-identify.

Asserting Indigenous needs and priorities

Deer and Brown both served in the US federal government—the former between 1993 and 1997 during Bill Clinton's administration and the latter between 1989 and 1993 during the George H.W. Bush administration. Both emphasized the importance of appreciating the role of federal government and the need for helping professionals to be skilled in working within this context.

Deer stressed that Native people and helping professionals must understand the dominant culture and how power is exerted if they wish to make a difference. She herself has worked closely with Senators, and noted that helping professionals must become familiar with politics, lobbying, and networking. They must appreciate the vast, far-reaching power of federal government and learn that congressional aides control much of the access to elected representatives. These aides make recommendations to Senators, often passing along their own biases. It is also crucial to understand how congressional committees and caucuses function and the influence they exert over the formation of policy.

Deer noted that while the existing treaties are far from perfect, they have yet to be improved upon and are crucial to the survival of American Indian Peoples. She emphasized that a variety of major policies continue to influence the wellbeing of Indigenous communities, including termination, relocation, and PL 280 (the transfer of legal jurisdiction from tribes to states, explained further below). She also noted that racism and sexism still permeate all levels of government.

Structural racism

Stereotypes and bigoted attitudes can affect how people are treated by service providers and researchers. Bias can lead to Native people experiencing differential treatment, diminished respect, and dehumanizing actions. This goes beyond individual biases and includes complicity of societal institutions, such as the Public Health Service, the Bureau of Indian Affairs, and the Indian Health Service. As an example, widespread sterilization programs were implemented without informed consent. These resulted in the sterilization of up to 42 percent of Native women of childbearing age (Chenault, 2011). Similarly, the Indian Health Service and the Bureau of Indian Affairs conducted research studies with American Indian children attending boarding schools without parental consent until well into the 1970s. Both of these agencies acted in violation of the federal trust responsibility by neglecting to provide minimal oversight and allowing researchers to engage in unethical practices (Chenault, 2011).

Societal institutions, such as legal structures and educational systems, are seen as authoritative and shape social norms in ways that reinforce symbolic violence against Indigenous Peoples. Likewise, consumer products and sports associations mirror attitudes that are codified in centuries of laws and policies that systematically depict Native people as inferior, incapable, and uncivilized. Bigoted terminology, imagery, and behavior are so normalized in US society that they are largely invisible and unwittingly supported by other marginalized people and potential allies (Robertson, 2015). Holidays like Columbus Day may be emotional triggers for Native people suffering from historical trauma, particularly as others remain oblivious to their racial connotations. Indigenous people offer counter-narratives and decolonizing tactics, such as speaking out in ways that demonstrate resilience and empowerment. These counter-narratives balance continued oppression and trauma (Robertson, 2015).

Deer noted that many Christian religions have been relentless in trying to undermine Indigenous traditions, identity, and spirituality—a process that seems destined to continue. Religious figures often disparage others in the belief that they alone have a monopoly on truth. American Indians have long borne the brunt of these efforts as Christian leaders strive to turn them into replicas of White people.

Contemporary racism is a direct descendant of overt colonial racist discourses that continue to evoke false memories of colonizers as simple settlers. Narratives of noble pioneers and bloodthirsty savages were used to legitimize colonization, slavery, and the genocide of Indigenous Peoples. Similar narratives continue to resonate and provide a foundation for contemporary views and actions. A case in point is the continued use of caricatures of Indigenous Peoples as sports mascots. Studies have documented that non-Native people believe mascots reflect the characteristics of actual American Indian people (Robertson, 2015). This type of sanctioned racism is the foundation of contemporary power and societal structures. All of the major national sports leagues use racist team names, imagery, and mascots that negatively affect the wellbeing of Native people (Steinfeldt et al., 2010). Obliviousness to the impact of appropriated names, stereotypes, and distorted images on contemporary Native people is enshrined in American society and goes well beyond sports teams. For example, car manufacturers have appropriated names like Cherokee, Dakota, and Winnebago without seeking approval. Likewise, advertising uses stereotypical logos like the Land o' Lakes Indian maiden and names like Eskimo Pie. Military weapons and codewords include Apache, Chinook, Geronimo, and Blackhawk. There is little appreciation in wider society that these names reinforce stereotypes of American Indian people as ferocious and warlike (Robertson, 2015).

Many states struggle with offensive Native names for geographic features as well as sports teams. American Indian references once went largely unnoticed, but now some lawmakers are starting to acknowledge that many of them are racist, stereotypical, and demeaning. In 2014, Oregon became the first state to require tribal permission to use any name associated with a tribe. This followed a 2012 Oregon Board of Education rule banning public school use of Native mascots, names, or images. Wisconsin, on the other hand, has passed legislation making it more difficult for school districts to change race-based logos and mascots. Both California and Washington, DC, have passed resolutions calling for a change in the name of the latter's NFL team, but this has met substantial opposition and has yet to happen (Salazar, 2014).

The implications of individual bias

Racism continues to be a significant factor in the lives of many American Indians. This is particularly prevalent in areas where Native people have a visible presence. For example, 36 percent of Native Americans living in majority Native areas avoid calling the police because of fear of discrimination. This fear is shared by 22 percent of American Indians overall and 14 percent of those living in areas where they are a minority. Nearly half of American Indians living in a majority Native area report unfair treatment by the courts, as do 32 percent of all American Indians, and 22 percent of those living in areas where they are a minority (Edwards, 2017).

Racism need not be blatant to be damaging. Indeed, people may be unaware of their own biases yet think and feel more negatively about those who are different from themselves. However, bias may be changed by what people see or read. To test this notion, researchers in a state where 8.8 percent of the population was American Indian employed the Implicit Associations Test (IAT) with college students who read news stories about American Indians facing obstacles (Sternadori, 2017). Some of the participants read stories about successful American Indians while others read about tragic events, such as murder and suicide. All of the participants demonstrated a decrease in negative attitudes but attitudinal change was statistically significant only among those who read about tragic events. Opportunities for interactions with American Indians likely mitigated the participants' prejudice. Likewise, positive stories about Native Americans probably had limited effect because media content is generally less influential when populations have personal experiences with a group.

American Indians continue to experience overt as well as covert racism in everyday media and discourse, while many non-Native people remain oblivious to this fact. Invisibility can be a covert manifestation of racism that serves to maintain White privilege (Robertson, 2015). Native people encounter daily racist images, language, and behaviors without social recourse. This is normalized and institutionally sanctioned, making it invisible:

> While minstrel shows have long been castigated as racist, Americans are socialized into *playing* Indian. Columbus Day celebrations, Halloween costumes, and Thanksgiving reenactments stereotype Indigenous Peoples as a much-distorted, monolithic culture. That is, other groups assert racial power over Indigenous Peoples by relegating indigeneity (complex understandings and representations of Indigenous identity) to racist archetypes and cultural caricatures.
>
> *(Robertson, 2015, p. 114; emphasis in original)*

Online forums share information and spread ideas. They are a powerful, increasingly popular form of communication reflective of prevailing attitudes and beliefs. A study of online forum comments examined content on the University of North Dakota's (UND) "Fighting Sioux" nickname (Steinfeldt et al., 2010). The researchers found that many forum participants expressed disbelief that anyone would react negatively to the UND mascot. Many posts reflected assertions of power and privilege, including assertions that mascots honored Native people. The researchers noted that sports fans who believe a hyper-aggressive, inaccurate, stereotypic image honors American Indians remain oblivious to how they impose their own attitudes and norms upon Native people. Many of the comments trivialized the issue of mascots, denigrated Native people, and demonstrated the respondents' ignorance about Native cultures. They displayed disdain, promoted stereotypes, and demonstrated overt racism. Indeed, the forum contained some racially virulent posts, despite the best efforts of online editors to monitor content. While many blatantly and aggressively racist posts were censored, others made it past the overwhelmed editors.

Overt stereotypes and racism toward Native Americans persist. In the Midwest, where gaming has facilitated economic prosperity and cultural revitalization, a newer, more subtle form of racism and novel microaggressions have arisen, sustaining White racial dominance perceived to be under threat (Senter & Ling, 2017). One study found that Indigenous cultural revitalization and economic prosperity did not change White people's views of Native Americans, including racism, stereotypes, overt hostility, and microaggressions (Senter & Ling, 2017).

Racial discrimination has multiple, significant implications for wellbeing. In addition to psychological consequences and limited life opportunities, it is associated with higher blood pressure (Thayer et al., 2017). Internalized oppression fed by external stereotypes and biases also has a significant impact on Native people. Indigenous young people accept stereotypes and distortions as true and inevitable (Chenault, 2011). In addition to internalizing negative representations of themselves, some Native people confront and belittle each other. The author Sherman Alexie recounted how he felt like responding when he believed another Native person was challenging him about his Native credentials:

> My name is Sherman Alexie. Yes, I have an Indian name. But I ain't going to share it with you. I learned a long time ago that the only way to keep something sacred is to keep it private. So, yeah, you might think I reveal everything, but I keep plenty of good and bad stuff all to myself. On my mother's side, I was born into the Clan of Busted Promises and Dynamite and White Man's Hydroelectric Concrete. On my father's side, I was born into the Clan of Sniper and Head Shot and Posthumous Bronze Star and Purple Heart. On my mother's side, I was born into the Clan of Rivers Flowing with Wild Salmon Ghosts. On my father's side, I was born into the Clan of Bloody and Broken Lungs. And all of us Spokanes and Coeur d'Alenes, after the Grand Coulee Dam, have been born into the Clan of Doing Our Best to Re-create and Replicate the Sacred Things That Were Brutally Stolen From Us. My name is Sherman Alexie and I was born from loss and loss and loss and loss and loss and loss and loss and loss and loss and loss and loss and loss. And loss.
>
> *(Alexie, 2017, p. 141)*

Socioeconomic status

Poverty remains a substantial issue for many Native Americans. Centuries of government-sponsored control and disempowerment cannot easily be alleviated by new policies. Contemporary economic disadvantage follows a course set in motion by historical events and traumas, including experiences of control, exclusion, and discrimination (Davis, Roscigno & Wilson, 2016; Walls & Whitbeck, 2012).

Overall, the Native American poverty rate is 28.4 percent, but poverty is particularly an issue for those living on reservations (Mauer, 2017). There are clear geographic patterns of concentrated disadvantage derived from historical and political forces that led to removal and isolation. In particular, the Gila River, Rosebud, Standing Rock, Spirit Lake, and Pine Ridge reservations all had poverty rates over 50 percent between 2008 and 2012. Local labor markets and limited opportunities perpetuate poverty (Davis et al., 2016). Meanwhile, college education has less influence on earnings on reservations than in urban areas (Mauer, 2017).

Poverty is a longstanding issue in Indian Country. While casinos make a small difference in terms of reducing poverty, history is the primary factor in shaping how geography, labor markets, and economic development either reduce or reinforce inequality (Davis et al., 2016). Contemporary poverty is a result of historically accumulated disadvantage, beginning with forced relocation to isolated rural areas with poor-quality land far from job opportunities and forced dependence on state paternalism. Allotment laid the foundation for entrenched deprivation and concentrated poverty (Davis et al., 2016). Limited resources and opportunity structures on reservations, including lack of employment, contribute to high rates of poverty (Mauer, 2017; Moghaddam, Momper & Fong, 2013). Discrimination has also been identified as a barrier for Native-owned businesses. Native Americans experience labor market marginality and exclusion:

> Taking into account group history is vital for explaining the rigidity of racial inequality. Forced relocations and failed assimilation programs do not simply hold historical relevance. Two centuries of quixotic government interventions thrust American Indians into a rigid, durable pattern of inequality that has withstood dramatic migratory shifts and the first Native-led economic boom of the contemporary era.
>
> *(Davis et al., 2016, p. 24)*

Reservations and reserves across North America were established in remote areas that were often devoid of resources. This lack of sustainable resources contributes to contemporary hardships, including high poverty and unemployment rates. Isolated contexts compound issues of access and exacerbate educational and health disparities. The historical and structural contexts of oppressed communities led to cumulative disadvantage and a chain of adversity across the lifespan. In addition, the BIA failed to deliver adequate transitional assistance as part of the urban relocation program, resulting in the development of a chronically disadvantaged urban Native community (Moghaddam et al., 2013). Deer critiqued this program for relocating American Indian people without appropriate orientation, preparation, or support.

The Indian Relocation Act led to a major population shift, but rather than eliminating poverty, it merely shifted it to urban settings. Between 2007 and 2011, American Indian poverty rates in cities with significant Indigenous populations, such as Denver, Tucson, and Phoenix, exceeded 28 percent. In Minneapolis and

Rapid City, South Dakota, the Native poverty rate exceeded 48 percent. Urban poverty cannot be explained by isolation; it is more likely attributable to difficulties many American Indians experience in the labor market (Davis et al., 2016). Persistent racial discrimination is at least partially to blame. American Indians in urban areas are 20 percent more likely to be underemployed than non-Hispanic Whites. Similar disparities can be found in Canada, including significant income disparities between Indigenous women living off-reserve and non-Indigenous women (Amnesty International, 2004).

Multiple factors contribute to socioeconomic status. American Indian poverty varies across communities but is pervasive throughout the United States, regardless of locality type. It is also notable that the poverty gap between Natives and Whites cannot be explained by the distribution of employment opportunities. Although Native-owned casinos have reduced poverty in some reservation communities over recent decades, substantial poverty remains, even where gaming enterprises flourish. While some Native people have built successful lives in urban areas, cities have not been the economic salvation proposed by many federal policy makers. All of this points to persistent, pervasive labor market discrimination as a key factor in Native poverty, especially in industries largely owned and controlled by Whites (Davis et al., 2016).

In 2013, 235 tribal governments had gaming operations, grossing over $28 billion, but the overall impact remains unclear. For some tribes, gaming has increased per capita income and reduced poverty. As a result, the Cherokee of Oklahoma have one of the strongest tribal economies in the country. However, while casinos do create job opportunities, enhance economies, and help alleviate poverty, they have not generated a widespread Indigenous economic renaissance. Rather than reducing socioeconomic disparities for Native people as a whole, gaming has helped create a much more complex poverty landscape (Davis et al., 2016).

Other policies that are seemingly unrelated to socioeconomic issues can impact poverty. For instance, an analysis of areas subject to PL 280 found that it led to increased crime and lowered incomes (Dimitrova-Grajzi, Grajzi & Guse, 2014). PL 280 is an externally driven, non-consensual transfer of jurisdiction. Enacted in 1953, this federal statute allowed states to assert jurisdiction over reservations, but it caused confusion, became an unfunded mandate for states, and reduced tribal autonomy. It now applies in some states but not in others, and certain reservations are exempt in states where it does apply. This jurisdictional complexity inhibits prosecutions and can foster a climate that allows crime to flourish. Furthermore, crime engenders uncertainty, discourages investment, and necessitates reallocation of resources. Therefore, this drastic change in the legal order initiated a chain of events that stifled economic development (Dimitrova-Grajzi et al., 2014).

Development

Indigenous sovereignty and nationhood offer opportunities for development. As Deer noted, land and resources are always significant issues. In the past, resources like timber have been an incentive for outsiders to take Indigenous land, as evidenced in the Menominee termination. Today, other resources, like carbon credits (see below), are sought by outsiders who are willing to pay money, often to the detriment of tribal sovereignty. On the other hand, Indigenous Peoples can assert sovereignty and make choices to pursue development on their own terms. With federal support for self-determination and economic development, they can implement a variety of development projects to mitigate poverty (Mauer, 2017).

Development is usually discussed within an international context, but it has applications for Indigenous populations within settler societies, too. After decades of state-led economic development, Native Americans remain among the poorest people in the United States, with less than half the median income according to the 2000 census. In addition, Native communities often lack an adequate infrastructure, including water, sewerage, and telecommunication systems (Mathers, 2012).

The creation of dependency has been proposed as a possible explanation for continuing poverty among Indigenous Peoples in spite of the financial and human resources that have been expended on development. Another likely cause is that planners lack relevant knowledge to stimulate economic growth. Mathers (2012) suggests that so-called state handouts are inconsistent with entrepreneurship and lead to long-term economic stagnation. However, this argument fails to recognize that federal governments in the United States and Canada have incurred treaty obligations and that funding for Indigenous development is not the same as that for international development. They recommend a bottom-up instead of a top-down approach that draws on local knowledge as relevant for both Indigenous and international contexts. While affirmation of local knowledge is important, framing development in terms of top-down or bottom-up reinforces hierarchical, colonial dynamics, rather than a decolonized, government-to-government perspective. It is also important to recognize that undermined authority and lack of control over resources are substantial barriers to development.

Forcible displacement and human rights violations often occur in the wake of an unsustainable, unidimensional model of economic development that ignores the rights of Indigenous Peoples, low-income communities, and the natural world. This is prevalent in many parts of the world, including the Amazon region, which is home to some 390 Indigenous Peoples. Colonization, territorial occupation, and resource extraction have had an enormous and synergistic impact in this region. Indigenous and other marginalized Peoples struggle to retain their territory and subsistence practices, while industrialized agriculture and extractive projects, occupy ever more of their lands. States have prioritized economic growth based on these unsustainable practices, leading to human rights violations and displacement or even annihilation of Indigenous and impoverished communities (REPAM PanAmazon Ecclesial Network, 2018).

An ability to control fate is linked with human development frameworks. Many Arctic communities exist within wealthy nation states but remain economically troubled (Kimmel, 2014). The Human Development Report for the Arctic, published in 2004, calls for recognition of the unique history and attributes of this region. Arctic communities must be able to control their own fates, promote their own cultural viability, and be able to continue to practice subsistence lifestyles drawing on the resources of the natural environment. Successful development requires that Native people have property rights and empowered local governments. While Alaska emphasizes local self-governance, as noted earlier, the state's tribal governments lack authority. The state authorities have often been unwilling to work with these tribal governments, and have even litigated against them to prevent their exercise of some aspects of local self-governance (Kimmel, 2014).

Some American Indian tribes have no control over their own lucrative mineral resources. Policies that tout self-determination may, in fact, strengthen external control and undermine sovereign authority. For example, self-determination policies may require commercial contracts and leases to be negotiated by the Bureau of Indian Affairs, thus denying tribes the opportunity to act in their own interests. In terms of natural resources, Native Nations often export agricultural commodities, timber, minerals, energy, water, and forest products to non-Native society but seldom profit from their sale (Mauer, 2017).

Opportunities and new possibilities

Perhaps the most visible form of Indigenous economic development is casino gaming. This has been possible for tribes in states that otherwise prohibit gaming because their retention of some sovereignty has left them outside state legal frameworks, except when state law is expressly applied under the terms of PL 280.

Brown was Assistant Secretary of the Interior when the Gaming Act was passed, which meant he was responsible for approving the first 50–60 tribal–state gaming compacts. He noted that he is not a gambler himself and the growth of tribal gaming operations challenged his personal belief system. Watching the development of gaming from passage of the legislation to the present day, however, he quickly realized its tremendous economic potential. While not all tribes have developed gaming operations, and some have seen their projects fail, others have put the stream of income they can generate to very good use. For instance, Brown noted that some tribes have used gaming money to establish scholarships and tribal colleges while also improving health services, children's services, and law enforcement for their members. Used wisely, gaming profits return directly to the community and allow it to achieve far more than it could with meager federal funding alone. In acknowledgement of this fact, Brown now sits on the board of directors of his tribe's gaming enterprise.

Tribal economic development is often framed as a false choice between exploiting polluting energy resources or remaining in extreme poverty. In fact, it can be grounded within Indigenous spiritual principles and cultural identity in ways that promote thriving economies and ecosystems (Goldtooth, 2010). True empowerment and self-determination can empower tribes to abide by their own principles in support of both economic development and climate justice. Decolonization provides a solid foundation for clear thinking and culturally driven development that is grounded in traditional values. Indeed, reflecting on values and priorities should be a precursor to all thoughtful development and governance decisions.

Community change must be rooted in supporting the wellbeing of members. The first part of self-determination is the self. Indigenous Peoples must be guided by our own definitions of who we are and how we should live, grounded in relationships and responsibilities to our communities and the natural world:

> Before we can start rebuilding ourselves and achieve meaningful change in the areas of law and government, of economics and development, we must start to remember one important thing: our communities are made up of people. Our concern about legal rights and empowering models of national self-government has led to the neglect of the fundamental building blocks of the peoples: the women and men, the youth and the elders.
>
> *(Alfred, 2005, p. 31)*

Tribal economic development is one component of holistic Indigenous revitalization. This regeneration must be grounded in contemporary needs and times. In that sense, it will be different than pre-colonial and colonial models. Thoughtful reflections on traditions can lead to regeneration of cultural practices, political identities, and reorganization of personal and collective ideas of what it means to live as Indigenous Peoples (Alfred, 2005).

Indigenous entrepreneurship can be contentious if it is seen as individualistic and contrary to community cultural norms or more centralized economic development (Gallagher & Selman, 2015). Entrepreneurship, however, can be critical to building tribal economies and complementary to other forms of economic development. It can be implemented with a sense of commitment to community and linked to traditional practices and ways of life. Although entrepreneurs may have a variety of motivations, Indigenous entrepreneurs can be anti-colonial actors, protecting and strengthening the interests of Native people in ways that rebuild Indigenous economies and foster tribal self-determination. Prior to contact, many tribal communities participated in thriving trade networks. Drawing on this tradition, Indigenous entrepreneurs can establish a place in developing tribal economies (Gallagher & Selman, 2015).

The natural world

Indigenous identity is grounded within the natural world as being Indigenous is place specific. In spite of challenges including access to traditional territories and the differential legal status of land, Native people and communities remain connected to specific physical places that continue to provide foundations for their identity, culture, and survival (Shoemaker, 2017). Indigenous identity can be conceptualized as place based but not place bound. In other words, while Native identity is typically tied to a specific part of the natural world, being Indigenous links people to the entirety of the natural world and this broader connection provides a foundation for activism (Larsen & Johnson, 2017).

The centrality of place can shape individual wellbeing. There is a connection between Indigenous Peoples and their traditional territories—a sense of reciprocity in which each cares for the other. In this symbiotic relationship, the wellbeing of one is intertwined with the wellbeing of the other. For example, Indigenous people seeking educational or employment opportunities may feel literally *out of place*—that is, uncomfortable or lost when away from their tribal communities and homelands. In a poignant example that illustrates the close connection between sacred geography and Indigenous wellbeing, Griffin-Pierce (1997) quoted a Navajo professor at a major Southwestern university who declared, "when I am lonely the mountains call me."

The natural world is sacred, nurturing, and intertwined with Indigenous cultures, Peoples, and wellbeing. In simple terms, the Lakota word *waste'* (pronounced "wash-tay") means good, but it also signifies reverence, value, significance, and beauty. Ironically, the English word "waste"—despite having almost exactly the same spelling—is an apt description of the devastation left in the wake of environmental exploitation when the sacredness of the natural world is disregarded and the earth's bounty is extracted for profit.

In traditional Indigenous understandings, the earth is a living being with thoughts, feelings, and agency—an animate personality (Wiebe, 2016). Beyond a physical manifestation, each place possesses a spiritual dimension (Larsen & Johnson, 2017; Orr, 2018). The dominant society, on the other hand, is grounded in non-relational forms of being and knowing (Wiebe, 2016). From this perspective, the environment is seen as providing resources. Water and land are viewed as commodities to be used for the benefit of humankind, rather than relatives that deserve care.

The impact of environmental trauma

Given the intimate connections between Indigenous Peoples and the environment, an examination of trauma, both historical and contemporary, must include environmental losses and damage to the natural world. Colonization is steeped in the commodification of land, food, labor, forests, water, genes, ideas, and the privatization of knowledge. Such practices are unsustainable for both human beings and the natural world (Goldtooth, 2010).

Indigenous Peoples have experienced significant environmental trauma, including the loss of virtually all their land in the United States. The land losses that accompanied the establishment of reservations and allotment were world-changing events. Their magnitude must be understood in the context of the loss of animate, spiritual beings, rather than replaceable localities. The loss of sacred territories has led to substantial emotional trauma that cannot be remedied with financial reimbursement. For instance, the Lakota have refused all offers of compensation since the illegal seizure of the Black Hills as this land is considered irreplaceable (Lazarus, 1991; Ostler, 2010).

If land is at risk, so is everything else. People's origins are rooted in specific geography. The flooding of tribal land, as happened on Crow Creek Dakota territory after the diversion of the Missouri River, is invariably experienced as a cataclysmic event. Homelands that once nourished and sustained people with edible roots and medicine plants disappeared under water, changing the tribe's world forever (Fitzgerald, 2015). Other massive projects similarly flooded large tracts land, leaving a legacy of human and environmental destruction. There are many examples in Washington State, where dams were built in the 1930s as part of federal New Deal programs that promised economic recovery fueled by hydroelectric power. In particular, the Grand Coulee Dam blocked an ancient salmon migration that was crucial for the Native people of the inland Northwest. Interior Salish people, whose culture is intimately intertwined with and dependent upon wild salmon, are now spiritual orphans (Alexie, 2017). In New York State, Tuscarora land was taken by the Federal Power Commission to create the New York Power Authority. Likewise, the Seneca Nation lost one-third of the Allegany Reservation in the Southern Tier area of the state with construction of the Kinzua Dam. The same dam also destroyed the Corn Planter Tracks—land guaranteed under a treaty signed by George Washington and the last remaining reservation land in Pennsylvania (Haupton, 2015).

The environment is traditionally positive, sustaining, and meaningful for Indigenous Peoples, but it has been altered in ways that damage and hurt. For instance, the Seneca Nation's relationship to the Allegany River has been irrevocably altered. Kinzua once meant "good fishing place," but after this word was appropriated for the name of the dam it became synonymous with flooding and destruction. Seneca homes were condemned and burned. The school and the longhouse—the spiritual center of the community—were in the land seized by the Army Corps of Engineers. The best farmland was submerged (Haupton, 2015).

Many Indigenous communities have similar stories of loss. Cultural, spiritual, linguistic, and epistemological losses persist, decades after completion of Hydro-Quebec in Canada and the Pick–Sloan Project in the Missouri River Basin. Plants lost to the flooded landscape fade from memory, knowledge of their uses vanishes, and even their names disappear from everyday language. These losses are closely linked with health issues (Fitzgerald, 2015). When tribes are relocated from traditional territories, items that have been vital to their culture and wellbeing for centuries may no longer exist or must be purchased instead of gathered traditionally. Disrupting a river disrupts a way of life, stories, and land narratives, as well as means of transferring knowledge. Environmental disruption breaks a link in cultural transmission, causes trauma, and inhibits Indigenous sustainability. Assaults on the environment also exacerbate the perpetual moving and resettlement experienced by Native people. They are subjected to the repeated destruction of places where their ancestors were born and buried. This, in turn, destabilizes communal codes of behavior. What distinguishes us from other Peoples in the world is tenuous and possibly disappearing (Fitzgerald, 2015).

Environmental racism is a prominent component of uranium contamination in Native American communities. Thirty million tons of uranium were blasted from Navajo lands during World War II and the Cold War. Native people have been exposed to contaminants for three generations and many tribal members have died from related conditions. For example, Helen Nez saw seven of her ten children die of so-called Navajo neuropathy, a disorder linked to uranium contamination. The drinking water in the local spring contained at least five times the safe level of uranium (Morales, 2017).

Contemporary environmental threats

Hydroelectric projects threaten Indigenous Peoples around the world. For instance, the Chepete-Bala mega-hydroelectric dam project in Bolivia seems likely to displace Indigenous Peoples from the Moseten, Tsimane, Tacana, Esse Ejja, Leco, and Uchupiamona Nations as well as uncontacted Indigenous groups (Indigenous and Conserved Communities Area Consortium, 2018).

Much of the land that was retained by Native Americans has been subsequently subjected to degradation and contamination. Natural resources have been stripped, leaving nothing but toxic residues (Goldtooth, 2010). In one survey, 39 percent of Native Americans expressed the belief that legally sanctioned discrimination framed in laws and government policies is more devastating than individual prejudices (Morales, 2017). The sluggish decontamination of toxic tribal land is just one example of that sort of institutionalized discrimination. At the time of writing, of 500 abandoned mines on the Navajo Reservation, only nine had been decontaminated. Uranium mining is a primary source of radioactive groundwater and surface water. Dust and particulate matter from abandoned stockpiles enter the air and are deposited in both soil and water (Orescanin et al., 2011). The slow cleanup on the Navajo Reservation is grounded in the law itself, which prioritizes relationships between the Environmental Protection Agency (EPA) and the corporations that extract natural resources over the rights of the communities affected by the inevitable contamination. The Navajo see this as nothing short of institutionalized racism (Morales, 2017).

Uranium beyond the EPA maximum contaminant level has also been documented in well water on the Crow Reservation (Eggers et al., 2015). Tribal members worked with tribal college partners to develop a participatory research project to test the water, explain the results, and offer treatment options to reservation homeowners. In the past, Crow tribal members lived near natural water sources where clean water was readily available. Now, access to safe drinking water is elusive. By the 1960s, expanding agriculture had affected the quality of river water, so many families opted for piped well water instead. Rather than a positive development, however, this brought hardship. The groundwater in home wells was so high in dissolved solids as to be undrinkable. Widespread high alkalinity and excessive hardness in the water also rapidly ruined plumbing, hot-water heaters, and septic systems. Today, community members are increasingly concerned about contaminants and the associated health risks (Eggers et al., 2015).

Lack of access to safe drinking water is a concern in many Indigenous communities. More than a quarter of Native Americans believe that the quality of their drinking water is worse than in other places (Morales, 2017). Many Canadians take safe drinking water for granted and would be outraged if their water systems failed. First Nations communities, however, have faced years of boil-water advisories, with between 12 and 13 percent of reserves under these advisories at any given time (Chambers, 2017). Waterborne diseases are exceptionally prevalent. For example, poor water quality contributes to an infant mortality rate on the reserves that is four times the national average (Chambers, 2017).

In 2003, the Canadian government assessed First Nations water systems and reported that 218 of 740 are at high risk of contamination and causing human illness. In response, it issued a new First Nations Water Management Strategy to upgrade existing and build new facilities, monitor water, create sustainable maintenance plans, expand training, develop emergency responses, and launch a public awareness campaign. However, no funds were allocated to implement this plan and build the necessary infrastructure. Two years later, more than 1000 residents of the Kashechewan First Nation had to be evacuated due to an E. coli outbreak. Funding is a choice that reflects priorities. The poverty and preventable deaths in Indigenous communities are linked to differential treatment and discriminatory policies (Chambers, 2017).

Issues of environmental injustice plague many Indigenous communities. The Aamjiwnaang First Nation Reserve in Ontario is surrounded by Chemical Valley—the densest concentration of petrochemical plants in Canada. This Anishinaabek community lives in a perpetual state of emergency, subjected to regular leaks, spills, toxic emissions, and evacuations (Wiebe, 2016). The same doctrine of *terre nullius* that facilitated colonization of lands presumed to be "empty" or at best underutilized undergirds justifications of toxic waste and emissions on and near contemporary Native lands. Those who continue to dump toxic waste seem to believe that the land has already been wasted simply because it is occupied by Native Peoples (Wiebe, 2016).

In December 2017, in a move that many consider illegal, President Trump diminished the Bears Ears National Monument by 85 percent without consulting the affected Indigenous Peoples. The administration allowed an expedited planning process that did not allow for meaningful co-management practices with the local tribes (Utah Dine Bikeyah, 2018). This territory includes sacred, ceremonial, cultural, and medicinal resources, including more than 100,000 archeological sites. Documents leaked to the *New York Times* reveal the Trump administration met with uranium mining companies that advised them on exact locations where protections could be removed to serve their interests (Utah Dine Bikeyah, 2018).

The way the natural world is treated is creating multiple ongoing stressors and environmental challenges. The effects of climate change have led to more frequent and more devastating natural disasters. While these disasters affect everyone, they often have a disproportionate impact on Indigenous Peoples. For instance, the Tunica-Biloxi from Louisiana were heavily affected by a hurricane in 1938 and more recently by Hurricane Katrina (Klopotek, Lintinger & Barbry, 2008). Climate change is causing continuing loss of land through erosion for the Houma of coastal Louisiana at a rate of approximately 34 square miles per year (Billiot, 2017). Global warming has led to shrinking territories and food supplies for subsistence hunters in the Arctic, where sea ice is declining at a rate of 13.2 percent each decade (National Aeronautics and Space Administration, 2018).

Restoring balance in our communities

Brown emphasized that children and families provide the foundation for Indigenous communities. Therefore, all efforts to restore balance in these communities must support the wellbeing of children and families. He noted that support for parenting skills has the potential to address significant community challenges, such as high truancy rates and dropping out of school. Programs are needed to support models of healthy fatherhood. Parents need to be engaged with educational systems to prepare youth to build a positive future for themselves and their communities. He pointed out the difficulty the Havasupai have with finding a teacher to serve their remote community and lamented the lack of attention to the needs of children and families. This is just one example of a missed opportunity that is likely to have a continuing impact.

It is important to move beyond simply identifying colonization as an explanation for what happened to Native people. Empowerment is essential. Focusing solely on colonization facilitates "a narrative that in its use privileges the colonizer's power and inherently limits our freedom, logically and mentally imposing a perpetual colonized victim way of life and view on the world" (Alfred, 2005, p. 25).

Brown identified resilience and hope in the increasing number of Native people with college degrees who return to serve their tribal communities. Early in his career, he was aware of only one other American Indian with a doctorate in social work; now there is a strong cadre. He reflected on a time when he believed he knew every American Indian lawyer and doctor; now there are many. The early American Indian social workers that he hired had little understanding of sovereignty and often wanted to adopt state laws within tribal contexts. Now Indigenous social workers understand the importance of developing their own codes and standards in tribal communities. These social workers appreciate, and can help others understand, the importance of government-to-government relationships. There is also greater receptivity in the wider social environment. Early in Brown's career, many government leaders did not want to sit at the table with tribal leaders; now many value tribal input.

Decolonizing has a tangible impact. Critiquing dominant narratives can change thinking in ways that facilitate changing structures. Communities that have regained control of land and implement their own services have lower suicide rates, less reliance on social assistance, and lower unemployment rates (Nutton & Fast, 2015). Decolonization has fostered empowerment and the development of diverse, viable economic enterprises, cultural and language revitalization, and more effective management of natural resources and social service programs (Nutton & Fast, 2015).

Brown highlighted the decolonizing aspects of community-based participatory research (CBPR). Rather than older models of research in which projects were developed and implemented by external scholars, CBPR can be driven by tribal priorities. Tribal communities need not be passive. Instead, they should identify their own priorities and be active participants in choosing methodologies, analyzing data, and making publication decisions. Brown cited examples in which American Indian tribes and communities first assessed their own strengths and needs then approached universities for assistance, as needed.

Empowerment and decolonization in tribal communities involve nation building. This, in turn, strengthens communities, families, and community members. As tribal communities go through this process, some develop programs to help Indigenous men understand traditional beliefs and knowledge, thus altering dysfunctional gender dynamics that foster violence against women and children. Traditional teachings and re-socialization strategies are employed to recognize, confront, and heal from the legacy of colonization (Chenault, 2011).

Alternative, culturally based forms of justice and healing, such as the Navajo Peacemaker process, can replace sentences for domestic violence based on mainstream models of justice (Chenault, 2011). This method of resolving disputes is grounded in traditional Navajo values and practices but addresses contemporary legal issues, such as family reunification, elder abuse, divorce, domestic violence, and probate. (See www.navajocourts.org for further details.)

Supporting and reinvigorating traditional systems of justice can be far less expensive and more culturally affirming than attempting to replicate mainstream justice approaches. However, for traditional systems of justice to be effective, the oppressive ideologies, beliefs, and practices inherent in colonization must be understood and challenged. This is because internalized colonial attitudes can contaminate traditional systems with philosophies of domination. Rejection of these philosophies is essential for nation building and reclaiming traditional justice and peacemaking systems in tribal communities (Chenault, 2011).

Tribal colleges are institutions rooted in place that contribute to community building (Crazy Bull, 2015). They are often centers of tribal and community life, offering the education that is necessary for community development while enhancing human capital. They engage with communities, provide a foundation for community service, and can contribute to a cultural renaissance. They play a crucial role in supporting traditional tribal identity within the contexts of modern society and rebuilding tribal nationhood (Crazy Bull, 2015).

Tribal colleges work with tribal histories, traditional knowledge, and language revitalization to provide services for the whole community, including adult education and financial guidance. Grounded in a holistic, community-based philosophy, they offer wellness and prevention activities and engage with tribal communities to foster healthier lifestyles. They also offer technology and library access and are the only places in some communities with computers and internet access. They develop partnerships and conduct research to address community needs and priorities, foster entrepreneurship, and have an economic impact. A 2012

North Dakota study found tribal colleges directly contributed $48 million to their states' economies and had an overall economic impact of $142 million. They prompt students and community members to develop their skills and provide a gathering place for the creation of diverse strategic partnerships (Crazy Bull, 2015).

Brown emphasized the importance of understanding sovereignty and centering community in all initiatives serving Indigenous Peoples and communities. Tribal Nations have the authority to offer a range of social, health, legal, and other services. Some operate their own radio stations, delivering content that is relevant to their communities. Indigenous communities can provide education through these broadcasts, inform listeners about services, and challenge entrenched views, such as regarding violence against women (Chenault, 2011).

During her time as Assistant Secretary of the Interior, Deer traveled to many tribal communities to learn about the creative and empowering work being done at the grassroots level. Even when encountering multiple barriers, she noted the importance of "not taking 'no' for an answer." She highlighted the work of the Great Lakes Inter-Tribal Council as an example of hope and resilience. This consortium of tribal leaders united to gain leverage in working with federal, state, and local governments in the context of developing and implementing health and human service projects, economic development initiatives, and education programs.

Environmental activism is a central component of restoring balance in our communities. Access to clean water should be a fundamental right for everyone. Beyond its utility as a resource, it is important to understand the *meaning* of water for Indigenous Peoples. The spiritual, environmental, and social values of water outweigh its economic value. On the Six Nations Reserve in southern Ontario, Haudenosaunee elders and clan mothers teach that water depicts how each human being is linked to Mother Earth, just as unborn babies are surrounded by water within their mothers (Baird et al., 2015). Women have a special relationship with water as both are the source of all living things. It is important to look at how context, including culture, traditions, meanings, and values related to water, influences water management (Baird et al., 2015).

The central role that water plays in Indigenous understandings is reflected in sayings such as "water is life"—the mantra of those who sought to prevent the Dakota Access Pipeline from crossing under Lake Oahe. Protecting water is an important catalyst for continuing activism by Indigenous people and their allies. One such example is the Cattaraugus Creek Water Walkerz and their work near the West Valley nuclear site in New York State. This group of activists and their allies regularly hold public informational events and marches that call attention to issues of water protection (Western New York Peace Center, 2018).

The Indigenous Environmental Network monitors environmental threats, distributes information, and mobilizes activists. Its members believe that ongoing threats are rooted in the dominant society's economic paradigm and the quest for wealth accumulation, and that the race to exploit natural resources disregards the finite limits of those resources and the implications of increasing consumption and waste accumulation.

At the time of her interview for this book, Deer was heavily involved in educating the members of her tribe about the environmental impact and sovereignty implications of a proposed deal on carbon credits—a tradable certificate that allows emission of greenhouse gasses. Corporations often try to buy carbon credits from tribes who emit very little carbon dioxide and other greenhouse gasses in the hope of offsetting their emissions elsewhere. She noted that people who care about the land should not be swayed by the money that is offered in exchange for these credits. A group of Menominee leaders, including Deer, gathered many signatures in opposition to BP's proposal, and the tribe ultimately rejected the deal.

Trauma-informed applications

Deer and Brown both suggested that any number of grassroots community programs are probably observing the principles of trauma-informed care, although they were unable to cite any specific examples.

Applying a trauma-informed framework reminds us of the importance of safety, trustworthiness, choice, collaboration, and empowerment. Indigenous communities deserve to be free from poverty and have access to all of the basic necessities for a secure and dignified life. This includes freedom from racism and oppression at all levels, including structures and policies. Eliminating racism and discrimination is a necessary component of building trust. Settler societies and governments must abandon federal paternalism while upholding the responsibilities they have to Indigenous Peoples. Policies that micromanage Indigenous Nations and undermine their sovereignty must be dismantled. Indigenous Peoples must retain the freedom to participate in their own communities and have full access to the benefits of wider society. With recognition of sovereignty, tribal governments will be able to exercise options and choices based on their own priorities, cultures, values, and community needs.

All trauma-informed care must prioritize safety. Brown highlighted the detailed research and recommendations of the Attorney General's Advisory Committee on American Indian/Alaska Native Children Exposed to Violence (2014) and noted that this committee adopted a trauma-informed approach when gathering information about violence in Indigenous communities by ensuring counselors were available to provide support to everyone who testified.

Collaboration is another central component of trauma-informed care. There are potential roles for everyone in supporting Indigenous communities within their wider societal and environmental contexts. It is important to raise critical awareness, mobilize energy, and make a commitment to challenge oppression in order to effect social change (Chenault, 2011). Deer repeatedly emphasized the importance of advocacy. This is an important skill for helping professionals and everyone who is working to make a difference in American Indian communities. Deer, a lifelong advocate herself, noted that she is "eighty-two, still not through, and looking for a crew." Effecting change is rarely an individual endeavor. Rather, change happens through collaboration and synergy when people unite to make a difference.

Coalitions that include people from different backgrounds and a variety of skills can further collaboration and change. For instance, Indigenous academics and tribal leaders can partner with helping professionals, activists, and change agents. Academics can create space for Indigenous knowledge and affirm its importance in shaping policies, structures, institutions, discourses, and practices (Wiebe, 2016). Likewise, Larsen & Johnson (2017) call for a collaborative process of "walking with" in which academics and professionals support Indigenous communities in ways that follow the latter's priorities and avoid cultural appropriation by non-Indigenous people.

With recognition of sovereignty come restoration of government-to-government relationships and opportunities to build collaborations and partnerships. Abandoning racism and notions of superiority clears the way for collaborations between Indigenous and non-Indigenous people for the benefit of the world that we share. As Brown pointed out, community-based participatory research that identifies community needs and informs programs and policies to improve the wellbeing of communities and their members is an ideal example of trauma-informed collaboration.

Trust is another crucial element of trauma-informed care. It is also a central to federal government's dealings with tribes. Although shrouded in paternalism, the federal trust responsibility is the foundation of the US legal framework. However, this book has presented numerous examples of the violation of this trust relationship. The Attorney General's Advisory Committee on American Indian/Alaska Native Children Exposed to Violence (2014) report contains explicit recommendations for how the federal government should live up to its responsibilities with respect to securing and improving the wellbeing of American Indian children and communities. These responsibilities include providing adequate funding for tribal programs in child welfare and criminal and civil justice. The report emphasizes that treaties and trust responsibilities are mandatory, not discretionary, so they require base funding for tribes to use according to their own wishes.

Trust includes having full faith in tribal governments and communities to set their own priorities and manage their own programs. A healthy government-to-government relationship assumes both collaboration and the belief that each partner is equally competent and trustworthy. Although this trustworthiness is rarely borne out in practice, the environmental co-management partnerships cited above may provide positive models for the future.

Empowerment can lead to more functional communities and tribal governments, the reclamation of Indigenous values and teachings, and their application in contemporary contexts. In addition, it may lead to the restoration of cultures, languages, and lands. It can both foster and result from activism.

Greater consciousness among Indigenous Peoples can facilitate an emancipatory process of decolonization. Oppressive language can be recognized and challenged, and historical myths can be critiqued and balanced by counter-narratives that expose the brutality of colonization while engendering cultural pride and celebrating Indigenous survival and strength (Robertson, 2015).

Brown emphasized the extensive needs identified in the aforementioned report to the US Attorney General, which he helped to prepare. Establishing safety is imperative for community wellbeing. For that to happen, barriers that prevent tribal empowerment must be removed:

> We must transform the broken systems that re-traumatize children into systems where American Indian and Alaska Native (AI/AN) tribes are empowered with authority and resources to prevent exposure to violence and to respond to and promote healing of their children who have been exposed.
> *(Attorney General's Advisory Committee on American Indian/Alaska Native Children Exposed to Violence, 2014, p. 7)*

Empowering tribes, removing barriers grounded in colonial history and federal paternalism, and providing resources were all key recommendations in this report.

The trauma-informed principle of choice is highlighted as tribal communities seek to develop and implement governance models that meet their own needs rather than replicate mainstream models. Borrowing external models of governance has fallen short of meeting Indigenous needs (Alfred, 2005). American Indian communities face many choices as they determine how they should move forward. These choices, many of which were discussed earlier in this chapter, must be honored and supported by external service providers and activists. Indigenous communities have a right to make thoughtful decisions about forms of development that meet the needs of their people. They must have the right to exercise territorial control in ways they see fit, rather than be disempowered and subjected to external control.

Conclusion

This chapter has explored various aspects of wellness in American Indian communities, including contemporary sovereignty and governance, how the wider social and environmental context affects wellbeing, socioeconomic status, and development. Examples of resilience and hope for restoring balance in communities and trauma-informed care have been offered and infused with reflections from subject-matter experts Eddie Brown and Ada Deer. Many American Indian communities are immersed in a regenerative struggle, rites of resurgence, and reclaiming what it means to be Indigenous in today's world. These are examples of true decolonization as Native people refuse to be disconnected from their traditional values.

> There are many differences among the peoples that are indigenous to this land, yet the challenge facing all Onkwehonwe is the same: regaining freedom and becoming self-sufficient by confronting the disconnection and fear at the core of our existences under colonial domination. We are separated from the sources of our goodness and power: from each other, our cultures, and our lands. These connections must be restored.
> *(Alfred, 2005, p. 20)*

Brown noted that the realization of true wellness in American Indian communities rests on putting the tribes' interests first. All aspects of research and social service initiatives must be tied to the tribal base that prioritizes issues identified by specific communities. Understanding sovereignty requires recognition of the fact that American Indian Nations have the right and the ability to be self-governing, and this must not be undermined by anyone, including the federal government and human service professionals.

Deer stressed that American Indian Peoples' resilience is undeniable, simply because we are here today. In spite of centuries of colonization, oppression, and resulting trauma and disparities, that resilience persists. This must be recognized by human service professionals and embraced by Indigenous people themselves. She noted, "If you care about your tribe, you care about your people. You devote your energy, heart, mind, and soul." While recognizing the importance of allies, she emphasized that American Indian people are well positioned to make positive and lasting changes in their own communities.

CONCLUSION

This book has explored contemporary issues for Native American Peoples, with particular attention paid to trauma and resilience. A review of trauma theory, prevalence, and impact was offered at the beginning of the book, but it is important to note that trauma theory continues to evolve. In particular, research is exploring and refining what we know about historical trauma and interactions between historical and contemporary trauma. It is clear that trauma is common, particularly among Indigenous Peoples, and can have significant implications for wellbeing. It is also important to recognize the importance of resilience. Not all people who experience traumatic events suffer lasting negative effects.

Chapters 2 and 3 offered a brief review of the history and contemporary circumstances of Native Americans. These chapters described major US policies and legal decisions, and made comparisons between Native Americans and other Indigenous Peoples. Central to understanding trauma and resilience for Native Americans are understandings of sovereignty, colonization, and assimilation policies, particularly the impact of residential schools. It is imperative to recognize that contemporary Native Americans are diverse in both cultures and living circumstances. Some retain or have reclaimed traditional values and lifestyles, some fit comfortably in the American mainstream, and others negotiate both worlds simultaneously. Native Americans often experience racism, socioeconomic, health, and educational disparities, and frequently maintain strong connections to the natural world, grappling with what it means to be Indigenous in contemporary multicultural circumstances.

The subject-specific chapters focused on children and families, elders and veterans, education, health, and communities, on the understanding that these are not mutually exclusive categories and each area intersects with others. Each chapter described helping efforts, both effective and ineffective, with particular attention paid to innovative models and trauma-informed care. Resilience in spite of significant adversity was a theme across all of these chapters.

Chapters 4 and 5 emphasized the continuing importance of relationships and reciprocal roles in spite of the challenges and losses generated by colonization. Children and families remain the heart of Indigenous societies, while elders and veterans continue to be respected sources of guidance, even though they are often burdened with disparities from a lifetime of cumulative disadvantage. Experiences of grief and loss are common among many American Indian people, regardless of age. Traditional family structures have been disrupted by colonization processes in ways that have undermined gender roles, fostered internalized oppression, and led to violence and addiction. Culturally grounded, trauma-informed services can help restore balance.

Chapter 6 explored knowledge about and for Native people, including how education has historically devalued Indigenous cultures and ways of knowing. The educational context often continues to stigmatize and treat Native students differently, particularly in terms of discipline. This results in disparities in retention and graduation rates. There are, however, opportunities for change in curriculum content and the learning environment. A number of schools and libraries have started to transform academia by developing and implementing decolonized models.

Chapter 7 reported significant disparities in health and explained the need for positive change. In addition to commonly cited physical and mental health disparities, such as diabetes and PTSD, it is important to recognize that disparities in food security and dental care continue to affect Native Americans. The chapter presented examples of how Indigenous communities have used sovereignty and traditional values to address these issues. It is important to recognize that historical and structural factors play ongoing roles in determining wellness. Traditional perspectives on wellbeing and healing persist among many Native Americans, often alongside the use of mainstream health services. Treaty rights and federal policies play a significant role in health services, yet Native people continue to face discrimination and inadequate access to those services.

Chapter 8 offered a social and environmental context for examining issues of trauma and resilience among American Indians. In particular, contemporary nation-building and culturally grounded development efforts illustrate that Native people can be guided by traditional values. Barriers to self-governance, such as ongoing federal paternalism and lack of control over territories, were examined, as were the challenges of decolonizing governance structures. Finally, the chapter highlighted the importance of respecting the natural world and the ways in which Indigenous Peoples are seeking to restore balance.

This book is grounded within an understanding of the importance of Indigenous sovereignty, human rights, and social justice, and recognition of the continuing impact of colonial dynamics. This perspective has direct relevance for social workers and other helping professionals. There are significant commonalities among Indigenous Peoples, not least their shared experiences with colonial powers and the resilience that has facilitated their survival. Being Indigenous is intimately connected to traditional territories: "It is a way of being and knowing—and a politics of resistance and resurgence—grounded in the agency of place to teach the responsibility of land" (Larsen & Johnson, 2017, p. 3). International examples from various Indigenous Peoples are interspersed throughout the book. It is, however, crucial to recognize that the degree of diversity among Indigenous people is substantial within countries, tribes, and even families.

The book is also informed by the perspectives of experts who are both observers and participants in the topics covered in the various chapters. All have years of experience in their respective fields, and they have impressive credentials and qualifications that are recognized by the external world. However, the latter can be a double-edged sword. Eddie Brown revealed that being one of the few Native Americans with a doctorate in the 1970s opened doors for him to participate in the creation of a wide range of policies and programs. On the other hand, Lori Quigley recalled that her doctorate led to assumptions that she was the best person to address a host of issues relating to Native people that were well beyond her areas of expertise.

At least as important for the purposes of this book, all of these experts have credibility within Indigenous communities because of their work with and on behalf of those communities. Most are now elders with a wealth of accumulated knowledge as well as experts in their fields. Some are well known, while others have done much of their work behind the scenes, but all of their contributions are equally valid and valuable. This parallels our knowledge base: some efforts are more visible than others. For example, some models of trauma-informed care are widely known, but there are probably many more at the grassroots level that have received no public attention. These experts were able to identify a number of model services that have not been discussed in the scholarly literature. Indeed, because of the nature of their work, they are more likely to be aware of such programs than most scholars. As they all emphasized, however, community-based efforts and trauma-informed care are being continually developed. Below, I offer a brief summary of the experts who contributed to this book and the basis for their valuable insights.

When Edwin Gonzalez-Santin was interviewed for this book, he was on the cusp of retirement, having served as Director of the Office of American Indian Projects at Arizona State University's School of Social Work for several decades. He balances his time between working with tribes to help them build their capacity and evaluate their projects, working with funders and policy makers to insure support for meaningful programs, and teaching and mentoring American Indian students to provide high-quality services. All of these efforts are focused on serving American Indian children and families. He is well versed in the history and nuances of federal policies as well as the implementation of services in tribal communities. He has been a steadfast activist for American Indian children and families for over four decades, with a particular focus on the Indian Child Welfare Act. In his interview, he emphasized the importance of relationships (among American Indian people themselves as well as between tribal members and service providers) and the centrality of families in American Indian communities. He highlighted the strength and resilience of American Indian people in the face of continuing policies that threaten to destroy them.

At the time of her interview, Dr. Priscilla Day was semi-retired from her position at the University of Minnesota, Duluth, where she had worked for a quarter-century. She continues to direct the Center for Regional and Tribal Child Welfare, actively working as a consultant on American Indian family preservation. Her work to champion American Indian child welfare content at her university led to the College of Education and Human Services gaining a reputation as one of the best in the country for providing high-quality, tribally informed human services education. Her perspectives as a tribal member, mother, and grandmother complement her scholarly perspectives. She not only understands issues of American Indian children and families from a research perspective but draws on her own lived experience when affirming that they are indeed our hope for the future. In her interview, she emphasized the importance of recognizing diversity among American Indian individuals and communities. In spite of this diversity, however, she highlighted the common legacy of disparities left by trauma as well as resilience grounded in traditional spirituality, values, and family systems. She particularly noted the ongoing attacks on the Indian Child Welfare Act and internalized oppression as key issues.

Dr. Jordan Lewis has felt a strong connection with elders since early childhood, and his ongoing commitment to elders has been a guiding force throughout his career. Now at the mid-point of that career, he has already worked on federal policy, conducted notable research, and served as Director of the National Resource Center for Alaska Native Elders. As an Alaskan Native with a multi-disciplinary background that includes social work, community psychology, and gerontology, he has a multifaceted perspective on trends and issues related to Indigenous elders. His work will likely be a driving force in elders policy and services for decades to come. In his interview, he emphasized that elders can serve as leaders and play a crucial role in research projects and academia. He pointed out that becoming an elder is a demonstration of hope and resilience, and a stage to which many Native people aspire. Indeed, mainstream society could learn a great deal from Indigenous communities' perception and treatment of their elders.

Likewise, Dr. Suzanne Cross is both a tribal member and a researcher on Native American issues. As a young child, she was drawn to elders and spent much of her time with them. Now an elder herself, she has recently retired after years in academia but remains uniquely positioned to comment on the current circumstances of her fellow elders. Just as she learned from elders as a youth, readers can now learn from her experiences, both personal and professional. She points out that while the current generation of elders has experienced significant trauma, there is still considerable joy, resilience, and contentment among those who know their roots, live according to their cultures, and continue to pass on traditions.

At the mid-point of her career, Dr. Katie Johnston-Goodstar has established a well-deserved reputation for outstanding scholarship and a strong commitment to including youth voices in her work. She came to academia after a period working with disenfranchised youth, during which she helped them access education and empowered them to shape educational systems to meet their needs. Today, her research into the social climate in schools and how this impacts learning informs the work of both educators and helping professionals. It seems highly likely that it will continue to shape human services and education for Native Americans over the coming decades. Johnston-Goodstar reminds us to make space for youth and to remember that they are resilient, powerful, and experts on their own experiences, including the disenfranchisement they continue to experience in many school systems. In her interview, she emphasized that the impact of the social context of education is vastly underestimated and merits far more attention from helping professionals and policy makers.

Dr. Lori Quigley is an established scholar and educator at the top of her field. As a college administrator and researcher, she has held both gubernatorial and presidential appointments as well as national leadership positions in educational associations. She continues to be a strong advocate for Native Americans and remains active in her community. Her work has shaped all levels of education, nurturing Native faculty as well as students, and her long-term perspectives provide invaluable insights. In her interview, she emphasized that Indigenous experiences and knowledge need no external validation to be meaningful. She also noted that students learn less when they are forced to expend energy trying to fit into someone else's mold. We must recognize that educational settings, curricula, and educators all have a profound effect on Indigenous students.

Dr. Maria Yellow Horse Brave Heart, the preeminent social work scholar on historical trauma, was first drawn to this subject in the 1970s, and since then she has focused her career on developing historical trauma theory. As a clinician, she integrated this theory into her work and contributed to its empirical validation. Her perspectives are grounded in her identity as an Indigenous woman and her commitment to enhancing the health and wellbeing of Native people. As a senior scholar, she has made a vast contribution to the knowledge base. She maintains her clinical interests and connections to both reservation and urban Indigenous communities. In her interview, she stressed the importance of ancestral, familial, and environmental connections for many Indigenous people and the implications of these connections for experiencing trauma. While recognizing resilience, she noted that major traumatic events continue to occur regularly in many Native communities, so the ongoing impact of trauma must be acknowledged. The historical trauma framework acknowledges both past and current trauma, along with resilience and unresolved grief. Disparities result from ongoing oppression, rather than any deficit in Indigenous people.

Dr. Margaret Moss has held a variety of academic positions in the United States and Canada. As the first US Native American to hold both a doctorate in nursing and a law degree, she is frequently asked to speak about the challenges and disparities American Indians face in accessing adequate healthcare. She has personal experience of these disparities, with many close relatives dying prematurely of health complications, accidents, and violence. This, coupled with her scholarly background, has fueled her passion for advocacy and securing better services for Indigenous Peoples. Her award-winning book was the first US nursing text to focus on Native Americans. Now in the prime of her career, her experience in countless communities in North America and other parts of the world has given her a broad and varied perspective on all aspects of Indigenous health. In her interview, she emphasized the importance of recognizing structural determinants of health as the root cause of disparities. She also highlighted the degree of diversity among American Indians, and made the crucial point that Native people are often misidentified. Finally, she stressed that care providers must ask clients about their cultural background as a prerequisite to providing culturally competent services.

Ada Deer is a lifelong activist who continues to fight injustices perpetrated against her own tribe and other American Indian Peoples. Now an elder, she has accomplished many "firsts" for her tribe, for the social work profession, and in the US federal government. While she has held numerous leadership positions, such as Chair of the Menominee Tribe and Assistant Secretary of the Interior in the federal government, she has always recognized the importance of working in partnership and coalition with others. She is a prominent role model for many social workers, many American Indian people, and many women. Although now retired from academia, she remains a committed activist and a powerful catalyst to motivate others to work toward social change. Her breadth of experience makes her uniquely qualified to comment on a wide variety of American Indian issues, particularly those related to communities and macro-level change. In her interview, Deer emphasized the importance of understanding the federal context and how to work within government systems that create policy and/or serve American Indians. She noted the power of activism and the importance of persistence. It is possible to make a difference, even in the face of significant adversity.

Dr. Eddie Brown also has a broad range of experience as a researcher and administrator at tribal, state, and federal levels. As an American Indian social worker with a doctorate, he was uniquely positioned to influence policy and pave the way for other American Indians to work in the human service and policy fields. His career has intersected with some of the most significant federal policies affecting American Indian people and tribes over the last four decades. Now retired from academia and his administrative positions, he still works with his tribe. He has mentored countless American Indian and allied scholars who now work with and advocate on behalf of American Indian communities. His extensive background ideally positioned him to address issues affecting American Indian communities. He has been both a witness to and an active participant in shaping modern history and policy for American Indian people. Throughout his interview, he emphasized that helping professionals must understand sovereignty and its implications. After drawing attention to a recent report by the Attorney General's Advisory Committee on American Indian/Alaska Native Children Exposed to Violence (2014), which details the impact of violence on the lives of American Indian children, he emphasized that children are the future and that helping professionals who wish to make a difference in the lives of American Indians must understand and act on this report. Building strong communities starts with families.

I was privileged to hear the stories, thoughts, experiences, journeys, and perspectives of these experts. They are the elders to whom I turn as I seek to improve the service to Indigenous Peoples provided by my chosen profession of social work and allied disciplines. I hold each of them in great esteem. Even those I have known for decades or have interviewed for other projects were generous enough to share stories and perspectives that I found surprising, enlightening, and informative. I listened, smiling, as many of their words resonated with me and my own experiences. Sometimes I found myself grinning from ear to ear and nodding in recognition. Other times, I was chilled when the sorrow and pain of their stories took a personal turn as one of the experts spoke of my own cousin's death and attributed this to how systems had failed her.

We should listen to these words and those of other Native people not simply because of their academic credentials. Lived experience must be acknowledged and valued, too. There are many ways of knowing. Too often, Indigenous knowledge is neglected. Too often, we are told to use someone else's citation to document our assertions. We need to decolonize our ideas about what we know and how we know it to become open to learning and helping. We must recognize the importance of human rights and the role that trauma has played and continues to play in the lives of countless Indigenous people.

The words that can help us provide quality, culturally responsive, decolonized, trauma-informed helping services are presented in this book. While the chapters draw on scholarly literature, they also highlight the Indigenous perspectives of people who have dedicated their lives and careers to enhancing wellness. Indeed, perhaps this book should be considered Indigenous knowledge in the Trojan horse of an academic publication. It is just one source of information that may prove useful for helping professionals and educators. There are many other examples and opportunities if we look for them and listen, particularly at the grassroots level. We have two eyes, two ears, and one mouth. Each of us is challenged to reflect on which we use the most as we seek to learn about and address the needs and priorities of Native Peoples.

We are faced with an urgent question: "Where do we go from here?" We have a lot to learn from our elders. They are often well versed in the needs and strengths of the community and can help us understand what succeeded or failed in the past. It is notable, however, that Indigenous Peoples are often grounded in collective values that include non-hierarchical forms of leadership. Indeed, there are lessons to learn from all people—from the oldest to the youngest. Some of the experts interviewed for this book have now retired, while others are nearing that stage. Others, however, are in the prime of their careers, and I fully anticipate that they and their peers will continue to drive the development of culturally responsive, trauma-informed models that will shape our understanding of best practices across a variety of fields. We have much to learn from both community members and younger scholars.

The process of writing this book has been inspiring and affirming for me. It has pulled me in new directions and informed how I think and speak. I hope that it will do the same for you, the reader. As I consult the literature from a variety of academic disciplines for information on libraries, dental therapists, and environmental contamination, I work to synthesize this published knowledge with the perspectives and wisdom of experts' lived experiences as both professionals and Indigenous people. Within the reflections of these experts are calls to action. Helping professionals have the ability to make a difference.

This book began by noting that our ancestors left a trail of breadcrumbs for us to follow in order to find our way home. Likewise, Lakota teachings remind us that nothing is ever truly lost, as long as we can go up the hill—a reference to traditional ways of seeking guidance. Both reflect narratives of continuity and resilience in the face of adversity—ways of returning home after being lost. These can help us determine where we go from here.

Indigenous Peoples have always had ways of helping and restoring balance. Helping professionals may employ different methods but also work to cultivate wellness. In today's world, Native people can benefit from both. Our ancestors survived many challenges while attending to the wellbeing of future generations. We can and should do the same.

Wilma Mankiller successfully negotiated Indigenous and mainstream worlds throughout her life. Her life journey reflects many of the topics in this book. A social worker, activist, Indigenous woman, and Principal Chief of the Cherokee Nation, she noted the resilience that continues to permeate Indigenous communities in spite of adversity:

> We acknowledge the hardships of the past without dwelling on them every day. Instead, we look to the future with the same faith that kept us together this far. To be sure, some Indigenous languages have vanished while others are endangered. Some of the old ceremonies have been lost over time, and our communities are no longer as intact as they once were—but in most tribal communities, even the most troubled and acculturated, there are Indigenous people who continue to use ancient knowledge to inform their lives. Their relationship to and interdependence with every other living thing—humans, animals, the stars, the land—is held together by a common understanding of history, culture, and most importantly values. Traditional stories passed from generation to generation as well as ceremonies and rituals contribute to Indigenous people's understanding of their place in the universe.
>
> *(Mankiller, 2004, pp. 145–146)*

We draw on our strength for those generations yet to come. We remain Indigenous. We are resilient. We are empowered. We have allies. We have a future in which our children's children will reclaim balance and restore wellness for their descendants.

REFERENCES

Alcantara, C. & Spicer, Z. (2016). A new model for making Aboriginal policy? Evaluating the Kelowna Accord and the promise of multilevel governance in Canada. *Canadian Public Administration*, 59(2), pp. 183–203.

Alexie, S. (2017). *You Don't Have to Say You Love Me: A Memoir*. New York: Little, Brown and Company.

Alfred, T. (2005). *Wasase: Indigenous Pathways of Action and Freedom*. Peterborough, Ontario: Broadview Press.

American Foundation for Suicide Prevention. (2018). *Suicide Statistics*. https://afspp.org. Accessed February 1, 2018.

American Indian Law and Order Commission. (2015). *A Roadmap for Making Native America Safer*. www.aisc.ucla.edu. Accessed February 1, 2018.

Amnesty International. (2004). *Stolen Sisters: A Human Rights Response to Discrimination and Violence against Indigenous Women in Canada*. Ottawa. Amnesty International.

Amnesty International. (2009). *No More Stolen Sisters: The Need for a Comprehensive Response to Discrimination and Violence against Indigenous Women in Canada*. Ottawa: Amnesty International.

Arincorayan, D., Applewhite, L., Garrido, M., Cashio, V. & Bryant, M. (2017). Resilience-enhancing relationships: What we can learn from those with a history of adverse childhood experiences. *US Army Medical Department Journal*, July-September, pp. 25–32.

Attorney General's Advisory Committee on American Indian/Alaska Native Children Exposed to Violence. (2014). *Ending Violence so Children Can Thrive*. Washington, DC: US Department of Justice.

Baird, J., Plummer, R., Dupont, D. & Carter, B. (2015). Perceptions of water quality in First Nations communities: Exploring the role of context. *Nature and Culture*, 10(2), pp. 225–249.

Balestrery, J.E. (2012). Intersecting discourses on race and sexuality: Compounded colonization among LGBTTQ American Indian/Alaska Natives. *Journal of Homosexuality*, 59(5), pp. 633–655.

Balestrery, J.E. (2016). Indigenous elder insights about conventional care services in Alaska: Culturally charged spaces. *Journal of Gerontological Social Work*, 59(4), pp. 296–315.

Ball, J. (2010). Indigenous fathers' involvement in reconstituting "Circles of Care". *American Journal of Community Psychology*, 45, pp. 124–138.

Balsam, K.F., Huang, B., Fieland, K.C., Simoni, J.M. & Walters, K.L. (2004). Culture, trauma and wellness: A comparison of heterosexual and lesbian, gay, bisexual, and two-spirit Native Americans. *Cultural Diversity and Ethnic Minority Psychology*, 10(3), pp. 287–301.

Bassett, D., Buchwald, D. & Manson, S. (2014). Posttraumatic stress disorder and symptoms among American Indians and Alaska Natives: A review of the literature. *Social Psychiatry and Psychiatric Epidemiology*, 49, pp. 417–433.

Beals, J., Manson, S.M., Croy, C., Klein, S.A., Whitesell, N.R., Mitchell, C.M. & AI-SUPERPTF Team. (2013). Lifetime prevalence of posttraumatic stress disorder in two American Indian reservation populations. *Journal of Traumatic Stress*, 26, pp. 512–520.

Bender, A. (2018). Oil keeps flowing as corp misses deadline for DAPL environmental study. www.indianz.com/News/2018/04/09/albert-bender-oil-continues-to-flow-thro.aspp. Accessed August 1, 2018.

Berliner, L. & Kolko, D.J. (2016). Trauma informed care: A commentary and critique. *Child Maltreatment*, 21(2), pp. 168–172.

BigFoot, D.S. & Funderburk, B.W. (2011). Honoring children, making relatives: The cultural translation of parent–child interaction therapy for American Indian and Alaska Native families. *Journal of Psychoactive Drugs*, 43(4), pp. 309–318.

BigFoot, D.S. & Schmidt, S.R. (2010). Honoring children, mending the circle: Cultural adaptation of trauma-focused cognitive-behavioral therapy for American Indian and Alaska Native children. *Journal of Clinical Psychology in Session*, 66(8), pp. 847–856.

Billiot, S.M. (2017). How do environmental changes and shared cultural experiences impact the health of Indigenous Peoples in South Louisiana? Thesis, Washington University. https://openscholarship.wustl.edu/art_sci_etds/1080/. Accessed December 6, 2018.

Bjorum, E. (2014). "Those are our people and that's our family": Wabanaki perspectives on child welfare practices in their communities. *Journal of Public Child Welfare*, 8, pp. 279–303.

Bourgeois, R. (2018). Generations of genocide. In K. Anderson, M. Campbell & C. Belcourt (eds.), *Keetsahnak: Our Missing and Murdered Indigenous Sisters*. Edmonton: University of Alberta Press, pp. 65–88.

Braga, L.L., Mello, M.F. & Fiks, J.P. (2012). Transgenerational transmission of trauma and resilience: A qualitative study with Brazilian offspring of Holocaust survivors. *BMC Psychiatry*, 12, pp. 134–144.

Braine, T. (2016). North Dakota oil spill leaks more than 176,000 gallons of crude. *Indian Country Today*, December 15.

Braun, K.L. & LaCounte, C. (2015). The historic and ongoing issue of disparities among Native elders. *Generations*, 38(4), pp. 60–69.

Brave Heart, M.Y.H., Chase, J., Elkins, J. & Altshul, D.B. (2011). Historical trauma among Indigenous Peoples of the Americas: Concepts, research, and clinical considerations. *Journal of Psychoactive Drugs*, 43(4), pp. 282–290.

Brave Heart, M.Y.H. & Debruyn, M. (1998). The American Indian holocaust: Healing historical unresolved grief. *American Indian Alaska Native Mental Health Research*, 8(2), pp. 56–78.

Brave Heart, M.Y.H., Elkins, J., Tafoya, G., Bird, D. & Salvador, M. (2012). Wicasa Was'aka: Restoring the traditional strength of American Indian boys and men. *American Journal of Public Health*, 102(S2), pp. 177–183.

Brayboy, B.M.J., Fann, A.J., Castagno, A.E. & Solyom, J.A. (2012). Postsecondary education for American Indian and Alaska Natives. *ASHE Higher Education Report*, 37(5), pp. 1–140.

Brayboy, B.M.J. & Maughan, E. (2009). Indigenous knowledges and the story of the bean. *Harvard Educational Review*, 79(1), pp. 1–21.

Brokenleg, M. (2012). Transforming cultural trauma into resilience. *Reclaiming Children and Youth*, 21(3), pp. 9–13.

Brown, D.L. (2016). Daughters of the drum: Decolonizing health and wellness with Native American women. *AlterNative*, 12(2), pp. 109–123.

Browne, A.J., Varcoe, C., Lavoie, J., Smye, V., Wong, S.T., Krause, M., Tu, D., Godwin, O., Kahn, K. & Fridkin, A. (2016). Enhancing health care equity with Indigenous populations: Evidence-based strategies from an ethnographic study. *BMC Health Services Research, 16*, pp. 1–17.

Browne, C.V., Carter, P. & Gray, J.S. (2015). National resource centers focus on Indigenous communities. *Generations: Journal of the American Society on Aging*, 38(4), pp. 70–78.

Burnette, C. (2015). Historical oppression and intimate partner violence experienced by Indigenous women in the United States: Understanding connections. *Social Service Review*, 89(3), pp. 531–563.

Burnette, C.E. (2016). Historical oppression and Indigenous families: Uncovering potential risk factors for Indigenous families touched by violence. *Family Relations: Interdisciplinary Journal of Applied Family Studies*, 65, pp. 354–368.

Burnette, C.E. & Figley, C.R. (2017). Historical oppression, resilience, and transcendence: Can a holistic framework help explain violence experienced by Indigenous People? *Social Work*, 62(1), pp. 37–44.

Burnette, C.E., Roh, S., Lee, K.H., Lee, Y., Newland, L.A. & Jun, J.S. (2017). A comparison of risk and protective factors related to depressive symptoms among American Indian and Caucasian older adults. *Health & Social Work*, 42(1), pp. 15–23.

Buse, N.A., Burker, E.J. & Bernacchio, C. (2013). Cultural variation in resilience as a response to traumatic experience. *Journal of Rehabilitation*, 79(2), pp. 15–23.

Byers, L. (2010). Native American grandmothers: Cultural tradition and contemporary necessity. *Journal of Ethnic and Cultural Diversity in Social Work*, 19(4), pp. 305–316.

Campbell, E.D.C., Jr. (2000). Caught between two worlds. *American History*, 35(1), p. 18.

Carlson, K.T. (2010). Familial cohesion and colonial atomization: Governance and authority in a Coast Salish community. *Native Studies Review*, 19(2), pp. 1–42.

Carroll, C.R., Noonan, C., Garroutte, E.M., Navas-Acien, A., Verney, S.P. & Buchwald, D. (2017). Low-level inorganic arsenic exposure and neuropsychological functioning in American Indian elders. *Environmental Research*, 156, pp. 74–79.

Cavalieri, C.E. (2013). Situating psychotherapy with tribal peoples in a sovereignty paradigm. *Journal of Social Action in Counseling and Psychology*, 5(3), pp. 25–43.

Centers for Disease Control and Prevention (CDC). (2017). About the CDC-Kaiser ACE Study. www.cdc.gov/violenceprevention/acestudy/about.html. Accessed January 12, 2018.

Cerecer, P.D.Q. (2013). Independence, dominance, and power: (Re)examining the impact of school policies on the academic development of Indigenous youth. *Theory into Practice*, 52, pp. 196–202.

Chambers, L. (2017). Boil water advisories and federal (in)action: The politics of potable water in Pikangikum First Nation. *Journal of Canadian Studies*, 51(2), pp. 289–310.

Chaudhri, A. & Schau, N. (2016). Imaginary Indians: Representations of Native Americans in Scholastic Reading Club. *Children's Literature in Education*, 47, pp. 18–35.

Chenault, V.S. (2011). *Weaving Strength, Weaving Power: Violence and Abuse against Indigenous Women*. Durham, NC: Carolina Academic Press.

Cho, P., Geiss, L.S., Burrows, N.R., Roberts, D.L., Bullock, A.K. & Toedt, M.E. (2014). Diabetes-related mortality among American Indians and Alaska Natives, 1990–2009. *American Journal of Public Health*, 104(S3), pp. S496–S503.

Cladoosby, B. (2017). Indian Country leads national movement to knock down barriers to oral health equity. *American Journal of Public Health*, 107, pp. 81–84.

Clarren, R. (2017). Left behind: How punitive discipline, inadequate curriculums, and declining federal funding put Native American students at risk. *The Nation*, 305(4), pp. 12–25.

Cobb, N., Espey, D. & King, J. (2014). Health behaviors and risk factors among American Indians and Alaska Natives, 2000–2010. *American Journal of Public Health*, 104(S3), pp. S481–S489.

Coleman, J.A. (2016). Racial differences in posttraumatic stress disorder in military personnel: Intergenerational transmission of trauma as a theoretical lens. *Journal of Aggression, Maltreatment and Trauma*, 25(6), pp. 561–579.

Conte, K.P., Schure, M.B. & Goins, R.T. (2015). Correlates of social support in older American Indians: The Native Elder Care Study. *Aging and Mental Health*, 19(9), pp. 835–843.

Crazy Bull, C. (2012). TCUs preserve heritage, educate American Indians. *Diverse: Issues in Higher Education*, 29(21), p. 27.

Crazy Bull, C. (2015). Engaging life: TCUs and their role building community. *Tribal College Journal*, 27(1), pp. 20–24.

Cross, S.L., Brown, E.F., Day, P.A., Limb, G.E., Pellebon, D.A., Proctor, E.C. & Weaver, H.N. (2009). *Status of Native Americans in Social Work Higher Education*. Alexandria, VA: Council on Social Work Education.

Cross, S.L., Day, A.G. & Byers, L.G. (2010). American Indian grand families: A qualitative study conducted with grandmothers and grandfathers who provide sole care for their grandchildren. *Journal of Cross Cultural Gerontology*, 25, pp. 371–383.

Davis, J.J., Roscigno, V.J. & Wilson, G. (2016). American Indian poverty in the contemporary United States. *Sociological Forum*, 31(1), pp. 5–28.

Dennis, M.K. (2014). Layers of loss, death, and grief as social determinants of Lakota elders' behavioral health. *Best Practice in Mental Health*, 10(2), pp. 32–47.

Dennis, M.K. & Brewer, J.P. (2017). Rearing generations: Lakota grandparents' commitment to family and community. *Journal of Cross Cultural Gerontology*, 32, pp. 95–113.

d'Errico, P. (2013). Jeffrey Amherst and smallpox blankets. www.nativeweb.org/pages/legal/amherst/lord-Jeff.html. Accessed December 6, 2013.

Deschenie, T. (2006). Historical trauma. *Tribal College Journal*, 17(3), pp. 8–11.

Deters, P.B., Novins, D.K., Fickenscher, A. & Beals, J. (2006). Trauma and posttraumatic stress disorder symptomatology: Patterns among American Indian adolescents in substance abuse treatment. *American Journal of Orthopsychiatry*, 76(3), pp. 335–345.

Devon, H. (2016). The Standing Rock Police attack protestors again: "He just smiled and shot both my kneecaps". *Daily Beast*, November 21. www.thedailybeast.com/articles/2016/11/21/standing-rock. Accessed December 6, 2018.

Dill, E.J., Manson, S.M., Jiang, L., Pratte, K.A., Gutilla, M.J., Knepper, S.L., Beals, J. & Roubideaux, Y. (2015). Psychosocial predictors of weight loss among American Indian and Alaska Native participants in a diabetes prevention translation project. *Journal of Diabetes Research, 2016*, pp. 1–10.

Dimitrova-Grajzi, V., Grajzi, P. & Guse, J.A. (2014). Jurisdiction, crime, and development: The impact of Public Law 280 in Indian Country. *Law and Society Review*, 48(1), pp. 127–160.

Dionne, D. & Nixon, G. (2014). Moving beyond residential school trauma abuse: A phenomenological hermeneutic analysis. *International Journal of Mental Health and Addiction*, 12, pp. 335–350.

Dotremon, D. (2013). *Stolen Children: The Removal of Native American Children through Fostering out and Adoption*. National Association of African American Studies and Affiliates Conference Monographs, pp. 1681–1706.

Dubois, J. & Saunders, K. (2017). Rebuilding Indigenous Nations through constitutional development: A case study of the Metis in Canada. *Nations and Nationalism*, 23 (4), pp. 878–901.

Dunbar-Ortiz, R. (2014). *An Indigenous Peoples' History of the United States*. Boston: Beacon Press.

Duran, E. (2006). *Healing the Soul Wound: Counseling with American Indians and Other Native Peoples*. New York: Teachers College Press.

Durham, M. & Webb, S.S.N. (2014). Historical trauma: A panoramic perspective. *Brown University Child and Adolescent Behavioral Letter*, 30(10), pp. 4–6.

Echo-Hawk, W. (2013). *In the Light of Justice: The Rise of Human Rights in Native America and the UN Declaration on the Rights of Indigenous Peoples*. Golden, CO: Fulcrum Publishing.

Edwards, M. (2017). For Native Americans facing sexual assault, justice feels out of reach. *Morning Edition*, National Public Radio, November 14.

Eggers, M.J., Moore-Nall, A.L., Doyle, J.T., Lefthand, M.J., Young, S.L., Bends, A.L. & Camper, A.K. (2015). Potential health risks from uranium in home well water: An investigation by the Apsaalooke (Crow) Tribal Research Group. *Geosciences*, 5(1), pp. 67–94.

Ehlers, C.L., Hurst, S., Phillips, E., Gilder, D.A., Dixon, M., Gross, A., Lau, P. & Yehuda, R. (2006). Electrophysiological responses to affective stimuli in American Indians experiencing trauma with and without PTSD. *Annals of the New York Academy of Sciences*, 1071, pp. 125–136.

Eichstaedt, P.H. (1994). *If You Poison Us: Uranium and Native Americans*. Santa Fe, NM: Red Crane Books.

Ellinghaus, K. (2008). The benefits of being Indian: Blood quanta, intermarriage, and allotment policy on the White Earth Reservation, 1889–1920. *Frontiers: A Journal of Women's Studies*, 29(2/3), pp. 81–105.

Elm, J.H.L., Lewis, J.P., Walters, K.L. & Self, J.M. (2016). "I'm in the world for a reason": Resilience and recovery among American Indian and Alaska Native two-spirit women. *Journal of Lesbian Studies*, 20(3/4), pp. 352–371.

Estrada, A.L. (2009). Mexican Americans and historical trauma theory: A theoretical perspective. *Journal of Ethnicity in Substance Abuse*, 8(3), pp. 330–340.

Evans-Campbell, T. (2008). Historical trauma in American Indian/Native Alaska communities: A multilevel framework for exploring impacts on individuals, families, and communities. *Journal of Interpersonal Violence*, 23(3), pp. 316–338.

Evans-Campbell, T., Lindhorst, T., Huang, B. & Walters, K.L. (2006). Interpersonal violence in the lives of urban American Indian and Alaska Native women: Implications for health, mental health, and help-seeking. *American Journal of Public Health*, 96(8), pp. 1416–1422.

Fallot, R. & Harris, M. (2008). Trauma-informed approaches to systems of care. *Trauma Psychology Newsletter*, 3(1), pp. 6–7.

Federal Register. (2017). Indian entities recognized and eligible to receive services from the United States Bureau of Indian Affairs. *Federal Register*, 82(10), pp. 4915–4920.

Feinstein, R.A. (2015). White privilege, juvenile justice, and criminal identities: A qualitative analysis of the perceptions and self-identification of incarcerated youth. *Contemporary Justice Review*, 18(3), pp. 313–333.

Fitzgerald, S.J. (2015). *Native Women and Land: Narratives of Dispossession and Resurgence*. Albuquerque: University of New Mexico Press.

Fixico, D.L. (2013). *Indian Resilience and Rebuilding: Indigenous Nations in the Modern American West*. Tucson: University of Arizona Press.

Forbes-Boyte, K. (1999). Fools Crow versus Gullett: A critical analysis of the American Indian Religious Freedom Act. *Antipode*, 31(3), pp. 304–323.

Ford, A. & Hughes, C. (2017). Coming home, building community: Aiding elders on a Native American reservation. *American Libraries*, 48(6), pp. 26–27.

Forte, M.C. (2013). Carib identity, racial politics, and the problem of Indigenous recognition in Trinidad and Tobago. In M.C. Forte (ed.), *Who is an Indian? Race, Place, and the Politics of Indigeneity in the Americas*. Toronto: University of Toronto Press, pp. 172–193.

Foulds, H.J.A., Rodgers, C.D., Duncan, V. & Ferguson, L.J. (2016). A systematic review and meta-analysis of screen time behaviour among North American Indigenous populations. *Obesity Reviews*, 17(5), pp. 455–466.

Fox, M.J.T. (2005). Voices from within: Native American faculty and staff on campus. *New Directions for Student Services*, 109, pp. 49–59.

Fox, M.J.T., Lowe, S.C. & McClellan, G.S. (2005). Where we have been: A history of Native American higher education. *New Directions for Student Services*, 109, pp. 7–15.

Franklin, T.W. (2013). Sentencing Native Americans in US federal courts: An examination of disparity. *Justice Quarterly*, 30(2), pp. 310–339.

Fueshko, T.M. (2016). The intricacies of shell shock: A chronological history of the Lancet's publications by Dr. Charles S. Meyers and his contemporaries. *Peace and Change*, 41(1), pp. 38–51.

Gallagher, B. & Selman, M. (2015). Warrior entrepreneur. *American Indian Quarterly*, 39(1), pp. 73–94.

Gentry, M., Fugate, C.M., Wu, J. & Castellano, J.A. (2014). Gifted Native American students: Literature, lessons, and future directions. *Gifted Child Quarterly*, 58(2), pp. 98–110.

Gilliard, J.L. & Moore, R.A. (2007). An investigation of how culture shapes curriculum in early care and education programs on a Native American Indian reservation. *Early Childhood Education Journal*, 34(4), pp. 251–258.

Goldtooth, T.B.K. (2010). Earth Mother, pinons, and apple pie. *Wicazo Sa Review*, 25(2), pp. 11–28.

Gone, J.P. (2009). A community-based treatment for Native American historical trauma: Prospects for evidence-based practice. *Journal of Consulting and Clinical Psychology*, 77(4), pp. 751–762.

Goodkind, J., LaNoue, M., Lee, C., Freeland, L. & Freund, R. (2012). Feasibility, acceptability, and initial findings from a community-based cultural mental health intervention for American Indian youth and their families. *Journal of Community Psychology*, 40(4), pp. 381–405.

Goodkind, J.R., Ross-Toledo, K., John, S., Hall, J.L., Ross, L., Freeland, L., Coletta, E., Becenti-Fundark, T., Poola, C., Begay-Roanhorse, R. & Lee, C. (2010). Promoting healing and restoring trust: Policy recommendations for improving behavioral health care for American Indian/Alaska Native adolescents. *American Journal of Community Psychology*, 46, pp. 386–394.

Goodman, R. (2013). The transgenerational trauma and resilience genogram. *Counseling Psychology Quarterly*, 26(3/4), pp. 386–405.

Grande, S. (2018). Aging, precarity, and the struggle for Indigenous elsewheres. *International Journal of Qualitative Studies in Education*, 31(3), pp. 168–176.

Grayshield, L., Rutherford, J.J., Salazar, S.B., Mihecoby, A.L., & Luna, L.L. (2015). Understanding and healing historical trauma: The perspectives of Native American elders. *Journal of Mental Health Counseling*, 37(4), pp. 295–307.

Griffin-Pierce, T. (1997). "When I am lonely the mountains call me": The impact of sacred geography on Navajo psychological well being. *American Indian and Alaska Native Mental Health Research*, 7(3), pp. 1–10.

Hansen, K.B., Jepsen, K. & Jacquelin, P.L. (eds.). (2017). *The Indigenous World 2017*. Copenhagen: International Workgroup for Indigenous Affairs.

Harjo, S.S. (2017). Vampire policy is bleeding us dry—blood quantums, be gone! In K. Ratterree & N. Hill (eds.), *The Great Vanishing Act: Blood Quantum and the Future of Native Nation*. Golden, CO: Fulcrum Publishing, pp. 77–79.

Harrington, B.G. & Chixapkaid [Pavel, D.M.]. (2013). Using Indigenous educational research to transform mainstream education: A guide for P-12 school leaders. *American Journal of Education*, 119(4), pp. 487–511.

Hartmann, W.E. & Gone, J. P. (2014). American Indian historical trauma: Community perspectives from two Great Plains medicine men. *American Journal of Community Psychology*, 54, pp. 274–288.

Haupton, L.M. (2015). *The Iroquois Struggle for Survival: World War II to Red Power*. Syracuse: Syracuse University Press.

Hedrick, C. (2016). Returning the warrior spirit: Native men's wellness gatherings. *News from Native California*, 29(4), pp. 49–51.

Herman, L. (2010). Engaging images of evil: An imaginal approach to historical trauma. *ReVision*, 31(1), pp. 44–52.

Hill, D.L. (2006). Sense of belonging as connectedness, American Indian worldview, and mental health. *Archives of Psychiatric Nursing*, 20(5), pp. 210–216.

History Matters. (n.d.). "Kill the Indian and save the man": Capt. Richard H. Pratt on the education of Native Americans. http://historymatters.gmu.edu/d/4929/. Accessed October 17, 2013.

Holm, T. (2017). Strong hearts, wounded souls revisited: The research, the findings, and some observations of recent Native veteran readjustment. *Wicazo Sa Review*, 32(1), pp. 118–128.

Hudson, W. (2017). Native American leaders in higher education. *Diverse: Issues in Higher Education,* *34*(21), pp. 11–13.

Huffman, T. (2010). *Theoretical Perspectives on American Indian Education: Taking a Look at Academic Success and the Achievement Gap*. Blue Ridge Summit, PA: AltaMira Press.

Hughes, R.W. (2017). Pueblo Indian water rights: Charting the unknown. *Natural Resources,* 57(1), pp. 219–261.

Iacoviello, B.M. & Charney, D.S. (2014). Psychosocial facets of resilience: Implications for preventing posttrauma psychopathology, treating trauma survivors, and enhancing community resilience. *European Journal of Psychotraumatology*, 5, pp. 1–10.

Indian Country Today. (2017). Breaking: DAPL approval illegal, judge finds. *Indian Country Today*, June 14.

Indigenous and Conserved Communities Area Consortium. (2018). Self-determination and resistance to destructive development in ICCAs. Paper presented at the United Nations Permanent Forum on Indigenous Issues, New York, April 17.

Iliceto, P., Candilera, G., Funaro, D., Pompili, M., Kaplan, K.J. & Markus-Kaplan, M. (2011). Hopelessness, temperament, anger and interpersonal relationships in Holocaust (Shoah) survivors' grandchildren. *Journal of Religion and Health*, 50, pp. 321–329.

Indian Health Service. (2018a). Health topics. www.ihs.gov/forpatients/healthtopics/. Accessed February 14, 2018.

Indian Health Service. (2018b). Suicide prevention. www.ihs.gov/suicideprevention/. Accessed February 1, 2018.

Indianz.com. (2017). Federal recognition Bill for six tribes in Virginia inches another step forward. www.indianz.com/News/2017/09/13/federal-recognition-bill-for-six-tribes.aspp. Accessed September 15, 2017.

Iroquois White Corn. (2018). Welcome to Ganondagan. www.iroquoiswhitecorn.org. Accessed February 9, 2018.

Jernigan, V.B.B., Duran, B., Ahn, D. & Winkleby, M. (2010). Changing patterns in health behaviors and risk factors related to cardiovascular disease among American Indians and Alaska Natives. *American Journal of Public Health*, 100(4), pp. 677–683.

Jernigan, V.B.B., Wetherill, M.S., Hearod, J., Jacob, T., Salvatore, A.L., Cannady, T., Grammar, M., Standridge, J., Fox, J., Spiegel, J., Wiley, A., Noonan, C. & Buchwald, D. (2017). Food insecurity and chronic diseases among American Indians in rural Oklahoma: The THRIVE study. *American Journal of Public Health*, 107(3), pp. 441–446.

Johnston-Goodstar, K. (2013). Indigenous youth participatory action research: Re-visioning social justice for social work with Indigenous youth. *Social Work*, 58(4), pp. 314–320.

Johnston-Goodstar, K., Piescher, K. & LaLiberte, T. (2016). Critical experiential learning in the Native American community for Title IV-E students: A pilot evaluation. *Journal of Public Child Welfare*, 10(3), pp. 310–326.

Johnston-Goodstar, K. & VeLure Roholt, R. (2017). "Our kids aren't dropping out, they're being pushed out": Native American students and racial microaggressions in schools. *Journal of Ethnic and Cultural Diversity in Social Work*, 26(1–2), pp. 30–47.

Jones, L. (2008). The distinctive characteristics and needs of domestic violence victims in a Native American community. *Journal of Family Violence*, 23, pp. 113–118.

Kahn, C.B., Reinschmidt, K., Teufel-Shone, N., Ore, C.E., Hensen, M. & Attakai, A. (2016). American Indian elders' resilience: Sources of strength for building a healthy future for youth. *American Indian and Alaska Native Mental Health Research*, 23(3), pp. 117–133.

Kanu, Y. (2006). Getting them through the college pipeline: Critical elements of instruction influencing school success among Native Canadian high school students. *Journal of Advanced Academics*, 18(1), pp. 116–145.

Kaufman, C.E., Kaufmann, L.J., Shangreau, C., Dailey, N., Blair, B. & Shore, J. (2016). American Indian veterans and VA services in three tribes. *American Indian and Alaska Native Mental Health Research*, 23(2), pp. 64–83.

Kaufmann, L.J., Richardson, W.J., Floyd, J. & Shore, J. (2014). Tribal Veterans Representative (TVR) Training Program: The effect of community outreach workers on American Indian and Alaska Native veterans' access to and utilization of the Veterans Health Administration. *Journal of Community Health*, 39, pp. 990–996.

Kelly, U., Boyd, M.A., Valente, S.M. & Czekanski, E. (2014). Trauma-informed care: Keeping mental health settings safe for veterans. *Issues in Mental Health Nursing*, 35, pp. 413–419.

Kiel, D. (2017). Bleeding out: Histories and legacies of "Indian blood". In K. Ratterree & N. Hill (eds.), *The Great Vanishing Act: Blood Quantum and the Future of Native Nation*. Golden, CO: Fulcrum Publishing, pp. 80–97.

Kimmel, M. (2014). Fate control and human rights: The policies and practices of local governance in America's Arctic. *Alaska Law Review*, 31(2), pp. 179–210.

King, D. (2017). Red Lake Nation College dedicates memorial to veterans. *Tribal College Journal*, 29(2), p. 2.

Kipp, W. (2004). *Viet Cong at Wounded Knee: The Trail of a Blackfeet Activist*. Lincoln: University of Nebraska Press.

Klopotek, B., Lintinger, B. & Barbry, J. (2008). Ordinary and extraordinary trauma: Race indigeneity, and Hurricane Katrina in the Tunica-Biloxi history. *American Indian Culture and Research Journal*, 32(2), pp. 55–77.

Kostelecky, S.R., Hurley, D.A., Manus, J. & Aguilar, P. (2017). Centering Indigenous knowledge: Three Southwestern tribal college and university library collections. *Collection Management*, 42(3/4), pp. 180–195.

Kramer, B.J., Creekmur, B., Cote, S. & Saliba, D. (2015). Improving access to noninstitutional long-term care for American Indian veterans. *Journal of the American Geriatrics Society*, 63(4), pp. 789–796.

Kramer, B.J., Creekmur, B., Mitchell, M.N. & Saliba, D. (2018). Expanding home-based primary care to American Indian reservations and other rural communities: An observational study. *Journal of American Geriatrics Society*, 66(4), pp. 818–824.

Kristianto, B. (2013). The notion of the body and the path to healing. *International Journal of Religion and Spirituality in Society*, 2, pp. 41–52.

LaDuke, W. (2005). *Recovering the Sacred: The Power of Naming and Claiming*. Cambridge, MA: South End Press.

Lajimodiere, D. (2012). A healing journey. *Wicazo Sa Review*, 27(2), pp. 5–19.

Lane, D.C. & Simmons, J. (2011). American Indian youth substance abuse: Community-driven interventions. *Mount Sinai Journal of Medicine*, 78, pp. 362–372.

Larsen, S.C. & Johnson, J.T. (2017). *Being Together in Place: Indigenous Coexistence in a More than Human World*. Minneapolis: University of Minnesota Press.

LaVallie, D.L., Wolf, F.M., Jacobsen, C., Sprague, D. & Buchwald, D.S. (2012). Health numeracy and understanding of risk among older American Indians and Alaska Natives. *Journal of Health Communication*, 17(3), pp. 294–302.

Lawrence, B. (2013). Federally unrecognized Indigenous communities in Canadian contexts. In M.C. Forte (ed.), *Who is an Indian? Race, Place, and the Politics of Indigeneity in the Americas*. Toronto: University of Toronto Press, pp. 71–91.

Layton, L. (2013). In Montana, an Indian reservation's children feel the impact of sequester's cuts. *Washington Post*, March 21.

Lazarus, E. (1991). *Black Hills White Justice: The Sioux Nation versus the United States 1775 to the Present*. New York: HarperCollins.

Leavitt, P.A., Covarrubias, R., Perez, Y.A. & Fryberg, S.A. (2015). "Frozen in time": The impact of Native American media representations on identity and self-understanding. *Journal of Social Issues*, 71(1), pp. 39–53.

Lee, J.H. (2017). Establishing applicable water quality standards for surface waters on Indian reservations. *Emory Law Journal*, 66(4), pp. 965–1006.

Legal Information Institute. (n.d.). 362 US 99 (80 S.Ct. 543, 4 L.Ed. 2d 584) Federal Power Commission, Petitioner, v. Tuscarora Indian Nation. Power Authority of State of New York, Petitioner, v. Tuscarora Indian Nation. www.law.cornell.edu/supremecourt/text/362/99. Accessed October 25, 2017.

Lewington, J. (2017). Truth and education. *Maclean's*, 130(10), pp. 52–56.

Lewis, J., Gonzalez, M., Burnette, C., Benally, M., Seanez, P., Shuey, C., Nez, H., Nez, C. & Nez, S. (2015). Environmental exposures to metals in Native communities and implications for child development: Basis for the Navajo Birth Cohort Study. *Journal of Social Work in Disability and Rehabilitation*, 14(3/4), pp. 245–269.

Lewis, J.D. (2012). Towards a unified theory of trauma and its consequences. *International Journal of Applied Psychoanalytic Studies*, 9(4), pp. 298–317.

Lewis, J.P. (2016). American Indian/Alaska Native elders: A growing demographic that is changing how we view aging. *Journal of Gerontological Social Work*, 59(4), pp. 277–280.

Lewis, J.P. & Allen, J. (2017). Alaska Native elders in recovery: Linkages between Indigenous cultural generativity and sobriety to promote successful aging. *Journal of Cross-Cultural Gerontology*, 32(2), pp. 209–222.

Lindsay, R. (2016). Navajo code talker remembered as a "warrior". *Christian Science Monitor*, September 7.

Linton, K.F. (2015). Interpersonal violence and traumatic brain injuries among Native Americans and women. *Brain Injury*, 29(5), pp. 639–643.

Linton, K.F. & Kim, B.J. (2014). Traumatic brain injury as a result of violence in Native American and Black communities spanning from childhood to older adulthood. *Brain Injury*, 28(8), pp. 1076–1081.

Littletree, S. & Metoyer, C.A. (2015). Knowledge organization from an Indigenous perspective: The Mashantucket Pequot Thesaurus of American Indian Terminology project. *Cataloging and Classification Quarterly*, 53(5/6), pp. 640–657.

Lock, M. (2015). Comprehending the body in the era of the epigenome. *Current Anthropology*, 56(2), pp. 151–177.

Low, M. & Shaw, K. (2011). First Nations' rights and environmental governance: Lessons from the Great Bear Rainforest. *BC Studies*, 172, pp. 9–33.

Lucero, N.M. & Bussey, M. (2015). Practice-informed approaches to addressing substance abuse and trauma exposure in urban Native families involved with child welfare. *Child Welfare*, 94(4), pp. 97–117.

Lyte, B. (2017). Native Hawaiians again seek political sovereignty with a new constitution. *Washington Post*, November 5.

Machado, T.D., Salum, G.A., Bosa, V.L., Goldani, M.Z., Meaney, M.J., Agranonik, M., Manfro, G.G. & Silveira, P.P. (2015). Early life trauma is associated with decreased peripheral levels of thyroid-hormone T3 in adolescents. *International Journal of Developmental Neuroscience*, 47, pp. 304–308.

Maduram, I.K. (2011). The significance of cultural center and text in shaping Native American students' cultural identity. *Journal of Global Intelligence and Policy*, 4(4), pp. 19–25.

Maldonado, J., Bennett, T.M.B., Chief, K., Cochran, P., Cozzetto, K., Gough, B., Redsteer, M.H., Lynn, K., Maynard, N. & Voggesser, G. (2016). Engagement with Indigenous peoples and honoring traditional knowledge systems. *Climatic Change*, 135, pp. 111–126.

Mankiller, W. (2004). *Every Day is a Good Day: Reflections by Contemporary Indigenous Women*. Golden, CO: Fulcrum Publishing.

Mann, C.C. (2005). *1491: New Revelations of the Americas before Columbus*. New York: Vintage Books.

Manson, S.M., Beals, J., Klein, S.A., Croy, C.D. & AI-SUPERPFP Team. (2005). Social epidemiology of trauma among 2 American Indian reservation populations. *American Journal of Public Health*, 95(5), pp. 851–859.

Marass, P. (2017). Balancing the fishes' scales: Tribal, state, and federal interests in fishing rights and water quality in Maine. *Vermont Law Review*, 41(4), pp. 853–890.

Marker, M. (2009). Indigenous resistance and racist schooling on the borders of empires: Coast Salish cultural survival. *Paedagogica Historica*, 45(6), pp. 757–772.

Maschi, T., Viola, D. & Morgen, K. (2014). Unraveling trauma and stress, coping resources, and mental well-being among older adults in prison: Empirical evidence linking theory and practice. *The Gerontologist*, 54(5), pp. 857–867.

Mathers, R.L. (2012). The failure of state-led economic development on American Indian reservations. *Independent Review*, 17(1), pp. 65–80.

Mauer, K.W. (2017). Indian Country poverty: Place-based poverty on American Indian territories, 2006–2010. *Rural Sociology*, 82(3), pp. 473–498.

McCrea, K.T., Guthrie, D. & Bulanda, J.J. (2016). When traumatic stressors are not past, but now: Psychosocial treatment to develop resilience with children and youth enduring concurrent, complex trauma. *Journal of Child and Adolescent Trauma*, 9, pp. 5–16.

McMillan, M. & Rigney, S. (2016). The place of the First Peoples in the international sphere: A logical starting point for the demand for justice by Indigenous Peoples. *Melbourne University Law Review*, 39, pp. 981–1002.

McQuaid, R.J., Bombay, A., McInnis, O.A., Matheson, K. & Anisman, H. (2015). Childhood adversity, perceived discrimination, and coping strategies in relation to depressive symptoms among First Nations adults in Canada: The moderating role of unsupportive social interactions from ingroup and outgroup members. *Cultural Diversity and Ethnic Minority Psychology*, 21(3), pp. 326–336.

Means, R. & Wolf, M. (1996). *Where White Men Fear to Tread: The Autobiography of Russell Means*. New York: St. Martin's Press.

Meza, N. (2015). Indian education: Maintaining tribal sovereignty through Native American culture and language preservation. *Brigham Young University Education and Law Journal*, 1, pp. 353–366.

Migchels, E. (2018). Indigenous Students' Council calls for autonomous governing body, student council reacts. *The Sheaf*, March 2. www.thesheaf.com/2018/03/02/indigenous-students-council-calls-for-autonomous-governing-body-student-council-reacts/. Accessed December 3, 2018.

Mihesuah, D.A. (2006). Indigenizing the academy. *Wicazo Sa*, 21(1), pp. 127–138.

Mitchell, C. (2013). Sequester cuts already hitting Minnesota's reservation schools. *Star Tribune*, March 19.

Moghaddam, J.F., Momper, S.L. & Fong, T. (2013). Discrimination and participation in traditional healing for American Indians and Alaska Natives. *Journal of Community Health*, 38, pp. 1115–1123.

Mohatt, N.V., Thompson, A.B., Thai, N.D. & Tebes, J.K. (2014). Historical trauma as public narrative: A conceptual review of how history impacts present-day health. *Social Science and Medicine*, 106, pp. 128–136.

Momper, S.L., Dennis, M.L. & Mueller-Williams, A.C. (2017). American Indian elders share personal stories of alcohol use with younger tribal members. *Journal of Ethnicity and Substance Abuse*, 16(3), pp. 293–313.

Morales, L. (2017). For some Native Americans, uranium contamination feels like discrimination. *You, Me, and Them: Experiencing Discrimination in America*, National Public Radio, November 14.

Morgan, H. (2010). Teaching Native American students: What every teacher should know. *Education Digest*, 75(6), pp. 44–47.

Morgan, R. & Freeman, L. (2009). The healing of our people: Substance abuse and historical trauma. *Substance Use and Misuse*, 44, pp. 84–98.

Myhra, L.L. (2011). "It runs in the family": Intergenerational transmission of historical trauma among urban American Indians and Alaska Natives in culturally specific sobriety maintenance programs. *American Indian and Alaska Native Mental Health Research*, 18(2), pp. 17–40.

Myhra, L.L. & Wieling, E. (2014). Psychological trauma among American Indian families: A two-generation study. *Journal of Loss and Trauma*, 19, pp. 289–313.

National Aeronautics and Space Administration. (2018). Global climate change: Vital signs of the planet. https://climate.nasa.gov/vital-signs/arctic-sea-ice/. Accessed July 15, 2018.

National Congress of American Indians. (2018). Education. www.ncai.org/policy-issues/education-health-human-services/education. Accessed January 19, 2018.

Navajo Nation & Office of the President and Vice President. (2018). President Begaye signs agreement with ASU to strengthen support of Navajo social service programs. Press release, September 18.

Nebelkopf, E., King, J., Wright, S., Schweigman, K., Lucero, E., Habte-Michael, T. & Cervantes, T. (2011). Growing roots: Native American evidence-based practices. *Journal of Psychoactive Drugs*, 43(4), pp. 263–268.

Nelson, L.A., Noonan, C.J., Goldberg, J. & Buchwald, D.S. (2013). Social engagement and physical and cognitive health among American Indian participants in the Health and Retirement Study. *Journal of Cross-Cultural Gerontology*, 28(4), pp. 453–463.

Neumann, D. (2017). UTTC honors WWI Native servicemen. *Tribal College Journal*, 29(2), pp. 13–14.

Nicolai, S.S. & Saus, M. (2013). Acknowledging the past while looking to the future: Conceptualizing Indigenous child trauma. *Child Welfare*, 92(4), pp. 55–74.

Noe, T.D., Kaufman, C.E., Kaufmann, L.J., Brooks, E. & Shore, J.H. (2014). Providing culturally competent services for American Indian and Alaska Native veterans to reduce health care disparities. *American Journal of Public Health*, 104(S4), pp. S548–S554.

Norris, T., Vines, P.L. & Hoeffel, E.M. (2012). *The American Indian and Alaska Native Population: 2010*. Washington, DC: United States Census Bureau.

Nutton, J. & Fast, E. (2015). Historical trauma, substance use, and Indigenous Peoples: Seven generations of harm from a "big event". *Substance Use and Misuse*, 50, pp. 839–847.

Nu'uhiwa, B.S. (2013). Government of the people, by the people, for the people: Cultural sovereignty, civil rights, and good Native Hawaiian governance. *Asia-Pacific Law and Policy Journal*, 14(3), pp. 57–106.

O'Brien, S. (1991). A legal analysis of the American Indian Religious Freedom Act. In C. Vecsey (ed.), *Handbook of American Indian Religious Freedom*. New York: Crossroad, pp. 27–43.

Odani, S., Armour, B.S., Graffunder, C.M., Garrett, B.E., & Agaku, I.T. (2017). Prevalence and disparities in tobacco product use among American Indian/Alaska Natives—United States, 2010–2015. *Morbidity and Mortality Weekly Report*, 66(50), pp. 1374–1378.

Orescanin, V., Kollar, R., Nad, K., Mikelic, I.L. & Kollar, I. (2011). Characterization and treatment of water used for human consumption from six sources located in the Cameron/Tuba City abandoned uranium mining area. *Journal of Environmental Science and Health*, 46(6), pp. 627–635.

Orr, E. (2018). Empowerment models for social work practice with Aboriginal and Torres Strait Islander communities to inform cultural competence and ethical practice in Australian social work. Thesis, La Trobe University, Graduate Research School, Melbourne.

Ortman, J.M., Velkoff, V.A. & Hogan, H. (2014). *An Aging Nation: The Older Population in the United States: Population Estimates and Projections*. Washington, DC: United States Census Bureau. www.census.gov/prod/2014pubs/p25-1140.pdf. Accessed December 6, 2018.

Ostler, J. (2010). *The Lakotas and the Black Hills: The Struggle for Sacred Ground*. New York: Penguin Books.

Patrick, D. (2013). Inuitness and territoriality in Canada. In M.C. Forte (ed.), *Who is an Indian? Race, Place, and the Politics of Indigeneity in the Americas*. Toronto: University of Toronto Press, pp. 52–70.

Peacock, T. (2011). I share a dream: How can we eliminate racism? *Tribal College Journal*, 23(1), 14–18.

Pearce, M.E., Jongbloed, K.A., Richardson, C.G., Henderson, E.W., Pooyak, S.D., Oviedo-Joekes, E., Christian, W.M., Schechter, M.T. & Spittal, P.M. (2015). The Cedar Project: Resilience in the face of HIV vulnerability within a cohort study involving young Indigenous people who use drugs in three Canadian cities. *BMC Public Health*, 15(1), pp. 1–12.

Pember, M.A. (2016). Intergenerational trauma: Understanding Natives' inherited pain. https://indiancountrymediannetwork.com. Accessed February 13, 2017.

Pihama, L., Reynolds, P., Smith, C., Reid, J., Smith, L.T. & Nana, R.T. (2014). Positioning historical trauma theory within Aotearoa New Zealand. *AlterNative: An International Journal of Indigenous Peoples*, 10(3), pp. 248–262.

Pirkle, C., Murkle, G. & Lemire, M. (2016). Managing mercury exposure in northern Canadian communities. *Canadian Medical Association Journal*, 188(14), pp. 1015–1023.

Prussia, L. (2018). Relationship of the mind and body in the healing process: Somatic literacy and the role of connection with the natural environment. Presentation at the Social Work, Education, and Social Development Conference, Dublin, July 4–7.

Raffle, S. (2007). Native American education: A timeline. *American School Board Journal*, December, pp. 22–23.

Reinschmidt, K.M., Attakai, A., Kahn, C.B., Whitewater, S. & Teufel-Shone, N. (2016). Shaping a stories of resilience model from urban American Indian elders' narratives of historical trauma and resilience. *American Indian & Alaska Native Mental Health Research*, 23 (5), pp. 63–85.

REPAM PanAmazon Ecclesial Network. (2018). *Regional Report of Violation of Human Rights in the Amazonia: Weaving Networks of Resistance and Struggle in Colombia, Brazil, Ecuador, Peru and Bolivia*. www.comece.eu/dl/LqquJKJKKLklJqx4LJK/EN-REPAM_report_on_violation_of_HR_in_the_Amazonia.pdf.

Rhoades, D.A., Wagener, T.L., Beebe, L.A., Ding, K., Dvorak, J., Hopkins, M. & Doescher, M.P. (2017). Electronic cigarette use among American Indian youth. *Tobacco Regulatory Science*, 3(3), pp. 315–324.

Rivera, H.H. & Tharp, R.G. (2006). A Native American community's involvement and empowerment to guide their children's development in the school setting. *Journal of Community Psychology*, 34(4), pp. 435–451.

Roberts, E.B., Butler, J. & Green, K.M. (2016). Identifying and understanding Indigenous ways of evaluating physical activity programs. *American Indian & Alaska Native Mental Health Research*, 23(5), pp. 34–58.

Robertson, D.L. (2015). Invisibility in the color-blind era. *American Indian Quarterly*, 39(2), pp. 113–153.

Roh, S., Burnette, C.E., Lee, K.H., Lee, Y., Easton, S.D. & Lawler, M.J. (2015). Risk and protective factors for depressive symptoms among American Indian older adults: Adverse childhood experiences and social support. *Aging & Mental Health*, 19(4), pp. 371–380.

Ryser, R., Korn, L. & Berridge, C.W. (2014). American Indian caregivers policy: A case study. *Fourth World Journal*, 13(1), pp. 107–138.

Salazar, M. (2014). What's in a name? *State Legislatures*, 40(9), p. 11.

Salazar, M. (2016). State recognition of American Indian tribes. *National Conference of State Legislatures*, 24(39). www.ncsl.org/research/state-tribal-institute/state-recognition-of-american-indian-tribes.aspx. Accessed September 15, 2017.

Sarche, M., Tafoya, G., Croy, C.D. & Hill, K. (2017). American Indian and Alaska Native boys: Early childhood risk and resilience amidst context and culture. *Infant Mental Health Journal*, 38(1), pp. 115–127.

Sawchuk, C.N., Russo, J.E., Roy-Byrne, P., Goldberg, J., Forquera, R. & Buchwald, D. (2017). Changes in physical activity barriers among American Indian elders: A pilot study. *American Indian & Alaska Native Mental Health Research*, 24(1), pp. 127–140.

Schimmel, J. (2005). Killing without murder: Aboriginal assimilation policy as genocide. *Lehigh Review*, 13(7), pp. 35–54.

Schmidt, R.W. (2011). American Indian identity and blood quantum in the 21st century: A critical review. *Journal of Anthropology*, 2011. www.hindawi.com/journals/janthro/2011/549521/. Accessed December 6, 2018.

Schure, M. & Goins, R.T. (2017). Psychometric examination of the Center for Epidemiologic Studies Depression Scale with older American Indians: The Native Elder Care Study. *American Indian & Alaska Native Mental Health Research*, 24(3), pp. 1–13.

Schure, M.B., Odden, M. & Goins, R.T. (2013). The association of resilience with mental and physical health among older American Indians: The Native Elder Care Study. *American Indian & Alaska Native Mental Health Research*, 20(2), pp. 27–41.

Senter, M.S. & Ling, D.A. (2017). "It's almost like they were happier when you were down": Microaggressions and overt hostility against Native Americans in a community with gaming. *Sociological Inquiry*, 87(2), pp. 256–281.

Sheppard, M. & Mayo, J.B. (2013). The social construction of gender and sexuality: Learning from two spirit traditions. *Social Studies*, 104(6), pp. 259–270.

Shoemaker, J.A. (2017). Complexity's shadow: American Indian property, sovereignty, and the future. *Michigan Law Review*, 115(4), pp. 487–552.

Shore, J.H., Orton, H. & Manson, S.M. (2009). Trauma-related nightmares among American Indian veterans: Views from the dream catcher. *American Indian & Alaska Native Mental Health Research*, 16(1), pp. 25–38.

Shreve, B. (2017). Serving those who served. *Tribal College Journal*, 29(2), pp. 10–11.

Siler, J.F. (2012). *Lost Kingdom: Hawaii's Last Queen, the Sugar Kings, and America's First Imperial Adventure*. New York: Grove Press.

Simonds, V.W., Goins, R.T., Krantz, E.M. & Garroutte, E.M. (2014). Cultural identity and patient trust among older American Indians. *Journal of General Internal Medicine*, 29(3), pp. 500–506.

Simonds, V.W., Omidpanah, A. & Buchwald, D. (2017). Diabetes prevention among American Indians: The role of self-efficacy, risk perception, numeracy and cultural identity. *BMC Public Health*, 17, pp. 1–11.

Singson, J.M., Tachine, A.R., Davidson, C.E. & Waterman, S.J. (2016). A second home: Indigenous considerations for campus housing. *Journal of College and University Student Housing*, 42(2), pp. 110–125.

Smith, M.K. (2003). A recovery story that heals. *Arctic Anthropology*, 40(2), pp. 83–86.

Smith, T. (2017/2018). Humboldt State University's legacy of supporting Native students. *News from Native California, 31*(2), pp. 26–29.

Song, S.J., Tol, W. & Jong, J.D. (2014). Indero: Intergenerational trauma and resilience between Burundian former child soldiers and their children. *Family Process*, 53(2), pp. 239–251.

Sprague, J.R., Vincent, C.G., Tobin, T.J. & Chixapkaid [Pavel, D.M.]. (2013). Preventing disciplinary exclusions of students from American Indian/Alaska Native backgrounds. *Family Court Review*, 51(3), pp. 452–459.

Stand with Standing Rock. (2016). *Stand with Standing Rock*. https://standwithstandingrock. net. Accessed November 23, 2016.

Steinfeldt, J.A., Foltz, B.D., Kaladow, J.K., Carlson, T.N., Pagano, L.A., Jr., Benton, E. & Steinfeldt, M. (2010). Racism in the electronic age: Role of online forums in expressing racial attitudes about American Indians. *Cultural Diversity and Ethnic Minority Psychology*, 16 (3), pp. 362–371.

Sternadori, M. (2017). Empathy may curb bias: Two studies of the effects of news stories on implicit attitudes toward African Americans and Native Americans. *Contemporary Readings in Law and Social Justice*, 9(2), pp. 11–27.

Stevens, S., Andrade, R., Korchmaros, J. & Sharron, K. (2015). Intergenerational trauma among substance-using Native American, Latina and White mothers living in the Southwestern United States. *Journal of Social Work Practice in the Addictions*, 15, pp. 6–24.

Stinson, J.D., Quinn, M.A. & Levenson, J.S. (2016). The impact of trauma on the onset of mental health symptoms, aggression, and criminal behavior in an inpatient psychiatric sample. *Child Abuse and Neglect*, 61, pp. 13–22.

Stocker, K. (2013). Locating identity: The role of place in Costa Rican Chorotega identity. In M.C. Forte (ed.), *Who is an Indian? Race, Place, and the Politics of Indigeneity in the Americas*. Toronto: University of Toronto Press, pp. 151–171.

Struthers, R. & Lowe, J. (2003). Nursing in the Native American culture and historical trauma. *Issues in Mental Health Nursing*, 24, pp. 257–272.

Suarez, E.B. (2013). The association between post-traumatic stress-related symptoms, resilience, current stress and past exposure to violence: A cross sectional study of the survival of Quechua women in the aftermath of the Peruvian armed conflict. *Conflict and Health*, 7 (1), pp. 1–20.

Substance Abuse and Mental Health Services Administration (SAMHSA). (2014). Understanding historical trauma when responding to an event in Indian Country. https://store. samhsa.gov/system/files/sma14-4866.pdf. Accessed January 12, 2017.

Substance Abuse and Mental Health Services Administration (SAMHSA). (2016). Behind the term: Trauma. https://calswec.berkeley.edu/sites/default/files/4-3_behind_the_term_ trauma.pdf. Accessed January 12, 2017.

Substance Abuse and Mental Health Services Administration (SAMHSA). (2017). Home page. http://samhsa.gov. Accessed January 12, 2017.

Swoyer, A. (2017). Supreme Court ruling against censoring the Slants' name bolsters Washington Redskins trademark case. *Washington Times*, June 19. www.washingtontimes.

com/news/2017/jun/19/washington-redskins-trademark-fight-aided-by-supre/. Accessed October 23, 2017.

Sykes, B.E., Pendley, J. & Deacon, Z. (2017). Transformative learning, tribal membership and cultural restoration: A case study of an embedded Native American service-learning project at a research university. *Gateways: International Journal of Community Research and Engagement*, 10, pp. 204–228.

Szlemko, W.J., Wood, J.W. & Thurman, P.J. (2006). Native Americans and alcohol: Past, present, and future. *Journal of General Psychology*, 133(4), pp. 435–451.

Taualii, M. (2017). (Re)building the Lahui (Hawaiian nation). In K. Ratterree & N. Hill (eds.), *The Great Vanishing Act: Blood Quantum and the Future of Native Nation*. Golden, CO: Fulcrum Publishing, pp. 173–188.

Thayer, Z.M., Blair, I.V., Buchwald, D.S. & Manson, S.M. (2017). Racial discrimination associated with higher diastolic blood pressure in a sample of American Indian adults. *Yearbook of Physical Anthropology*, 163(1), pp. 122–128.

Thompson, S. & Lozecznik, V. (2011). Harvesting hope in northern Manitoba: Can participatory video help rebuild Aboriginal food sovereignty? *Women and Environments International Magazine*, 88/89, pp. 10–13.

Tiedt, J.A. & Brown, L.A. (2014). Allostatic load: The relationship between chronic stress and diabetes in Native Americans. *Journal of Theory Construction & Testing*, 18(1), pp. 22–27.

Towne, S.D., Jr., Smith, M.L. & Ory, M.G. (2014). Geographic variations in access and utilization of cancer screening services: Examining disparities among American Indian and Alaska Native elders. *International Journal of Health Geographics*, 13(1), pp. 1–25.

Trask, H.K. (1993). *From a Native Daughter: Colonialism and Sovereignty in Hawaii*. Monroe, ME: Common Core Press.

Tsosie, R. (2012). Reconceptualizing tribal rights: Can self-determination be actualized within the US constitutional structure? *Lewis and Clark Law Review*, 15(4), pp. 923–950.

Tsosie, U., Nannauck, S., Buchwald, D., Russo, J., Trusz, S.G., Foy, H. & Zatzick, D. (2011). Staying connected: A feasibility study linking American Indian and Alaska Native trauma survivors to their tribal communities. *Psychiatry*, 74(4), pp. 349–361.

Tucker, R.P., Wingate, L.R. & O'Keefe, V.M. (2016). Historical loss thinking and symptoms of depression are influenced by ethnic experience in American Indian college students. *Cultural Diversity and Ethnic Minority Psychology*, 22(3), pp. 350–358.

Turner, S.L. & Pope, M. (2009). North America's Native Peoples: A social justice and trauma counseling approach. *Multicultural Counseling and Development*, 37, pp. 194–205.

United Nations. (2008). *United Nations Declaration on the Rights of Indigenous Peoples*. www.un.org/development/desa/indigenouspeoples/declaration-on-the-rights-of-indigenous-peoples.html. Accessed December 6, 2018.

United Nations Human Rights Office. (n.d.). Acts of intimidation and reprisal for engaging with the United Nations on human rights. Handout distributed at the United Nations Permanent Forum on Indigenous Issues, New York, April 2018.

United Nations Population Fund. (2018). *Recommendations of the UN Permanent Forum on Indigenous Issues on Sexual and Reproductive Health and Rights & Gender Based Violence: Progress and Challenges*. www.un.org/development/desa/indigenouspeoples/wp-content/uploads/sites/19/2018/04/Executive-Summary.pdf. Accessed December 6, 2018.

University of Arizona Rogers College of Law. (2018). *Indigenous Resistance to the Dakota Access Pipeline: Criminalization of Dissent and Suppression of Protest*. Report prepared for the United Nations Special Rapporteur on the Rights of Indigenous Peoples, Victoria Tauli-Corpuz.

Utah Dine Bikeyah. (2018). Native wisdom speaks at Bears Ears National Monument: Will America listen? http://utahdinebikeyah.org/media-kit/booklet.pdf. Accessed December 3, 2018.

VeLure Roholt, R., Johnston-Goodstar, K. & Eubanks, D. (2016). The social determinants of Native youth gang involvement. *CURA Reporter*, spring, pp. 3–10.

Venables, R.W. (1990). Looking back at Wounded Knee 1890. www.dickshovel.com/ TwistedFootnote.html. Accessed December 6, 2013.

Venables, R.W. (2004). *American Indian History: Five Centuries of Conflict and Coexistence.* Santa Fe, NM: Clear Light Publishing.

Vernon, I.S. (2012). "We were those who walked out of bullets and hunger": Representation of trauma and healing in "solar storms". *American Indian Quarterly*, 31(1), pp. 34–49.

Von der Porten, S., De Loe, R.C. & McGregor, D. (2016). Incorporating Indigenous knowledge into collaborative governance for water: Challenges and opportunities. *Journal of Canadian Studies*, 50(1), pp. 214–243.

Walls, M.L. & Whitbeck, L.B. (2012). The intergenerational effects of relocation policies on Indigenous families. *Journal of Family Issues*, 33(9), pp. 1272–1293.

Walters, K. (2013). Indigenizing research: Demystifying indigenous knowledges and "western" science. Paper presented at Place, Belonging and Promise: Indigenizing the International Academy, University of British Columbia, Vancouver, May 7.

Wandler, H.A. (2017). Helping Native American veterans with VA claims: New opportunities for tribes and tribal colleges. *Tribal College Journal*, 29(2), pp. 34–35.

Warne, D. & Lajimodiere, D. (2015). American Indian health disparities: Psychosocial influences. *Social and Personality Psychology Compass*, 9/10, pp. 567–579.

Warren, J.W. (2013). The colour of race: Indians and progress in a centre-left Brazil. In M. C. Forte (ed.), *Who is an Indian? Race, Place, and the Politics of Indigeneity in the Americas.* Toronto: University of Toronto Press, pp. 218–233.

Washburn, K.K. (2017). What the future holds: The changing landscape of federal Indian policy. *Harvard Law Review*, 130, pp. 200–232.

Waziyatawin & Yellow Bird, M. (2012). Introduction: Decolonizing our Minds and Actions. In Waziyatawin & M. Yellow Bird, *For Indigenous Minds Only: A Decolonization Handbook.* Santa Fe, NM: School for Advanced Research Press, pp. 1–14.

Weaver, H.N. (2000). Balancing culture and professional education: American Indians/ Alaska Natives and the helping professions. *Journal of American Indian Education*, 39(3), pp. 1–18.

Weaver, H.N. (2011). A cruel and surreal result: Restrictions on indigenous spirituality in the land of the free. In J. Schiele (ed.), *Social Welfare Policy: Regulation and Resistance among People of Color.* Los Angeles: Sage, pp. 329–346.

Weaver, H.N. (2012). Urban and indigenous: The challenges of being a Native American in the city. *Journal of Community Practice*, 20, pp. 1–19.

Weaver, H.N. & Congress, E.P. (2009). Indigenous people in a landscape of risk: Socially just social work responses. *Journal of Ethnic and Cultural Diversity, 18*(1/2), pp. 166–179.

Westermeyer, J. & Canive, J. (2013). Posttraumatic stress disorder and its comorbidities among American Indian veterans. *Community Mental Health Journal*, 49(6), pp. 704–708.

Western New York Peace Center. (2018). Cattaraugus Creek Water Walkerz Nuclear Free Water Walk Earth Day: Run, walk, paddle! www.wnypeace.org/wp/event/Cattaraugus-creek-wa ter-walkerz-nuclear-free-water-walk-earth-day-run-walk-paddle/. Accessed August 30, 2018.

Whitbeck, L.B., Adams, G.W., Hoyt, D.R. & Chen, X. (2004). Conceptualizing and measuring historical trauma among American Indian people. *American Journal of Community Psychology*, 33(3/4), pp. 119–130.

White House Initiative on American Indian and Alaska Native Education, US Department of Education. *Tribal Colleges and Universities.* https://sites.ed.gov/whiaiane/tribes-tcus/ ttribal-colleges-and-universities/. Accessed January 11, 2018.

Whitesell, N.R., Beals, J., Big Crow, C., Mitchell, C.M. & Novins, D.K. (2012). Epidemiology and etiology of substance use among American Indians and Alaska Natives: Risk, protection, and implications for prevention. *American Journal of Drug and Alcohol Abuse*, 38 (5), pp. 376–382.

Whitney, E. (2017). Native Americans feel invisible in US health care system: You, me, and them: Experiencing discrimination in America. *Morning Edition*, National Public Radio, December 12.

Wiebe, S.M. (2016). *Everyday Exposure: Indigenous Mobilization and Environmental Justice in Canada's Chemical Valley*. Vancouver: UBC Press.

Wildcat, D.R. (2009). *Red Alert! Saving the Planet with Indigenous Knowledge*. Golden, CO: Fulcrum Publishing.

Wilkins, D.E. & Wilkins, S.H. (2017). Blood quantum: The mathematics of ethnocide. In K. Ratterree & N. Hill (eds.), *The Great Vanishing Act: Blood Quantum and the Future of Native Nation*. Golden, CO: Fulcrum Publishing, pp. 210–227.

Wilson, C., Pence, D.M. & Conradi, L. (2013). Trauma-informed care. In *Encyclopedia of Social Work*. Oxford: Oxford University Press.

Wilson, D. (2018). Indian Health Service observes heart health month. www.ihs.gov/news room/ihs-blog/february2018/indian-health-service-observes-heart-health-month/. Accessed February 14, 2018.

Zonana, K. (2016). American Indians and Stanford researchers come together to prevent diabetes. *Stanford Medicine*, 33(3), pp. 10–52.

INDEX